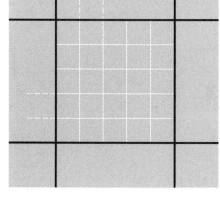

Fundamentals
of Special
Radiographic Procedures

third edition

ALBERT M. SNOPEK, B.S., R.T.(R)

Chairman
Radiologic Technology Department
Middlesex County College
Edison, NJ

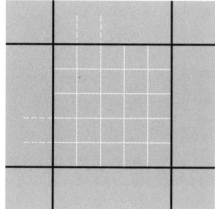

Fundamentals of Special Radiographic Procedures

third edition

W.B. SAUNDERS COMPANY
Harcourt Brace Jovanovich, Inc.
Philadelphia   London   Toronto   Montreal   Sydney   Tokyo

W. B. SAUNDERS COMPANY
Harcourt Brace Jovanovich, Inc.

The Curtis Center
Independence Square West
Philadelphia, Pennsylvania 19106

Library of Congress Cataloging-in-Publication Data

Snopek, Albert Michael, 1942–

Fundamentals of special radiographic procedures / Albert M.
Snopek.—3rd ed.

p.   cm.

Includes index.

ISBN 0-7216-3441-9

1. Radiography, Medical—Technique.   I. Title.

RC78.S66   1992

616.07′57—dc20   92-3759
                                                        CIP

Editor: Lisa A. Biello
Designer: Ellen Bodner-Zanolle
Production Manager: Peter Faber
Manuscript Editors: Allison Esposito and Amy Norwitz
Illustration Specialist: Cecelia Roberts
Indexer: Kathleen Cole

Fundamentals of Special Radiographic Procedures, 3rd edition   ISBN 0–7216–3441–9

Printed in Mexico.

Last digit is the print number: 9   8   7   6   5   4   3   2   1

To All My Girls:

my wife, Deborah,
and my children,
Beth Ann
Cheryl
Danielle
Julianne
Kristin
Shawna
also
to Barbara, in memoriam

Preface

This text discusses the basic concepts of special procedure radiography with reference to seven fundamental categories—anatomy, indications and contraindications, procedures, contrast media, patient care, equipment, and patient positioning. The text was not designed to be an atlas of positions, and most of the positions used during these procedures are variations on basic radiographic positioning. The discussion of the specialized equipment and its operation also assumes that the reader has knowledge of the fundamental physical principles of radiography.

The third edition has been expanded to include two chapters that were recommended by educators and practitioners who used the second edition. These are "Principles of Angiography" (Chapter 9) and "Venous Angiography" (Chapter 11). "Principles of Angiography" discusses concepts common to all angiographic procedures, including methods of catheter introduction and preprocedural and postprocedural patient care. Specific principles of patient care have also been added to discussions of all nonangiographic special procedures.

Sections on computed tomography, magnetic resonance imaging, and digital radiography have been expanded and included in the beginning of the text. These chapters present the basic principles underlying these modalities, discuss the computer hardware necessary for the successful operation of the procedures, and illustrate state-of-the-art equipment. In current practice, these modalities have been integrated with specialized diagnostic and interventional procedures as a routine part of a patient's diagnostic workup. Whenever applicable, reference has been made to these ancillary modalities as they apply to the specific procedures being discussed.

Some of the procedures and techniques presented in the text have become obsolete in most of the institutions in the United States. Discussions of these concepts have been kept in the text, but they have been minimized. Their presentation is still significant and can provide the reader with a historical perspective as well as a sufficient amount of information to obtain a basic understanding of the methods used for these procedures. Pneumoencephalography and ventriculography have been consolidated and included within the discussion of myelography.

Suggested readings have been included at the end of each chapter to aid the radiographer in obtaining more detailed information on specific aspects of each procedure or modality presented. Students and practitioners are urged to use the suggested readings as a springboard for further research.

Diagnostic special procedures have been overshadowed by interventional studies in recent years. Chapters on interventional studies have been updated and expanded to include current techniques and equipment. The section of the text devoted to interventional radiography has been divided into vascular and nonvascular procedures. The discussion of these procedures follows the pattern set in the section of the text covering the diagnostic procedures. The reader is presented with a discussion of the basic techniques and equipment necessary for these procedures.

In July 1991, the American Registry of Radiologic Technologists administered the first cardiovascular–interventional technology examination to provide a mechanism for recognizing the special competency of the individuals who have mastered this area of radiography. The information in this textbook covers the basic concepts of these specialty areas; however, preparation for the cardiovascular–interventional technology examination must also include practical experience in the specialty.

I hope that the third edition will provide a helpful reference manual for students and practicing radiographers seeking information about the basics of diagnostic and interventional special procedures as well as information pertinent to the ancillary modalities such as digital radiography, computed tomography, and magnetic resonance imaging.

I would like to take this opportunity to thank all of those people who have helped to bring the third edition to completion. The updated materials relating to the equipment were graciously provided by the various manufacturers. A list of names and addresses of the manufacturers is provided in the Appendix to help the reader obtain additional information on any of their products.

I would also like to give special thanks to my father, whose foresight in guiding my choice of careers made all of this possible.

ALBERT M. SNOPEK
EDISON, NJ

Contents

1 Design and Equipment

one
The What, Where, and How of Special Procedures 2

two
Image Recording Systems 15

three
Automatic Injection Devices 38

four
Contrast Media 66

five
Catheters and Accessories 77

2 Special Modalities

six
Digital Subtraction Angiography 96

seven
Computed Tomography 110

eight
Magnetic Resonance Imaging 133

3 Angiography

nine
Principles of Angiography 156

ten
Aortography 169

eleven
Venous Angiography 179

twelve
Femoral Arteriography 193

thirteen
Renal Angiography 202

4   Cardiac Catheterization

fourteen
Selective Angiocardiography 214

5   Neuroradiography

fifteen
Cerebral Angiography 232

sixteen
Central Nervous System Radiography 251

6   Other Special Procedures

seventeen
Hysterosalpingography 276

eighteen
Lymphangiography 285

nineteen
Bronchography 299

twenty
Arthrography 309

twenty-one
Sialography 320

7   Interventional Radiography

twenty-two
Vascular Interventional Procedures 330

twenty-three
Nonvascular Interventional Procedures 351

8   Special Techniques

twenty-four
Xeroradiography 372

twenty-five
Serial Magnification in Special Procedures 381

twenty-six
Subtraction 390

Appendix 399

Index 405

1 Design and Equipment

one

The What, Where, and How of Special Procedures

SPECIAL PROCEDURE ROOM AND SUITE
 DESIGN
INTERVENTIONAL RADIOGRAPHY ROOM
 AND SUITE DESIGN

ADDITIONAL DESIGN
 CONSIDERATIONS

Special procedure radiography had its beginnings soon after the discovery of x-radiation by Roentgen. It was noted that the introduction of certain substances into various organs of the body provided an amazing demonstration of their anatomic features. In the early 1900s, special procedure radiography was limited to areas such as the gallbladder, gastrointestinal tract, and genitourinary tract. As more complicated procedures were developed, these early procedures became the routine diagnostic contrast procedures performed daily in modern radiology departments.

A special procedure can be defined as a radiographic method of demonstrating certain anatomic features that lack natural contrast with surrounding structures by the instillation of a substance to produce structural contrast. This definition encompasses all contrast studies done today. Some have become routine procedures and can be performed without specialized radiographic equipment. Other procedures, especially those involving the vascular and nervous systems, are designated as special radiographic procedures.

In addition to specialized equipment, vascular and neuroradiographic procedures require a highly trained team of individuals to execute the techniques required to successfully obtain the most accurate diagnostic information. The radiographer is an integral part of this team and is responsible for understanding the operation of the equipment, making the preparations for the procedure, and assisting the physician during the examination.

Some special procedures can be performed in routine diagnostic radiographic rooms. However, vascular, neuroradiographic, and interventional procedures require a special room (or rooms) that is equipped to perform these examinations. This room should be designated the special procedure room or suite, or the interventional radiography room or suite, and its size, location, and construction should be given special consideration when this area is planned.

SPECIAL PROCEDURE ROOM AND SUITE DESIGN

Unlike the routine diagnostic radiographic room, the special procedure suite must serve various purposes. It must be designed so that it can be used for minor surgery as well as for special diagnostic radiography. It should also be equipped with cardiac monitoring devices and emergency materials for institutions in which a large number of cardiovascular catheterization procedures are performed.

In institutions in which many special procedures are performed, the special procedure suite should consist of several radiographic rooms. At least two specialized rooms should be available—one equipped for neuroradiography, and one equipped for cardiovascular radiography. These rooms will differ in the type of equipment required for the various special procedures.

Before discussing equipment, consideration should be given to the planning or layout of the special procedure suite. In addition to a team of personnel, a wide variety of specialized equipment is necessary for special procedure radiography. At times, the procedures may pose a risk to the patient, and severe, if not fatal, reactions may occur. These considerations require a room that is considerably larger than a routine radiographic room. The room should be a minimum of 400 ft² (37.16 m²); more complex vascular special procedure rooms should be 600 ft² (55.74 m²) (this does not take into consideration the control, monitoring, preparation, and dressing rooms).[1]

The control room must be larger than a routine radiographic room to accommodate the specialized equipment. The console of most three-phase radiographic units is larger than that of single-phase machines. The control booth should be adjacent to or in the special procedure suite and should be designed to permit an unobstructed view of the entire suite. It should be adequately protected from radiation hazards, yet it must afford rapid access to the suite. In general, the special procedure control booth should be a minimum of 50 to 75 ft² (4.645 to 6.9677 m²) to provide ample room for the placement and operation of the equipment.

In some sophisticated cardiovascular catheterization special procedure suites, a cardiac monitoring room is necessary to house the equipment required for cardiac testing. This room should also be protected from radiation hazards. Its size will depend on the amount and type of monitoring equipment available to the institution. It should also give an unobstructed view of the radiographic room and have free communication with the other major areas in the special procedure suite.

The preparation (prep) room is an important addition to the special procedure suite. It provides necessary storage space for the smaller pieces of equipment that are essential to the examinations. It can also be designed and equipped to function as a scrub room, if necessary. The prep room should contain a work area that may be used for making the catheters required during the procedure. This may be important only in larger teaching institutions in which research is performed. Most smaller hospitals use disposable catheters almost exclusively, which diminishes the importance of this area. If nondisposable catheter and needles are used, the prep area should have facilities for cleaning this equipment adequately after the procedure before it is repackaged for sterilization. In summary, the prep room should provide ample work space to allow the technologist to prepare and clean the equipment before and after the procedure.

If a large number of special procedures are done on an outpatient basis, dressing and waiting rooms should be provided adjacent to the suite for the comfort and convenience of the patient.

Figures 1–1 and 1–2 illustrate some possible special procedure suite layouts for vascular and neuroradiographic procedures.

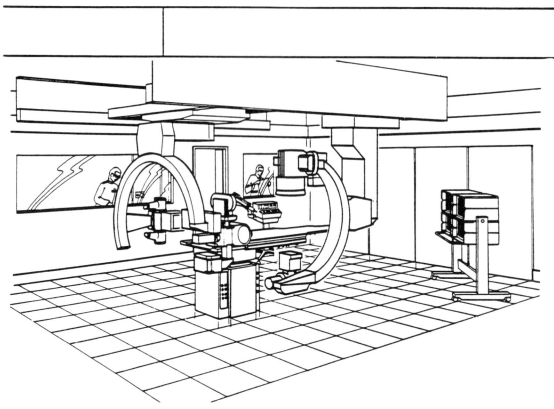

Figure 1–1. Dedicated cardiovascular suite setup. (From CGR Medical Corporation.)

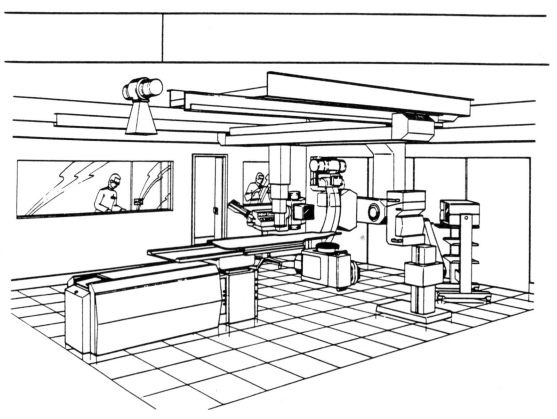

Figure 1–2. Vascular room with specialty for neuroradiology. (From CGR Medical Corporation.)

INTERVENTIONAL RADIOGRAPHY ROOM AND SUITE DESIGN

The need for a dedicated interventional radiography room is determined by the numbers and types of procedures performed. Vascular interventional procedures are usually performed in the general special procedure suite. Its design and equipment make it ideal for use during diagnostic angiography as well as for interventional radiographic procedures.

Nonvascular interventional studies may also be performed in the angiography suite, but the room design is usually too sophisticated for this type of radiography, which does not require the elaborate recording equipment necessary for vascular studies. The nonvascular interventional procedures need a slightly more sophisticated room design than is provided by a general fluoroscopic room. As the number of interventional examinations increases, especially in the larger hospitals, dedicated interventional radiography rooms will become necessary to prevent the disruption of the normal work flow in either a special-purpose fluoroscopic room or a special procedure suite.

The design of the interventional radiography room is very similar to that of the special procedure suite. Vascular interventional procedures can be performed in the angiography suite, and unless the number of these procedures interferes with the normal work flow of these rooms, a dedicated room will not be necessary. The nonvascular interventional room will require some modification of the basic special procedure room design. Basic interventional radiography room design considerations may be summarized as follows:

Radiographic room
  400 to 600 ft² (37.16 to 55.74 m²) minimum size
  Doorways, 4 ft (1.2 m) minimum width
  Patient holding and monitoring area, 96 ft² (8.91 m²) minimum size
  Adequate radiation protection
  View boxes for review of films
  Vertical wall-mounted chest changer
  Ceiling-mounted television monitors
  Biplane fluoroscopic and radiographic capabilities desirable
  90° to 90° floating top table
  Three-phase generation, 800 to 1000 mA capacity
Control room
  50 to 75 ft² (4.645 to 6.9677 m²) minimum size
  Optimal viewing of procedural area
  Adequate radiation protection
Laboratory and work areas
  Size dependent on equipment, 50 to 75 ft² (4.64 to 6.96 m²) minimum size
  View boxes
  Storage cabinets
  Laboratory table with staining facilities for bacteriologic and/or pathologic specimens
  Scrub basin

The interventional radiography room should be close to the special procedure area as well as to the ultrasonography and computed tomography (CT) rooms. Room size should be comparable to that of the basic angiography suite, a minimum of 400 to 600 ft² (37.16 to 55.74 m²). Doorways should be at least 4 ft (1.2 m) wide to accommodate stretchers, beds, and any extra-wide equipment that may be necessary.

Adjacent to the interventional suite should be a patient holding and monitoring area that will be used to hold patients before and after the procedure as well as to house any preprocedural or postprocedural monitoring equipment. The room should comfortably allow two isolated stretchers or beds. An appropriate room size is about 100 ft² (9.29 m²). It can be equipped with a centralized supply of oxygen if funding allows.

The control room area is equal in size and capacity to that used for general angiography, affording the occupants optimum viewing of the procedure as well as maximum radiation protection.

Ideally, a laboratory and workroom should be part of the interventional suite. The size of this room will depend on the type of equipment used. Space should be provided for a laboratory table with facilities to process cytologic samples obtained by needle aspiration or brush biopsy. This area can also be used as a viewing room, storage center, and scrub room, if size and design permit.

The design and construction of dedicated vascular and nonvascular interventional radiography suites will depend on the amount of funding allotted to the project, the types of procedures performed, and the personal preferences of the staff involved in the design process.

ADDITIONAL DESIGN CONSIDERATIONS

Film processing will usually be done in the general radiographic darkroom. In some institutions in which the special procedure or interventional radiography suite is located far from a darkroom facility, it may be necessary to provide a darkroom adjacent to the suite for the rapid development of the radiographs. This may be also be desirable when the case load is great enough to conflict with the processing requirements of the routine diagnostic department.

The special procedure or interventional radiography room must be constructed with its ultimate operation in mind. Electric wiring should be arranged so that the floors are virtually free of any type of obstruction that may be hazardous to the patient or personnel during the procedure or in an emergency situation. The power supply and wiring requirements for any particular special procedure room will vary with the equipment used. If new installations are planned, consultation with the manufacturers of desired equipment will be essential. If some procedures are to be done in areas in which combustible or explosive substances are used for general anesthesia, the wiring should adhere to specific codes governing electric connections in hazardous locations. The National Fire Code* (The National Fire Prevention Association Handbook, No. 56) lists the requirements for installation and use of permanent and mobile x-ray apparatus in hazardous locations.*

The construction of the room should allow for ease of cleaning after a procedure. Because many special procedures require surgical techniques, the physical construction of the floors and walls should be the same as that of an operating room. These surfaces should be tiled or finished with a smooth material to permit proper cleaning.

If new facilities are planned, provision should be made for equipping the room with a centralized supply of oxygen. Outlets should be strategically placed so that oxygen may be easily and quickly supplied to the patient.

The specialized equipment necessary for the suite will vary according to the types of procedures to be done, the personal preferences of the radiologist, and the budget of the institution. Certain essential pieces of equipment, however, are found in all modern special procedure rooms; these include the x-ray generator, controls, and tube; a system to record the events of the procedure; and some type of automatic injector. The equipment for each of these categories is manufactured by many companies, and all

---

*National Fire Codes: A Compilation of NFPA Codes, Standards, Recommended Practices and Manuals, Boston, The National Fire Prevention Association, 1978.

offer a selection of features suitable for large or small budgets. The ultimate choice of equipment should be made on the basis of the type and amount of special procedures to be performed. If optional features are not absolutely essential to the operation of the suite, they should be avoided if cost is a major consideration. However, it is unwise to compromise on the purchase of essential equipment. Image-recording systems and automatic injectors used during special procedures are discussed in Chapters 2 and 3.

The type of x-ray generator chosen should offer high performance with minimum ratings of 500 mA. In special procedure suites in which a great deal of vascular radiography is done, minimum ratings of 700 to 1000 mA should be considered because of the short exposure frequency required by vascular studies. Multiphase generation is required in these cases because it permits higher ratings (shorter exposure times) than the conventional single-phase equipment. In departments in which much cardiovascular radiography is performed, a constant potential generator is advantageous. This type of generator has capabilities for ratings up to 3000 mA and exposure times as short as 0.001 s. Major consideration should be given to the constant potential generator because it produces essentially monochromatic or homogeneous x-radiation, which effectively reduces the radiation dosage to the patient, and because its extremely short exposure times facilitate rapid sequence filming at rates above eight exposures per second, thus expanding the possibilities and uses of cineradiography.

The choice of a generator for special procedure radiography depends on the type and number of procedures being done. In all cases, however, the unit should supply a minimum rating of 500 mA if a nominal number of vascular procedures are performed and 1000 mA if a large number of varied cardiovascular studies are done.

The x-ray tube chosen for special procedure radiography must be capable of providing the detail necessary for adequate diagnosis yet must withstand the increased heat generated from rapid sequence exposures. In routine diagnostic radiography, it is rare for the tube rating to be exceeded during one procedure. During an angiographic procedure, however, it can easily occur, especially when a high exposure per second frequency is used. It is necessary for the technologist to adhere to the manufacturer's suggested exposure ratings. For this reason, a tube rating chart should be posted in the special procedure suite. Cooling charts should also be available to the technologist.

Heat units are the product of the multiplication of peak kilovoltage by milliamperage by time. The basic formula for heat units remains constant for all types of generation; however, multiphase-generated apparatus will produce a greater number of heat units than single-phase machines; therefore, the total number of heat units must be multiplied by a constant factor if multiphase generation is used. These factors are listed in Table 1–1. The formula is HU = kV peak × mA × t × C (where HU is heat units, kV peak is peak kilovoltage, t is time, and C is a constant). The tube rating chart must be for the specific tube installed in the special procedure room; specific charts are available for tubes for angiographic and cineradiographic studies. Figure 1–3 is an example of tube rating charts for the Varian A182/A282 series angiographic tube when used in a radiographic mode.

Angiographic tube rating charts relate peak kilovolts and milliamperage to determine the maximum kilowatts allowed for each exposure in a series. Figure 1–4*A* is a sample angiographic tube rating chart for the Varian A182/A282 series tube. To determine the

Table 1–1. CONSTANT FACTORS FOR HEAT UNIT CALCULATION

Type of Generation	Factor
Single-phase	1
Three-phase (6-pulse)	1.35
Three-phase (12-pulse)	1.41

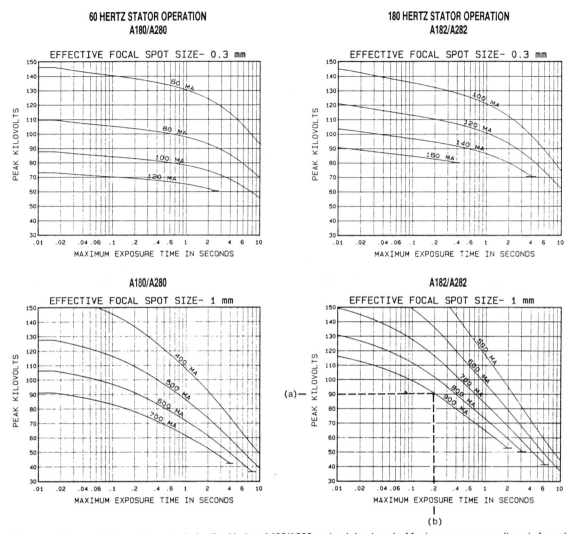

Figure 1–3. Sample tube rating charts for the Varian A182/A282 series tube inserts. Maximum exposure time is found by drawing a line between the desired peak kilovoltage and milliamperes *(a)*. A vertical line *(b)* drawn to intersect this point also crosses the maximum exposure time that can be used for a single exposure. (From Varian Power Grid and X-ray Tube Products.)

maximum kilowatts or exposure time for each exposure in the series, the following procedure should be used (Fig. 1–4*B*):

1. Determine the number of exposures in the series (a). It is important not to underestimate the number.
2. Determine the exposure rate per second (b).
3. The point at which the exposure rate per second (b) and the exposure time (c) intersect indicates the maximum amount of kilowatts (kVp × mA) allowed per exposure.

Cineangiographic tube rating charts differ from those used for angiographic tubes. Cineangiographic tube rating charts are primarily used to determine the maximum amount of time the tube can be used under certain conditions. These charts are sometimes called percent duty factor curves (Fig. 1–5).

A282   1.0 mm   **10 Degrees   3 PHASE   150/180 HZ**

EXPOSURE RATE PER SECOND	TUBE LOAD (KW) AS A FUNCTION OF THE EXPOSURE TIME (SEC.) OF THE INDIVIDUAL RADIOGRAPHS OF THE SERIES															NUMBER OF EXPOSURES IN SERIES
	.010	.020	.030	.040	.050	.060	.080	.100	.120	.140	.160	.180	.200	.225	.250	
1	82.7	77.3	73.1	69.6	66.5	63.7	58.9	54.9	51.5	48.5	45.9	41.7	37.5	33.3	30.0	
2	82.1	76.4	71.9	68.1	64.8	61.8	56.8	52.6	49.1	46.0	43.3	41.0	37.5	33.3	30.0	
3	81.7	75.5	70.7	66.6	63.1	60.1	54.8	50.5	46.9	43.8	41.1	38.7	0.0	0.0	0.0	
4	81.2	74.8	69.8	65.6	62.0	58.8	53.5	49.1	44.9	41.8	0.0	0.0	0.0	0.0	0.0	20
8	79.7	72.3	66.5	61.8	57.8	54.3	0.0	0.0	0.0	0.0	0.0	0.0	0.0	0.0	0.0	
15	77.6	68.9	62.4	57.1	0.0	0.0	0.0	0.0	0.0	0.0	0.0	0.0	0.0	0.0	0.0	
30	74.5	64.2	0.0	0.0	0.0	0.0	0.0	0.0	0.0	0.0	0.0	0.0	0.0	0.0	0.0	
1	79.8	72.5	66.8	62.1	58.1	54.7	46.9	37.5	31.2	26.8	23.4	20.8	18.8	16.7	15.0	
2	79.2	71.5	65.6	60.7	56.6	53.0	46.9	37.5	31.2	26.8	23.4	20.8	18.8	16.7	15.0	
3	78.7	70.6	64.4	59.3	55.1	51.5	45.6	37.5	31.2	26.8	23.4	20.8	0.0	0.0	0.0	
4	78.2	69.8	63.5	58.3	54.0	50.4	44.4	37.5	31.2	26.8	0.0	0.0	0.0	0.0	0.0	40
8	76.4	67.1	60.1	54.5	50.0	46.2	0.0	0.0	0.0	0.0	0.0	0.0	0.0	0.0	0.0	
15	73.9	63.3	55.6	49.7	0.0	0.0	0.0	0.0	0.0	0.0	0.0	0.0	0.0	0.0	0.0	
30	70.0	57.7	0.0	0.0	0.0	0.0	0.0	0.0	0.0	0.0	0.0	0.0	0.0	0.0	0.0	
1	77.2	68.3	61.6	56.2	50.0	41.7	31.3	25.0	20.8	17.9	15.6	13.9	12.5	11.1	10.0	
2	76.6	67.3	60.4	54.9	50.0	41.7	31.3	25.0	20.8	17.9	15.6	13.9	12.5	11.1	10.0	
3	76.0	66.4	59.3	53.7	49.1	41.7	31.3	25.0	20.8	17.9	15.6	13.9	0.0	0.0	0.0	
4	75.5	65.7	58.5	52.8	48.1	41.7	31.3	25.0	20.8	17.9	0.0	0.0	0.0	0.0	0.0	60
8	73.7	63.0	55.2	49.3	44.6	40.7	0.0	0.0	0.0	0.0	0.0	0.0	0.0	0.0	0.0	
15	71.0	59.2	51.0	44.8	0.0	0.0	0.0	0.0	0.0	0.0	0.0	0.0	0.0	0.0	0.0	
30	66.8	53.5	0.0	0.0	0.0	0.0	0.0	0.0	0.0	0.0	0.0	0.0	0.0	0.0	0.0	
1	74.8	64.6	57.1	46.9	37.5	31.2	23.4	18.8	15.6	13.4	11.7	10.4	9.4	8.3	7.5	
2	74.2	63.7	56.0	46.9	37.5	31.2	23.4	18.8	15.6	13.4	11.7	10.4	9.4	8.3	7.5	
3	73.6	62.8	55.0	46.9	37.5	31.2	23.4	18.8	15.6	13.4	11.7	10.4	0.0	0.0	0.0	
4	73.1	62.1	54.2	46.9	37.5	31.2	23.4	18.8	15.6	13.4	0.0	0.0	0.0	0.0	0.0	80
8	71.2	59.5	51.3	45.1	37.5	31.2	0.0	0.0	0.0	0.0	0.0	0.0	0.0	0.0	0.0	
15	68.6	55.8	47.3	41.1	0.0	0.0	0.0	0.0	0.0	0.0	0.0	0.0	0.0	0.0	0.0	
30	64.2	50.3	0.0	0.0	0.0	0.0	0.0	0.0	0.0	0.0	0.0	0.0	0.0	0.0	0.0	
1	72.5	61.2	50.0	37.5	30.0	25.0	18.8	15.0	12.5	10.7	9.4	8.3	7.5	6.7	6.0	
2	71.9	60.4	50.0	37.5	30.0	25.0	18.8	15.0	12.5	10.7	9.4	8.3	7.5	6.7	6.0	
3	71.3	59.6	50.0	37.5	30.0	25.0	18.8	15.0	12.5	10.7	9.4	8.3	0.0	0.0	0.0	
4	70.8	58.9	50.0	37.5	30.0	25.0	18.8	15.0	12.5	10.7	0.0	0.0	0.0	0.0	0.0	100
8	69.0	56.4	47.9	37.5	30.0	25.0	0.0	0.0	0.0	0.0	0.0	0.0	0.0	0.0	0.0	
15	66.3	52.9	44.2	37.5	0.0	0.0	0.0	0.0	0.0	0.0	0.0	0.0	0.0	0.0	0.0	
30	62.0	47.6	0.0	0.0	0.0	0.0	0.0	0.0	0.0	0.0	0.0	0.0	0.0	0.0	0.0	
1	67.3	50.0	33.3	25.0	20.0	16.7	12.5	10.0	8.3	7.1	6.3	5.6	5.0	4.4	4.0	
2	66.8	50.0	33.3	25.0	20.0	16.7	12.5	10.0	8.3	7.1	6.3	5.6	5.0	4.4	4.0	
3	66.3	50.0	33.3	25.0	20.0	16.7	12.5	10.0	8.3	7.1	6.3	5.6	0.0	0.0	0.0	
4	65.8	50.0	33.3	25.0	20.0	16.7	12.5	10.0	8.3	7.1	0.0	0.0	0.0	0.0	0.0	150
8	64.1	50.0	33.3	25.0	20.0	16.7	0.0	0.0	0.0	0.0	0.0	0.0	0.0	0.0	0.0	
15	61.5	47.1	33.3	25.0	0.0	0.0	0.0	0.0	0.0	0.0	0.0	0.0	0.0	0.0	0.0	
30	57.3	42.3	0.0	0.0	0.0	0.0	0.0	0.0	0.0	0.0	0.0	0.0	0.0	0.0	0.0	
1	50.0	25.0	16.7	12.5	10.0	8.3	6.3	5.0	4.2	3.6	3.1	2.8	2.5	2.2	2.0	
2	50.0	25.0	16.7	12.5	10.0	8.3	6.3	5.0	4.2	3.6	3.1	2.8	2.5	2.2	2.0	
3	50.0	25.0	16.7	12.5	10.0	8.3	6.3	5.0	4.2	3.6	3.1	2.8	0.0	0.0	0.0	
4	50.0	25.0	16.7	12.5	10.0	8.3	6.3	5.0	4.2	3.6	0.0	0.0	0.0	0.0	0.0	300
8	50.0	25.0	16.7	12.5	10.0	8.3	0.0	0.0	0.0	0.0	0.0	0.0	0.0	0.0	0.0	
15	50.0	25.0	16.7	12.5	0.0	0.0	0.0	0.0	0.0	0.0	0.0	0.0	0.0	0.0	0.0	
30	47.6	25.0	0.0	0.0	0.0	0.0	0.0	0.0	0.0	0.0	0.0	0.0	0.0	0.0	0.0	

NOTES
1. (kW) of Exposure Equals mA x kV
   For example - 70 kV x 300 mA = 21 kW

A 2. Exposures less than .010 seconds will have a kW Rating sarr

Figure 1–4. *(A)* Sample angiographic tube rating chart for the Varian A182/A282 series tube insert. (From Varian Power Grid and X-ray Tube Products.)

Illustration continued on following page

A282 0.3 mm c **10 Degrees 3 PHASE 150/180 HZ**

EXPOSURE RATE PER SECOND	TUBE LOAD (KW) AS A FUNCTION OF THE EXPOSURE TIME (SEC.) OF THE INDIVIDUAL RADIOGRAPHS OF THE SERIES															NUMBER OF EXPOSURES IN SERIES
	.010	.020	.030	.040	.050	.060	.080	.100	.120	.140	.160	.180	.200	.225	.250	
1	11.8	11.6	11.4	11.2	11.1	11.0	10.8	10.6	10.5	10.3	10.2	10.0	9.9	9.8	9.6	20
2	11.8	11.5	11.3	11.2	11.0	10.9	10.7	10.5	10.4	10.2	10.0	9.9	9.8	9.6	9.5	
3	11.8	11.5.	11.3	11.1	11.0	10.9	10.6	10.4	10.3	10.1	9.9	9.8	0.0	0.0	0.0	
4	11.8	11.5	11.3	11.1	10.9	10.8	10.6	10.3	10.2	10.0	0.0	0.0	0.0	0.0	0.0	
8	11.8	11.4	11.2	10.9	10.8	10.6	0.0	0.0	0.0	0.0	0.0	0.0	0.0	0.0	0.0	
15	11.7	11.3	11.0	10.7	0.0	0.0	0.0	0.0	0.0	0.0	0.0	0.0	0.0	0.0	0.0	
30	11.5	11.0	0.0	0.0	0.0	0.0	0.0	0.0	0.0	0.0	0.0	0.0	0.0	0.0	0.0	
1	11.8	11.4	11.2	11.0	10.8	10.7	10.4	10.1	9.9	9.7	9.5	9.3	9.1	8.9	8.7	a 40
2	11.8	11.4	11.2	11.0	10.8	10.6	10.3	10.0	9.8	9.6	9.4	9.2	9.0	8.8	8.6	
3	11.8	11.4	11.1	10.9	10.7	10.5	10.2	10.0	9.7	9.5	9.2	9.0	0.0	0.0	0.0	
4	11.7	11.4	11.1	10.9	10.7	10.5	10.2	9.9	9.6	9.3	0.0	0.0	0.0	0.0	0.0	
8	11.7	11.3	11.0	10.7	10.5	10.2	0.0	0.0	0.0	0.0	0.0	0.0	0.0	0.0	0.0	
15	11.6	11.1	10.7	10.4	0.0	0.0	0.0	0.0	0.0	0.0	0.0	0.0	0.0	0.0	0.0	
30	11.4	10.8	0.0	0.0	0.0	0.0	0.0	0.0	0.0	0.0	0.0	0.0	0.0	0.0	0.0	
1	11.7	11.3	11.0	10.8	10.6	10.4	10.0	9.7	9.4	9.2	8.9	8.7	8.5	8.2	8.0	60
2	11.7	11.3	11.0	10.7	10.5	10.3	10.0	9.6	9.3	9.1	8.8	8.6	8.3	8.1	7.8	
3	11.7	11.3	11.0	10.7	10.5	10.3	9.9	9.5	9.2	8.9	8.7	8.4	0.0	0.0	0.0	
4	11.7	11.3	10.9	10.7	10.4	10.2	9.8	9.4	9.1	8.8	0.0	0.0	0.0	0.0	0.0	
8	11.6	11.2	10.8	10.5	10.2	9.9	0.0	0.0	0.0	0.0	0.0	0.0	0.0	0.0	0.0	
15	11.5	11.0	10.5	10.2	0.0	0.0	0.0	0.0	0.0	0.0	0.0	0.0	0.0	0.0	0.0	
30	11.3	10.6	0.0	0.0	0.0	0.0	0.0	0.0	0.0	0.0	0.0	0.0	0.0	0.0	0.0	
1	11.7	11.2	10.9	10.6	10.4	10.1	9.7	9.3	9.0	8.7	8.4	8.2	7.9	7.6	7.4	80
2	11.6	11.2	10.8	10.6	10.3	10.1	9.6	9.2	8.9	8.6	8.3	8.0	7.8	7.5	7.2	
3	11.6	11.2	10.8	10.5	10.2	10.0	9.5	9.2	8.8	8.5	8.2	7.9	0.0	0.0	0.0	
4	11.6	11.1	10.8	10.5	10.2	9.9	9.5	9.1	8.7	8.4	0.0	0.0	0.0	0.0	0.0	
8	11.6	11.0	10.6	10.3	10.0	9.7	0.0	0.0	0.0	0.0	0.0	0.0	0.0	0.0	0.0	
15	11.5	10.9	10.4	10.0	0.0	0.0	0.0	0.0	0.0	0.0	0.0	0.0	0.0	0.0	0.0	
30	11.2	10.5	0.0	0.0	0.0	0.0	0.0	0.0	0.0	0.0	0.0	0.0	0.0	0.0	0.0	
1	11.6	11.1	10.7	10.4	10.1	9.9	9.4	9.0	8.6	8.3	8.0	7.7	7.4	6.7	6.0	100
2	11.6	11.1	10.7	10.4	10.1	9.8	9.3	8.9	8.5	8.2	7.9	7.6	7.3	6.7	6.0	
3	11.6	11.1	10.7	10.3	10.0	9.7	9.2	8.8	8.4	8.1	7.7	7.4	0.0	0.0	0.0	
4	11.6	11.0	10.6	10.3	10.0	9.7	9.2	8.7	8.3	8.0	0.0	0.0	0.0	0.0	0.0	
8	11.5	10.9	10.5	10.1	9.7	9.4	0.0	0.0	0.0	0.0	0.0	0.0	0.0	0.0	0.0	
15	11.4	10.7	10.2	9.8	0.0	0.0	0.0	0.0	0.0	0.0	0.0	0.0	0.0	0.0	0.0	
30	11.2	10.4	0.0	0.0	0.0	0.0	0.0	0.0	0.0	0.0	0.0	0.0	0.0	0.0	0.0	
1	11.5	10.9	10.4	10.0	9.6	9.3	8.7	8.2	7.8	7.1	6.3	5.6	5.0	4.4	4.0	150
2	11.4	10.8	10.3	9.9	9.6	9.2	8.6	8.1	7.7	7.1	6.3	5.6	5.0	4.4	4.0	
3	11.4	10.8	10.3	9.9	9.5	9.2	8.6	8.0	7.6	7.1	6.3	5.6	0.0	0.0	0.0	
4	11.4	10.8	10.3	9.8	9.5	9.1	8.5	8.0	7.5	7.1	0.0	0.0	0.0	0.0	0.0	
8	11.4	10.7	10.1	9.6	9.2	8.9	0.0	0.0	0.0	0.0	0.0	0.0	0.0	0.0	0.0	
15	11.2	10.5	9.9	9.3	0.0	0.0	0.0	0.0	0.0	0.0	0.0	0.0	0.0	0.0	0.0	
30	11.0	10.1	0.0	0.0	0.0	0.0	0.0	0.0	0.0	0.0	0.0	0.0	0.0	0.0	0.0	
1	11.1	10.2	9.5	8.9	8.4	7.9	6.3	5.0	4.2	3.6	3.1	2.8	2.5	2.2	2.0	300
2	11.1	10.1	9.4	8.8	8.3	7.9	6.3	5.0	4.2	3.6	3.1	2.8	2.5	2.2	2.0	
3	11.0	10.1	9.4	8.8	8.3	7.8	6.3	5.0	4.2	3.6	3.1	2.8	0.0	0.0	0.0	
4	11.0	10.1	9.4	8.7	8.2	7.8	6.3	5.0	4.2	3.6	0.0	0.0	0.0	0.0	0.0	
8	11.0	10.0	9.2	8.6	8.0	7.6	0.0	0.0	0.0	0.0	0.0	0.0	0.0	0.0	0.0	
15	10.8	9.8	9.0	8.3	0.0	0.0	0.0	0.0	0.0	0.0	0.0	0.0	0.0	0.0	0.0	
30	10.6	9.4	0.0	0.0	0.0	0.0	0.0	0.0	0.0	0.0	0.0	0.0	0.0	0.0	0.0	

NOTES
1. (kW) of Exposure Equals mA x kV
   For example - 70 kV x 300 mA = 21 kW
2. Exposures less than .010 seconds will have a kW Rating same as 0.10 seconds.

B

Figure 1–4 *Continued (B)* Angiographic tube rating chart used to determine the maximum allowed kilowatts per exposure in a series. (From Varian Power Grid and X-ray Tube Products.)

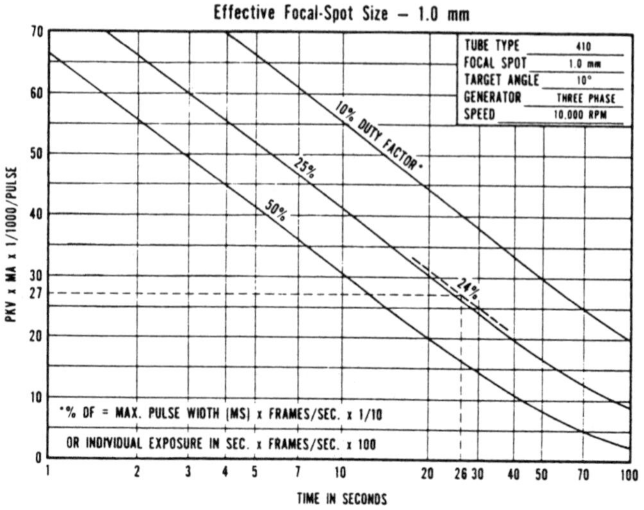

Figure 1–5. Sample percent duty factor curves illustrating how to determine the maximum length of time the tube can be run during cineangiography. (From Varian Power Grid and X-ray Tube Products.)

The percent duty factor can be calculated using the following formula:

$$\% \text{ DF} = \frac{\text{Maximum pulse duration (ms)} \times \text{frames/s}}{10}$$

where DF is duty factor.

Each chart is constructed with the power level (kVp × mA × 1/1000) on the x axis. The peak power level is expressed in kilowatts and can be calculated for any combination of factors using the following formula:

$$P = \frac{\text{kVp} \times \text{mA}}{1000}$$

where P is peak power.

Given the following factors and using the formulae listed above and the percent duty factor curve for the Varian 410 1.0-mm rotating anode tube, the length of time that the tube can be run can be determined.

Focal spot size	1.0 mm
Maximum pulse duration	4 ns
Frames per second	60
Peak voltage	90 peak kW
Tube current	300 mA

$$\% \text{ DF} = \frac{4 \times 60}{10} = 24\%$$

$$P = \frac{90 \times 300}{1000} = 27 \text{ kW}$$

At the point at which 27 kW crosses a 24% duty factor line, the tube can be run for a maximum of 26 s.

Maximum detail must be obtained during vascular special procedures to effect a diagnosis. Because detail depends on focal spot size, the smallest possible focal spot should be used. Of course, the smaller the focal spot, the greater the restriction on the individual exposure values that can be used. One method used by tube manufacturers to increase the tube rating for a particular tube is to use a decreasing target angle, thereby maintaining the actual focal spot size but decreasing the effective focal spot size (Fig. 1–6). A problem inherent in this method of increasing tube ratings is that at

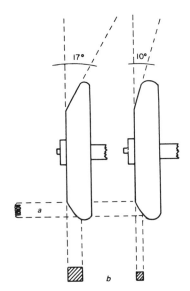

Figure 1–6. Target angle versus focal spot size. As the angle of the target face decreases, the effective focal spot size *(b)* is reduced. This permits increased tube loading with a corresponding change in filament size. In both situations, the actual focal spot size *(a)* remains unchanged. (From Culliman, J. E.: Illustrated Guide to X-ray Techniques. Philadelphia, J. B. Lippincott, 1972.)

steeper target angles, film coverage becomes critical (Fig. 1–7). The chart shows that if 14 × 14 in (35 × 35 cm) coverage is important, the source-image distance (SID) has to be increased over the standard 40 in when the 7° anode angle tube is used. This tube, however, is useful for work requiring a radiographic field size of less than 10 × 12 in (25 × 30 cm) at a 40-in SID. Such a tube could have considerable use for magnification arteriography, cineradiography, and image intensification, in which smaller field sizes are used continually.

The film coverage can be calculated for any combination of target angle and SID with the following formula[2]:

$$C = D_{fs-f} \times \tan TA \times 2$$

where C is dimension of one side of a square coverage pattern (in), D_{fs-f} is SID (in) (focal spot–film distance), and tan TA is tangent of the target angle. (Table 1–2 lists the tangents for various target angles.)

The formula can easily be applied to any combination of tube angle and SID. For example, using a Varian A182/A282 series rotating anode tube with a 10° target angle at an SID of 38 in, the dimension of one side of the square coverage pattern would be calculated as follows:

$$C = 38 \times 0.17633 \times 2$$

$$C = 13.40108 \text{ in}$$

Therefore, the maximum amount of coverage on the film would be 13 × 13 in. Figure 1–8 lists coverage for a variety of SID and target angles.

Some other factors influencing tube ratings are the size, thickness, and speed of rotation of the target. The special procedure x-ray tube should allow a combination of these factors to produce the high tube ratings necessary for vascular radiography.

Table 1–2. TANGENTS FOR VARIOUS TARGET ANGLES

Target Angle	Tangent
7°	0.12278
10°	0.17633
12°	0.21256
16°	0.28674

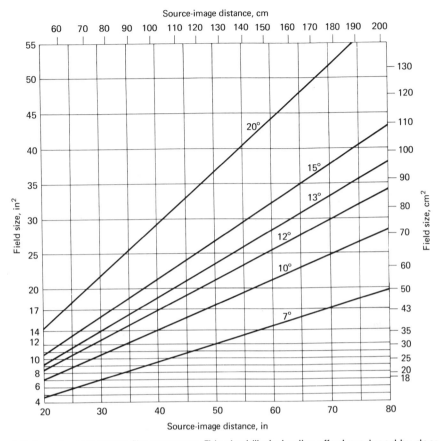

Figure 1–7. Target angle versus film coverage. This chart illustrates the effect produced by decreasing the target angle. As the target angle becomes steeper, the area of film coverage at a specific source-image distance (SID) is decreased. For example, the film coverage for a tube possessing a 10° target angle is 14 × 14 in at an SID of 40 in, whereas that for a tube with a 7° target angle is less than 10 × 10 in at the same SID. (From Varian Power Grid and X-ray Tube Products.)

FOCAL-SPOT-TO-FILM DISTANCE		DIMENSION "C" FOR VARIOUS TARGET ANGLES (in)			
(in)	(cm)	7°	10°	12°	16°
100	254	24.6	35.3	42.5	57.4
80	203.2	19.7	28.2	34.0	45.9
72	182.9	17.7	25.4	30.6	41.3
60	152.4	14.7	21.2	25.5	34.4
48	121.9	11.8	16.9	20.4	27.5
44	111.7	10.8	15.5	18.7	25.2
42	106.7	10.3	14.8	17.9	24.1
40	101.6	9.8	14.1	17.0	22.9
38	96.5	9.3	13.4	16.2	21.8
34	86.4	8.4	12.0	14.5	19.5
30	76.2	7.4	10.6	12.8	17.2

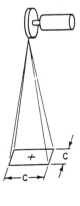

Figure 1–8. Film coverage for various target angles and source-image distances. (From Varian Power Grid and X-ray Tube Products.)

The ultimate choice of an x-ray tube for the special procedure suite will depend on the types of procedures to be done and the equipment with which it will be used. If a rapid sequence changer capable of 8 to 12 exposures per second is used, the tube must be able to withstand the increased heat that is generated.

SUMMARY

Special procedure rooms should be given careful consideration when they are being planned. The rooms should be larger than routine diagnostic radiographic rooms to provide the special procedure team with ample space in which to function effectively during the examination or in an emergency. The increased room size is also required to house the specialized equipment necessary for the examinations. Additional areas should be planned adjacent to the radiographic area to provide work and storage areas to facilitate preparation for the procedure. A dressing room should be provided for the convenience of outpatients.

The essential equipment required for a special procedure suite includes the generator, console, x-ray tube, and recording and automatic injection devices. These should be chosen on the basis of the types of procedures to be done, physician preference, and budget requirements. Compromises should not be made on the purchase of essential equipment, but optional features should be chosen on the basis of procedural requirements.

REFERENCES

1. Scott, W. G.: Planning Guide for Radiographic Installations, 2nd ed. Baltimore, Williams & Wilkins, 1966.

2. Information Bulletin 3780, Varian Power Grid and X-ray Tube Products, Salt Lake City, Utah, 1978.

SUGGESTED READINGS

Brateman, L., el al.: Transparent protective barrier for fluoroscopy during angiography, Am. J. Roentgenol., *133*:954, 1979.

Brinker, R. A.: Radiology Special Procedure Room. Baltimore, University Park Press, 1973.

Chesney, O. N.: X-Ray Equipment For Student Radiographers. Philadelphia, F. A. Davis, 1971.

Hudenberg, R.: Planning the Community Hospital. New York, McGraw-Hill, 1977.

Ullrich, H. M.: Technical possibilities to reduce radiation exposure during angiography, Ann. Radiol., *22*:331, 1979.

Watson, J. C.: Patient Care and Special Procedures in Radiologic Technology, 3rd ed. St. Louis, C. V. Mosby, 1969.

Wheeler, T. E.: Hospital Design and Function. New York, McGraw-Hill, 1964.

two

Image Recording Systems

RAPID SERIAL FILM CHANGERS
Roll Film Changers
Cut Film Changers
RAPID SEQUENCE CASSETTE CHANGERS
BASIC OPERATIONAL CONSIDERATIONS
BIPLANE OPERATION
INDIRECT IMAGING SYSTEMS

Image Intensification
Videotape System
Videodisc System
Laser Imaging Systems
Photofluorographic Systems
    Serial Spot Film Cameras
Cinefluorographic Systems

As with conventional radiography, during special procedures there must be a system to capture the images produced during the studies. The system must be capable of displaying the images during the procedure as well as providing a permanent copy for archiving and future analysis. In conventional radiography, the image is recorded on x-ray film, which is then processed, viewed, and filed to provide permanent storage. Generally speaking, the images produced in this manner are "passive" and are not meant to demonstrate motion or changes in the anatomic part during the procedure.

Conventional fluoroscopy can capture the images on x-ray film, cinefilm, or magnetic tape while displaying the images of the study on a television monitor for viewing in real time during the procedure. The advantages of this system are that changes can be recorded as they happen, analyzed during the procedure, and kept for future use.

In general, special procedures are dynamic studies. They are designed to demonstrate physiological sequences, such as the passage of a bolus of contrast medium through a portion of the vascular system. These sequences last only a few seconds, and if any abnormality is present, it might be visible for only a fraction of a second. Several systems are used to record these images—rapid serial changers, magnetic recording devices, laser optical (videodisc) devices, large-format serial spot filming devices, cinefluorography, and digital image storage devices.

Radiographic systems can be designed with one or more of these recording media incorporated into the design.

RAPID SERIAL FILM CHANGERS

As their name implies, rapid serial film changers are used to record a sequential series of images that occur during the special procedure. These are recorded on radiographic film, which is processed in the usual manner to provide the finished image. These types of systems produce a series of static images representing the changes that developed during the procedure. The disadvantage to this type of system is that the dynamic nature of the pathological or physiological process cannot be demonstrated.

Rapid serial changers are produced by a variety of manufacturers. However, all systems have several elements in common; once you are familiar with their operation, you can use almost any brand. This book describes the basic operational features of each type of rapid serial changer rather than presenting an exhaustive description of every brand available.

Rapid serial film changers can be one of two varieties—those that transport cut film, and those that transport roll film. Each is fully automatic, and each has advantages and disadvantages, which should be understood to appreciate the potential of each unit.

Roll Film Changers

The operation of a rapid serial roll film changer can be compared with that of a movie projector. The concept of rapid serial roll film changers is not new to the field of radiography. The first roll film changer was developed in 1925; since then, many refinements and improvements have been made. These systems have in large part been replaced by the smaller cut film serial changers. There are many roll film devices still in use; however, the manufacture of these devices has essentially been discontinued. Existing units are still being serviced by manufacturers, and their operating and design characteristics should be considered.

Roll film changers have four major parts: (1) changer and mounting stand; (2) supply magazine; (3) receiving magazine; and (4) program selector.

Additional components that may be found in the roll film changer are a drag brake, frictionless roller, and level. These accessory items can be considered essential to the roll film changer but may take different forms or be referred to by different names by different companies. Detailed information about these components can be obtained from the operational instructions furnished by the manufacturer.

The mounting stand is the support upon which the changer rests. It can be a simple support device with manual adjustments or a sophisticated piece of equipment adjusted by an electric drive. It usually has some means of anchoring the changer to the floor to minimize shifting movements during operation of the changer. Some mounting stands are made to hold the changer permanently in only one axis, either vertical or horizontal, while others allow movement of the changer into either of these positions.

To understand the operation of the roll film changer, it is necessary to understand the function and operation of each of its four major parts.

FILM CHANGER AND MOUNTING STAND ASSEMBLY. This is the drive portion of the roll film changer. It houses the mechanism necessary to transport the film from the supply magazine to the receiving magazine. The transport mechanism consists of three chain drives—main, supply, and receiving—which are driven by the main drive reactor and by the Geneva drive mechanism. The perforating wheels, which are devices used to meter the length of film advanced for each exposure, are on the two sides of the pressure plate toward the receiving end of the unit. When one frame is advanced for exposure, the perforating wheels make one complete revolution. This allows precisely 11 in (27.5 cm) of film to be advanced in the changer. Contained within the changer are a manually operated knife, intensifying screens and grid, and pressure plate; these ensure proper transport and exposure of the film.

Manual Knife. The manually operated film cutoff knife is usually at the receiving end of the changer body. It can be operated only when the changer is in its normal stop position. Its function is to cut the film for removal from the changer. This enables the radiographer to check a scout film or remove a portion of the film to be developed without exposing the entire roll.

Intensifying Screens and Grid. As in a regular cassette, the roll film changer is supplied with two intensifying screens, which can be par speed, high speed, or super speed screens. It is good practice to perform preventive maintenance at each loading. Check the screens for cleanliness, and when necessary, clean with a commercial cleanser. This not only lengthens screen life but also ensures artifact-free studies. An 8:1 linear grid is usually supplied as standard equipment in single-plane changers. If biplane changers are used, they may be equipped with 12:1 103-line linear grids. Available as an option is a 5:1 linear grid. This may be added to create a crossed grid with the effective cleanup of a 13:1 linear grid. (It can also be used in biplane studies in which a great amount of secondary radiation fog is produced.)

Pressure Plate. This component provides the screen contact necessary for good-quality radiographs. In the normal stop position, the pressure plate is closed (screens closed position). After the exposure, the pressure plate is opened (screens opened position), and the film is allowed to pass between the screens to the receiving magazine. The pressure plate is activated by the main drive chain. The basic operation of all roll film changers is similar in that film is moved from a supply magazine through an exposure field and into a receiving magazine (Fig. 2–1). The pressure plates ensure optimum screen contact while the exposure is being made.

SUPPLY MAGAZINE. This is a light-tight container that, depending on the brand of film changer chosen, can accommodate from 50 to 80 ft (15 to 24 m) of film. It is usually in an accessible location on the changer and is easily transported to and from the darkroom under normal lighting conditions.

RECEIVING MAGAZINE. This is also easily accessible and can be transported to the darkroom under normal lighting conditions without the risk of penetration of the film by light. Care must be exercised in the use of these components because light leaks may develop from rough handling.

PROGRAM SELECTOR. This may be considered the heart of the variable speed film changers. It operates the film changer during single or serial exposures and establishes the film rate (number of films per second) and the duration of each phase. According to the brand, the program stations can be varied from a minimum of one or two exposures per second to a maximum of 12 exposures per second.

The programmer can control one (single-plane) or two (biplane) film changers. When

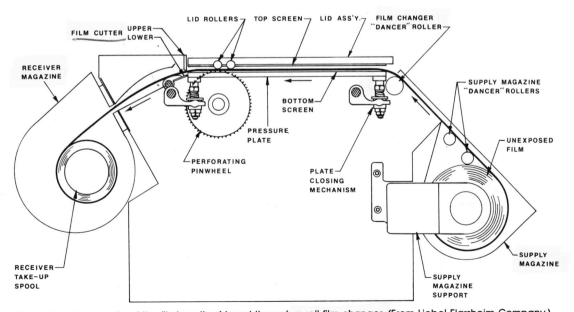

Figure 2–1. Schematic of the film's path of travel through a roll film changer. (From Liebel-Flarsheim Company.)

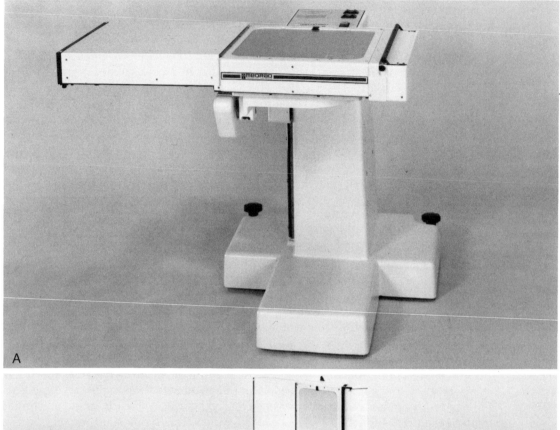

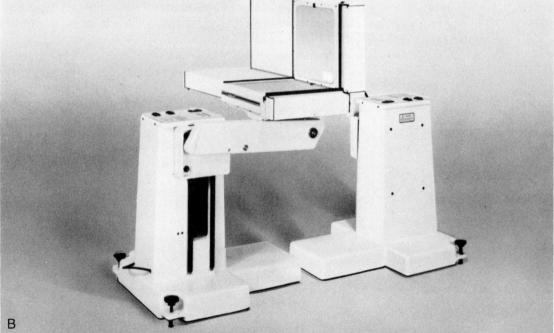

Figure 2–2. *(A)* The Medrad Omniplane rapid sequence changer and stand prepared for single-plane operation. (B) The Medrad Omniplane rapid sequence changer and stand prepared for biplane operation. (From Medrad, Inc.)

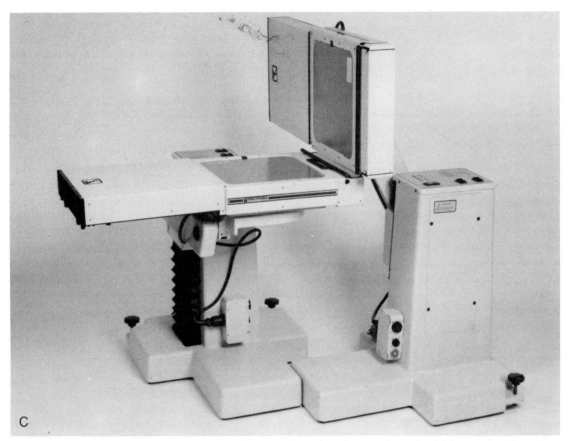

Figure 2–2 *Continued (C)* Two Medrad Omniplane changer systems set up for biplane operation. (From Medrad, Inc.)

used in the biplane mode, the program selector can provide either simultaneous or alternate exposure patterns.

The film-changing system can be controlled either directly by the switch on the program selector or indirectly through a triggering device located in an automatic pressure injector. The film changer can be programmed to provide a single film or "scout mode" for single radiographs. This is usually necessary to confirm proper exposure and positioning before the procedure or to provide a base film for conventional subtraction techniques.

Cut Film Changers

Rapid serial cut film changers rapidly transport single sheets of film of a specific size. The 14- × 14-in (35.6- × 35.6-cm) and the 10- × 12-in (25- × 30-cm) sizes are most often used. These units are usually available as single-plane changers; however, two units on different mounting stands may be combined for biplane operation (Fig. 2–2C).

The cut film changer is similar to a roll film changer in that it also comprises four major components: (1) changer and mounting stand assembly; (2) supply magazine; (3) receiving cassette; and (4) program selector.

FILM CHANGER AND MOUNTING STAND ASSEMBLY. The cut film changer, unlike the roll film changer, transports film by means of roller systems (Fig. 2–3). This type of changer is similar to an automatic processor in some respects. The film moves

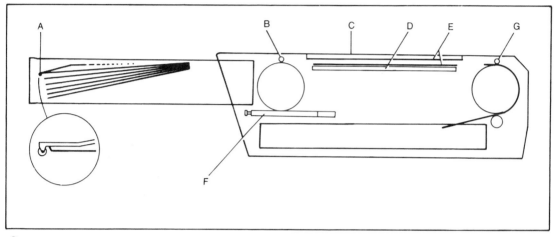

a

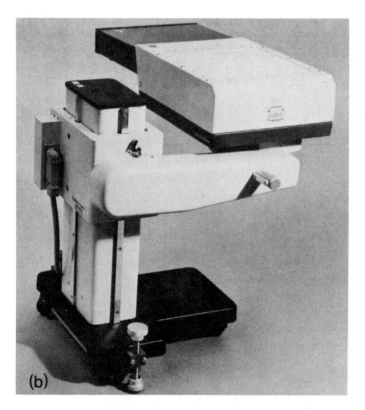

(b)

Figure 2–3. (*a*) Schematic of the Puck cut film changer showing the transport mechanism and major component parts: film puller *(A)*; feed-in rolls *(B)*; compression plate of CFRP *(C)*; pressure table *(D)*; intensifying screens *(E)*; marking rod *(F)*; feed-out rolls *(G)*. (From Siemens Corporation.) (*b*) The Puckwop 24/35 universal stand and Puck cut fim changer.

between roller systems, which transport the film to a compression table; this device is similar to the pressure plates of the roll film changer.

Compression Table. The compression table contains the intensifying screens. High-speed screens are supplied as standard equipment with the cut film changer. The compression table supplies the necessary screen contact for optimum radiography and is located directly beneath the exposure field of the changer. After the exposure, the compression table is lowered, and the film is transported between a rubber-covered wheel and a roller to the receiving cassette.

Exposure Field. The exposure field is equipped with a specially sized 8:1 focused grid. The grid can be replaced by removing the clips from around the frame of the exposure field.

Mounting Stand. The two basic mounting stands are made for horizontal or vertical changers. They come equipped with either hand- or foot-operated locking devices to ensure the stability of the changer.

The more sophisticated cut film changers, such as the Medrad Omniplane film changer system and the Siemens-Elema Puck cut film changer, can be either floor mounted or attached directly to the image intensifier on the C-arm system (Fig. 2–4). The Siemens-Elema Puck cut film changer can also be constructed as a built-in model in a radiographic table.

When the units are attached to a C-arm, conversion from one mode to another can be easily done in a minimal amount of time. With the proper component package, a changeover time of 6 s is possible when converting from TV fluoroscopy to serial radiography.

SUPPLY MAGAZINE. The supply, or loading, magazine is a stainless-steel box that can be easily carried to and from the darkroom. The film-loading capacity of the supply magazine varies with the manufacturer and model. When the magazine is properly inserted into the changer, the lids and small ports at the lower front of the magazine are opened automatically after the magazine carriage is advanced.

RECEIVING CASSETTE. The receiving cassette, a stainless-steel container with a light-tight lid, is a carrying case for the exposed films that are transported through the changer. When the cut film changer is prepared for use, the receiving cassette must be inserted with the lid open. To remove the receiving cassette from the changer, the lid must be closed. This is accomplished by depressing the button adjacent to the handle on the receiving cassette, although the receiving magazine of some units will automatically open when inserted into the changer body and automatically close when the magazine is removed.

PROGRAM SELECTOR. The program selector is similar in operation to that of the roll film changer. It can adapt the film changer to the exposure frequencies required for various special radiographic examinations.

The program selector for the Puck cut film changer is a microcomputer-based unit (Fig. 2–5A). It can store 19 individual programs in its memory, and these can be changed as required. The program selector allows a 40-s program duration. The display panel lists all information necessary for a specific program, even listing errors that must be corrected before beginning the procedure. A selector button is available on some models to control program selector operation for either single-plane or biplane radiography.

The Medrad Omniplane film changer program system can be supplied with one of two types of program selectors. The basic Omniplane 200 selector is microprocessor based and can store as many as 49 predefined programs with as many as 15 levels, with an unlimited program time. The more advanced system, Omniplane 300, is capable of controlling both the film changing system and the Mark V injection system. It has the same capabilities as the Omniplane 200 but adds an extra measure of safety as the injection system will be shut down if the routine is aborted for any reason. Both of the

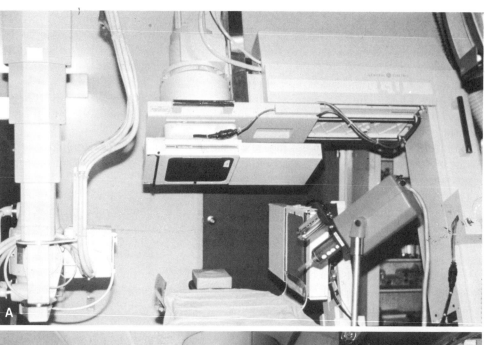

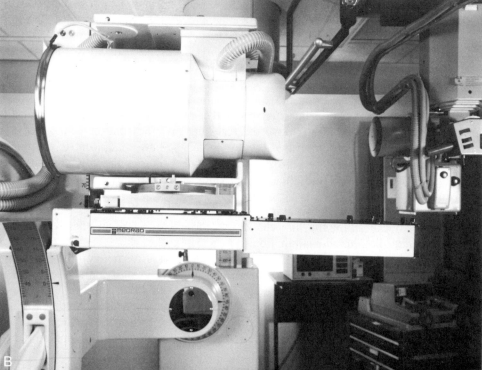

Figure 2–4. *(A)* Photo of the Medrad Omniplane rapid sequence changer attached to an image intensification system. *(B)* The Medrad Mark V automatic injector head attached to the radiographic table. (From Medrad, Inc.)

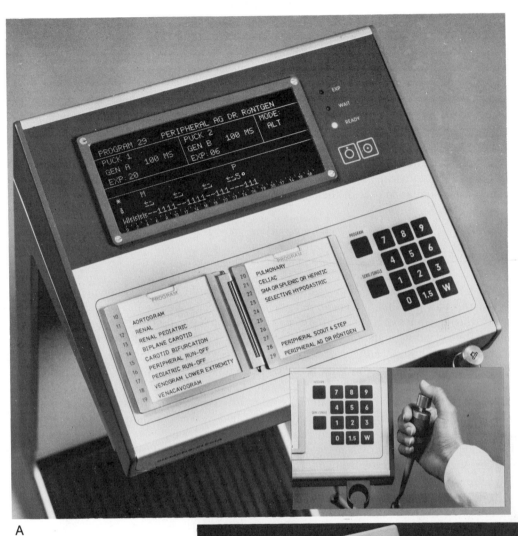

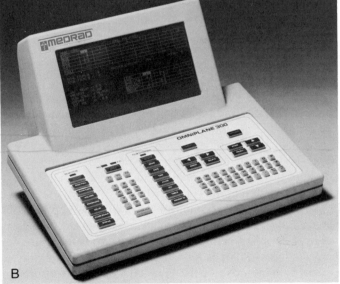

Figure 2–5. *(A)* Close-up photograph of the Puck film changer operator's console; insert shows programming pad and trigger switch. (From Siemens Corporation.) *(B)* Photograph of the Medrad Omniplane 300 combination film changer and automatic injector programmer. (From Medrad, Inc.)

programmers are self-diagnostic and come equipped with a dual-position hand switch that controls both the rotor and the x-ray exposure. The combination programmer, the Omniplane 300, has a printer that can provide written documentation of the injection and film changer parameters (Fig. 2–5B).

A hand switch containing a selector switch for single or serial operation is connected to the program selector.

An automatic cut film changer is also available for peripheral angiography, with an exposure frequency of two exposures per second. This unit is controlled by a punch card that is inserted into the program selector and coordinates and initiates the exposure frequency, injection, and operation of auxiliary equipment necessary to the procedure. An interesting feature of this unit is the central radiotransparent opening, through which television fluoroscopy may be used to position the patient and place the catheter. Its operation is similar to that of the cut film changer previously described.

RAPID SEQUENCE CASSETTE CHANGERS

Unlike the rapid sequence changers already discussed, the cassette changer does not transport the film through a specialized mechanism. It is a simple device for moving cassettes through an exposure field. In some rapid sequence cassette changers, the cassettes are loaded with standard 11- × 14-in (27.5- × 35.0-cm) cut film, eliminating the necessity of using specially sized film and intricate darkroom procedures.

Cassette size varies with the type of unit. The units currently in use are provided with cassettes ranging in size from 30 × 120 cm (12 × 47 in) to 35 × 90 cm (14 × 36 in). The rapid sequence cassette changer is primarily used for peripheral angiography and abdominal aortography. These units are controlled by a wall-mounted programmer that allows individual selection of time delays between each film.

The transport mechanism varies by manufacturer. However, in all cases, the unexposed cassettes are protected from the radiation beam during the examination. These systems are usually used with specially constructed step-tables. The table top is designed to shift in a stepwise fashion to expose different portions of the patient as the contrast agent moves through the blood vessels.

BASIC OPERATIONAL CONSIDERATIONS

The changers we have discussed have certain common features. They all have a period of time during which the film or cassette is in motion and a period of time during which no motion is occurring. It is logical to assume that the radiograph must be produced during the stationary period. Every rapid sequence changer, however, has a stationary period of a different length. This is usually less than 50% of the cycle time. The total length of the stationary period cannot be used to produce an exposure because certain delays are inherent in the x-ray apparatus. These delays are called *zero time* and *phase-in time* (Fig. 2–6).

The zero time is constant for any particular apparatus. Therefore, an adjustment can be made for this delay in the changer mechanism. The delay is caused by the operational time of the relays and contactors in the x-ray exposure control.

The phase-in time is related to the point at which the exposure contactor is closed in relation to the cycle of the line voltage. The exposure can be initiated only when the cycle of the line voltage passes through zero. It can be seen that this delay can vary from zero (no delay) to a maximum delay of one cycle of line frequency (1/60 s).

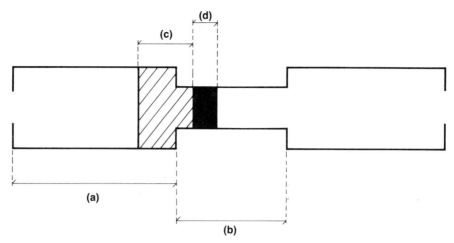

Figure 2–6. Schematic of a typical film cycle period. *(a)* Transport time; *(b)* stationary period; *(c)* zero time; *(d)* phase-in time.

Because the actual amount of delay cannot be determined, the only compensation would be to deduct the maximum delay from the total stationary period. If the maximum exposure time that could be used were to be *calculated,* this deduction would be a necessity. However, most manufacturers give maximum exposure times at different picture frequencies in their instruction manuals.

Each changer is equipped with a grid and intensifying screens. The selection of these items should be made carefully, with consideration given to the amount of recorded detail required, the limitations of the equipment, and the procedures that will be performed. A review of the basic physical principles underlying the actions of grids and intensifying screens is helpful in choosing accessories compatible with the above parameters. (For a detailed presentation of the physical principles of grids and intensifying screens, consult the Suggested Readings at the end of this chapter.)

BIPLANE OPERATION

A discussion of rapid sequence changers would not be complete without consideration of their use for biplane operation. The term *biplane* as applied to rapid sequence radiography is defined as simultaneous radiography in two planes (Fig. 2–7).

When rapid sequence changers are used for biplane radiography, certain technical difficulties arise. The most important factor, scatter, necessitates the use of special crossed grids in the vertical changer. This grid should absorb the scatter radiation produced in a biplane setup that strikes the vertical changer. The linear grid in the horizontal changer cannot absorb the scattered radiation, especially during çerebral angiography, and crossed grids are usually unacceptable here because tube angles are frequently used. This causes an increase in the density of the film in the horizontal changer. These factors should be considered when choosing the technical parameters for biplane operation. If single-plane study is required on the same patient, an adjustment in technique will be necessary to compensate for this effect.

We can see, therefore, that during biplane studies, it is necessary to use different exposure factors in each of the two planes. This is possible only if the x-ray tubes are supplied with separate generators, thus providing flexibility of technical factors for each tube. If, however, the x-ray tubes are connected in parallel on one generator, the selection of these factors will be severely compromised, and technical adjustments for the increased scatter radiation to one plane will be limited.

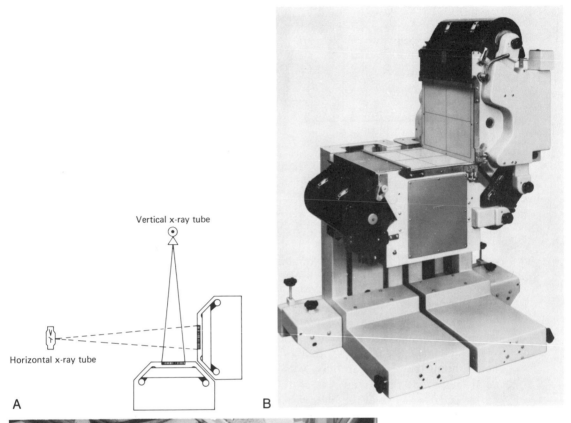

Vertical x-ray tube

Horizontal x-ray tube

A

B

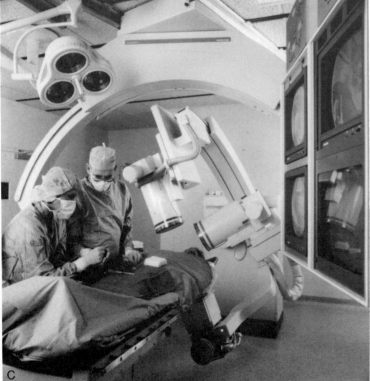

C

Figure 2–7. (A) Schematic of tube and film changers set up for biplane radiography; (B) photograph of two rapid sequence roll film changers positioned for biplane radiography; (C) photograph of Siemens microprocessor-controlled BICOR biplane cardiac imaging system consisting of two independent C-arm imaging units and a height-adjustable ceiling-suspended patient table. (A and B from Liebel-Flarsheim Company; C from Siemens Corporation.)

INDIRECT IMAGING SYSTEMS

Rapid serial radiographic systems produce the image through the direct interaction of the x-radiation with the screen/film system. Indirect imaging systems, however, record the image using the information produced at the output phosphor of an image intensification device. Indirect imaging systems include videotape recorders, videodisc recorders, digital recording systems, serial spot filming devices, and cinefluorographic systems. Videotape, videodisc, and digital recording systems use an electronic signal to produce the image, whereas the serial spot filming devices and cinefluorographic units (photofluorographic systems) capture the image directly from the output phosphor of the image intensifier (I.I.). A basic knowledge of the operation of image intensification systems is essential to understanding the principles of the indirect image recording devices. A brief review of these principles follows.

Image Intensification

An I.I. is used to increase the brightness of the image. This is accomplished with the I.I. tube (Fig. 2–8). The input side of the I.I. tube is coated with a phosphor layer, usually cesium iodide, that produces the image as a direct result of the action of the remnant radiation. Photoemissive material is coated on the substrate opposite the phosphor layer; this material converts the visible light image into an electron image. The electrons making up the image are accelerated across the I.I. tube by an electron lens system and are focused to strike the output side of the tube.

The output side of the I.I. tube is also coated with a phosphor, which converts the electron image to a smaller, corresponding light image. The image at the output side of the I.I. tube is brighter. This results from the process of reducing the size of the image and the acceleration of the electrons.

A television camera is attached directly to the output side of the I.I. tube via a special lens system or fiberoptic disc, and the images produced can be transmitted to a television monitor as well as a magnetic tape recorder or videodisc recorder. The use of an image distribution device will also allow the attachment of a serial spot filming

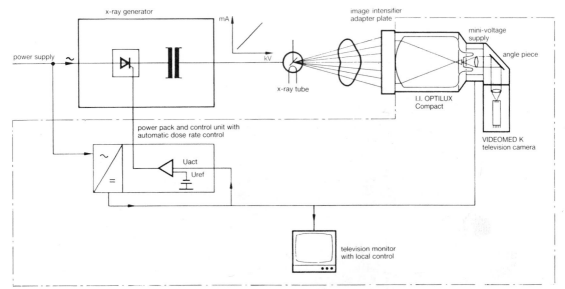

Figure 2–8. Schematic of the functional principles underlying an image-intensification system (the Siemens SIRECON Compact D, D-2 system. (From Siemens Corporation.)

device, a cinefluorographic unit, or both to the system. For more detailed information, consult the Suggested Readings at the end of the chapter.

Videotape System

The videotape recorder (Fig. 2–9) can be used with the image intensification and television monitoring systems to indirectly record the images produced during the study. Depending on its construction, the system can be used to record the entire procedure or only short segments for continuous playback during the examination.

The video image is recorded on a strip of magnetic tape. The width and length of this strip varies depending on the type of unit. Magnetic tape (videotape) is composed of a base coated with an emulsion of particles that can be magnetized. A variety of compounds are used for the base and the emulsion; however, Mylar (polyester) is often used in the construction of the base, and ferric (iron) oxide or chromium dioxide is used in the emulsion. Videotapes should be stored away from strong magnetic fields such as those found in magnetic resonance imaging (MRI) areas.

The recording and playback processes are accomplished through the video head (Fig. 2–10). The output signal from the television camera moves through a wire coiled in the video head. This creates a magnetic field that affects the particles in the emulsion on the magnetic tape. The particles are magnetized in accordance with the magnetic fields produced in the video head. In the playback mode, the reverse sequence of events happens, and the resultant electronic image is directed to a television monitor.

Usually, the videotape recorder is also capable of recording an audio track. This is an advantage if the physician wants a running commentary of the procedure to accompany the images. The videotape can be reused to record other examinations if it is not archived.

Videodisc System

The magnetic videodisc is made of a rigid material, shaped like a phonograph record, and coated with an emulsion of magnetic particles similar to magnetic tape. The image

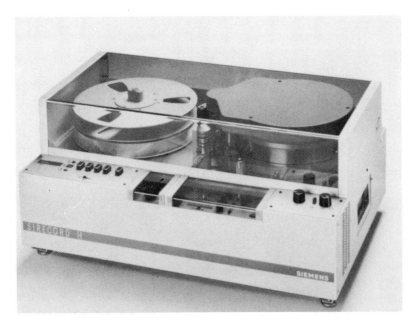

Figure 2–9. Photograph of the Siemens SIRECORD H videotape recorder. (From Siemens Corporation.)

Dimensions (mm)

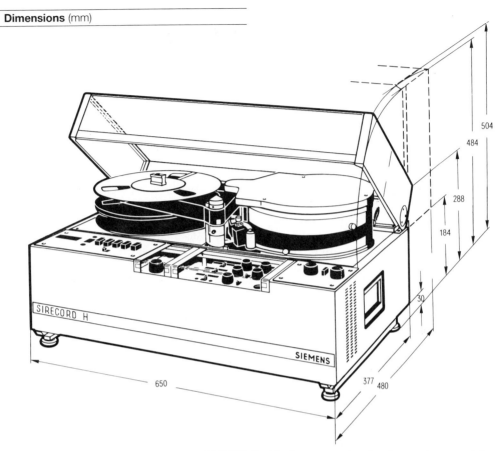

Figure 2–10. Schematic drawing of the SIRECORD H videotape recorder showing a close-up of the recording head. (From Siemens Corporation.)

is produced and played back by differential magnetization of the particles in the emulsion. The process is similar to that described in the discussion of magnetic tape recording. In this type of system, the disc rotates at high speed while the information is both magnetically recorded and viewed by a stationary head.

Laser Imaging Systems

The laser disc system stores the information on a rigid disc similar to the magnetic videodisc. In this type of system, the disc is coated with a reflective optical layer. During the procedure, the laser records the information on the disc by creating a series of microscopic, concentric depressions of varying shapes and distances on the surface of the disc.

The images are read by scanning the disc with the laser light. This light is reflected by the optical coating on the disc in varying degrees in relationship to the depressions in the disc. It is directed to a photodiode, which converts the light signal to an electrical signal. The electrical signal is then transmitted to a television monitor for viewing.

Lasers can also produce the image on special radiographic film. This type of unit uses an analog-to-digital conversion device to reformat the television image to digital data. A special infrared single emulsion film is scanned by the laser, which then transfers the digitized densities to the film emulsion. The film can be processed in the usual manner for viewing. This type of system can be interfaced with CT, MRI, or digital radiography units.

Photofluorographic Systems

This category includes the serial spot filming device and the cinefluorographic camera. These are attached to the I.I. by the image distribution unit (Fig. 2–11). This unit contains a beam-splitting mirror for diverting the optical image onto the lens of the photofluorographic device. The serial spot filming and cinefluorographic camera record the image from the output phosphor of the I.I. in the same way; that is, the light image from the output phosphor creates the image on the photofluorographic film.

The major difference in the two types of systems is the final product. The serial spot filming units produce images that are separated by a specific time interval and demonstrate the changes in the anatomy or pathology as a sequence of static events. These are usually cut from the roll of film and viewed in sequential order in the same manner as with conventional radiographic film.

The cinefluorographic units produce a rapid series of pictures similar to those of a home movie camera; when the film is processed, the images can be projected at the rate of speed at which they were acquired, showing the changes in the anatomy as they appear in motion.

SERIAL SPOT FILM CAMERAS

This type of unit is also called a *large-format*, *spot film*, or *rapid sequence* camera. Such cameras may be referred to by the size of film they use. The current film size formats are 70, 90, 100, and 105 mm; the most commonly used film formats are 100 and 105 mm. Spot film cameras are capable of recording from one to 12 pictures (frames) per second (fps) and can use either roll or cut film depending on the manufacturer and model.

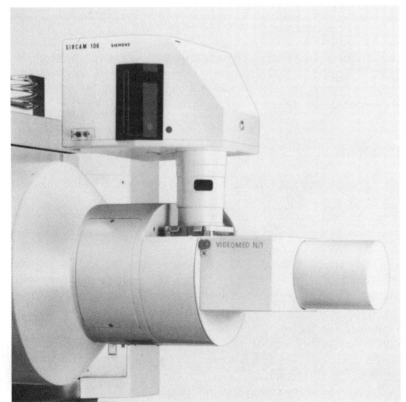

Figure 2–11. Photograph of an image-distribution system attached to the SIRECON 2 Image Intensifier showing the Siemens VIDEOMED N/1 TV camera and SIRCAM 106 100-mm cut film camera connected to the image-intensification unit by means of a dual-channel light-distribution system. (From Siemens Corporation.)

These cameras have certain elements in common: (1) lens system; (2) supply magazine; (3) film transport mechanism; (4) receiving or take-up magazine; and (5) cutoff knife (Fig. 2–12). These units also are capable of both recording patient data onto the film by means of an identification card that must be inserted before and sequentially numbering the frames in a sequence.

The serial spot filming devices do not contain a shutter. The image is produced on the I.I. by using a pulsed x-ray beam. When the beam is on, an image is recorded; when the beam is off, no image is produced on the output phosphor and therefore no image is recorded in the camera.

CINEFLUOROGRAPHIC SYSTEMS

The cine camera is similar in construction to a home movie camera (Fig. 2–13). It contains (1) lens system; (2) supply spool; (3) motor-driven film transport mechanism; (4) take-up spool; and (5) rotating shutter. Film sizes for the cine camera are 16 and 35 mm. The larger format is more popular because it produces a better-quality image.

The operation of the cine camera is also similar to that of a home movie camera. The film is passed in front of an aperture (hole) in synchronization with the shutter system; therefore, the film is in motion when the shutter is closed and stationary when the shutter is open. The image on the output phosphor of the I.I. tube can be produced

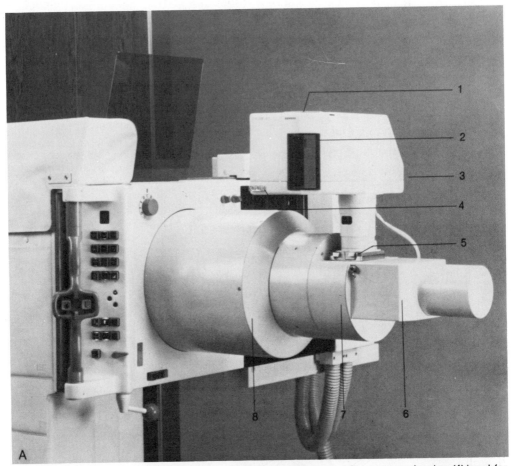

Figure 2–12. *(A)* Photograph of the Siemens SIRCAM 103 100-mm cut film camera showing *(1)* input for patient card; *(2)* receiving magazine; *(3)* cut film camera SIRCAM 103; *(4)* function and film quantity indicator; *(5)* connector for securing camera to light distributor; *(6)* TV camera; *(7)* two-channel light distributor; *(8)* image-intensifier unit SIRCAM 2. (From Siemens Corporation.)

Illustration continued on following page

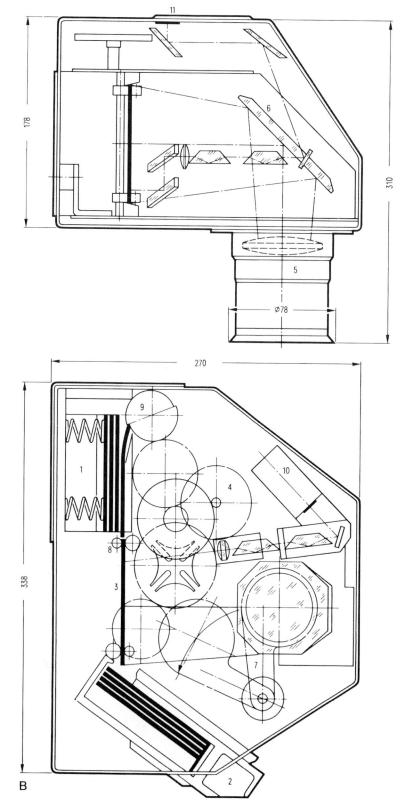

Figure 2–12 *Continued (B)* Schematic illustration of the Siemens SIRCAM 103 cut film serial changer showing *(1)* supply cassette; *(2)* receiving cassette; *(3)* film gate; *(4)* drive motor; *(5)* lens; *(6)* main mirror; *(7)* light guard; *(8)* transport rollers; *(9)* stepped roller; *(10)* exposure counter; *(11)* patient data exposed onto film. (From Siemens Corporation.)

B

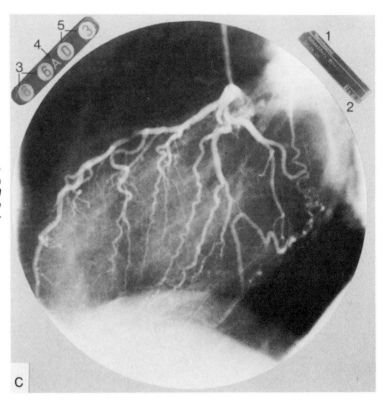

Figure 2–12 *Continued (C)* Photographic representation of a 100-mm x-ray with data: *(1)* patient data; *(2)* date; *(3)* patient number; *(4)* exposure plane; *(5)* consecutive film numbering. (From Siemens Corporation.)

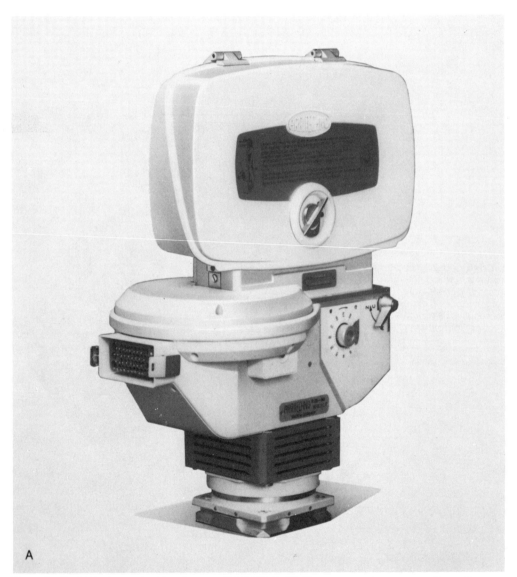

A

Figure 2–13. *(A)* Photograph of the Siemens ARRITECHNO 35, 35-mm x-ray cine camera. (From Siemens Corporation.)

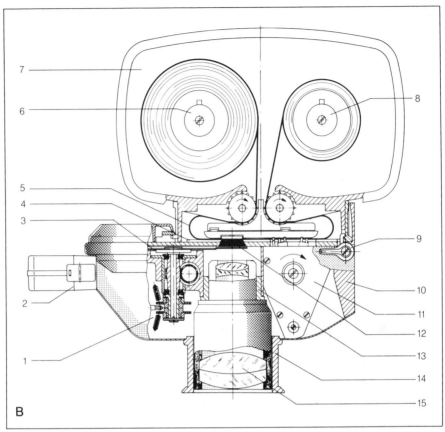

B

Figure 2–13 *Continued (B)* Schematic of the x-ray cine camera showing *(1)* electro-optical pulse generator; *(2)* camera plug; *(3)* shutter; *(4)* film track; *(5)* film loop; *(6)* supply spool; *(7)* cassette; *(8)* take-up spool; *(9)* cassette lock; *(10)* camera housing; *(11)* film driving mechanism; *(12)* aperture; *(13)* lens mount; *(14)* camera adapter; *(15)* lens. (From Siemens Corporation.)

by either a pulsed or a continuous x-ray beam. Modern cinefluorographic units use only the pulsed x-ray beam to produce the images. The pulsed format reduces the radiation dose to the patient, decreases the heat loading of the x-ray tube, and helps reduce motion artifacts, allowing very short exposure times.

The motor used to drive the transport mechanism is capable of varying speed settings. The speed of the motor will govern the number of frames per second that are exposed. The range of frames per second can be from eight to 200 depending on the film size used. Cinefluorography is usually accomplished at frame rates in excess of 16 fps to produce the effect of motion when the final images of the study are projected for viewing.

Cineradiographic film must be properly matched with the emission spectrum of the output phosphor of the I.I. The type of film used is either orthochromatic (yellow or green-blue sensitive) or panchromatic (orange, red, green, yellow, and violet sensitive). Film processing can be accomplished with a specialized processor that can handle film sizes ranging from 35 to 105 mm. If the department does not have a cineprocessor, the film can be developed in a conventional automatic processor if it is first attached to a suitable leader, such as a 14- × 17-in film.

Cinefluorographic units are used during cardiac catheterization to record the sequences in the coronary vasculature. They can be used in a single-plane setup or, if a C-arm is used, as a biplane system (Fig. 2–14).

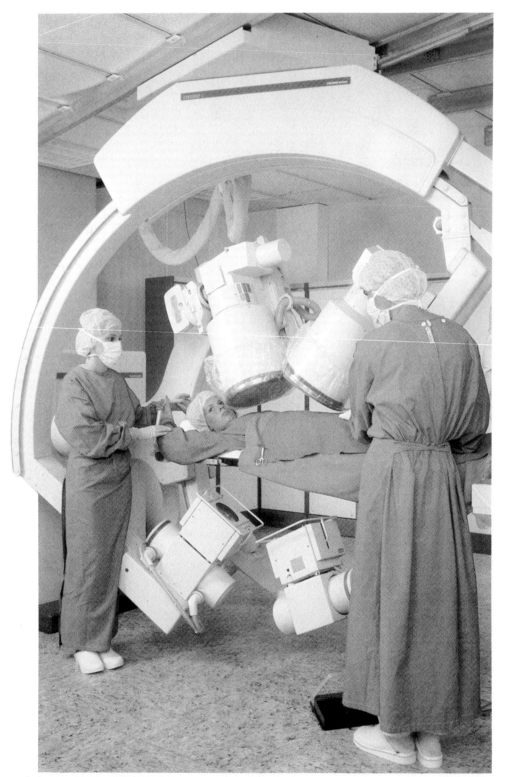

Figure 2–14. Photograph of the Siemens BICOR system set up for biplane cineradiography. (From Siemens Corporation.)

SUMMARY

Certain special procedures require that the image be recorded rapidly to capture the pathological or physiological processes being studied. To accomplish this, special image recording devices are necessary. There are two major categories of imaging devices: those that record the image directly, and those that record the image indirectly.

The large-film rapid sequence changers can be categorized as direct image recording systems and include the roll and cut film changers as well as the rapid sequence cassette changer. Despite the different forms of recording media (e.g., cut film, spot film, roll film) transported in this category, all of the changers have similar operational periods: the transport period (when the film is in motion), and the stationary period (when the film is stopped and exposed). Rapid sequence changers can be used in a single-plane or a biplane system. When these changers are used in a biplane system, technical error can occur if compensation is not made for the increased scatter radiation by the use of changes in exposure factors and high cleanup grid combinations.

The indirect image recording systems include the videotape recorder, videodisc systems, serial spot filming devices, and cinefluorographic systems. All of these devices record the image indirectly; that is, they capture the images from the output phosphor of an image intensification system. These devices can be further subdivided into those systems that record the images from the electrical signal generated by the television camera (videotape and videodisc recorders) and those systems that record the images directly from the output phosphor of the I.I. tube (serial spot filming and cinefluorographic cameras).

These recording systems can be used alone or in combination, depending on the configuration of the equipment.

SUGGESTED READINGS

INTENSIFYING SCREENS, GRIDS, AND FILM

Cullinan, J. E.: Illustrated Guide to X-Ray Techniques, 2nd ed. Philadelphia, J. B. Lippincott, 1980.

Curry, T. S., Dowdey, J. E., and Murray, R. C.: Christensen's An Introduction to the Physics of Diagnostic Radiology, 3rd ed. Philadelphia, Lea & Febiger, 1984.

Fuchs, A. W.: Principles of Radiographic Exposure and Processing, 2nd ed. Springfield, IL, Charles C Thomas, 1979.

Jacobi, C. A., and Paris, D. Q.: Textbook of Radiologic Technology, 6th ed. St. Louis, C. V. Mosby, 1977.

Ter-Pogossian, M. M.: The Physical Aspects of Diagnostic Radiology. New York, Harper & Row, 1969.

three

Automatic Injection Devices

AUTOMATIC INJECTORS
Basic Components
    Control Panel
    Syringe
    Heating Device
    High-Pressure Mechanism
Optional Components
    Arrhythmias
    Strip Chart Recorders and/or
      Oscilloscope Monitors
    Detachable Injector Head

Double-Syringe Assembly
    Safety Devices
Injector Operation
    Constant Flow Rate
    Constant Pressure
Injection Pressure
CT INJECTORS
LYMPHANGIOGRAPHIC INJECTORS
Syringe
Heating Device
Pressure Mechanism

Many special radiographic procedures require an injection of contrast medium under specific controlled conditions. It would be difficult to consistently perform these injections by hand. In the case of lymphangiography, for instance, the injection of the contrast medium must be made at a very slow rate with constant and even pressure, so a specialized automatic injector was designed. During angiographic procedures, the contrast medium is injected into the circulatory system. As it enters the bloodstream, the contrast medium is diluted. This dilution effect is dependent on the injection site; therefore, the site indicates the speed (rate of flow) of the injection. The larger the vessel, the greater the flow rate must be to maintain the proper concentration of contrast medium so that the desired anatomic features can be visualized radiographically. In some procedures, flow rates of 30 to 40 ml of contrast material per second are not uncommon.* Naturally, these injections must be performed with a mechanical device. The flow rate is controlled by many factors, such as the viscosity of the contrast medium, catheter length, catheter diameter, and injection pressure. The flow rate or injection speed can be increased or decreased by varying any of these parameters.

Automatic injectors can be classified by their mode of action; they may be electromechanical or air pressure activated. Most current injectors are designed for operation as either high- or low-pressure injectors, thereby broadening their usefulness in many types of angiographic procedures.

---

*Milliliters will be used throughout this text as the unit of measure for liquid and gas volumes.

AUTOMATIC INJECTORS

Basic Components

All automatic injectors have certain components in common; each is equipped with a control panel, syringe, heating device, and high-pressure mechanism.

CONTROL PANEL

Each of the automatic injection devices has a control panel that is used to set the parameters of the injection sequence (Fig. 3–1A and B). Depending on the unit and the optional equipment purchased, the control panel will appear more or less sophisticated. Almost all of the units available are digitally controlled and ergonomically designed for ease of use. Some of the systems allow the control panel to be removed from the unit and taken to the control area during the procedure (Fig. 3–1C). The controls and indicators present on the control panel will vary with the type of options available with the system. These controls are clearly marked for ease of operation. Each of the systems is supplied with an instruction manual that should be referred to if questions concerning operation or troubleshooting arise.

SYRINGE

In all automatic injectors, the syringe is removable. Disposable syringes are available for use with most automatic injectors; these are presterilized and can be installed easily. They are completely disposable, thereby eliminating the possibility of cross-contamination from reusable parts. Syringe capacity varies with brand. Table 3–1 lists the different syringe sizes available for some automatic injectors and indicates whether they are disposable or reusable. The reusable syringes can be readily autoclaved.

Handle the syringe with care when preparing for a procedure or sterilization because any abnormality can cause failure under operating conditions. Reusable syringes must be disassembled for sterilization; the manufacturer's instructions and recommendations should be followed to avoid the possibility of damage. It is wise to have extra syringes

Table 3–1. SYRINGE CAPACITY OF AUTOMATIC INJECTORS

Manufacturer	Injector	Type of Hydraulic System	Syringe Capacity (ml)	Syringe Material	Reusable	Disposable
Cordis	Injector I	Electromechanical	40	Plastic		X
Cordis	Injector II		100	Plastic		X
Medrad	Mark II	Electromechanical	65	Polypropylene		X
			130	Polypropylene		X
Medrad	Mark III	Electromechanical	65	Polypropylene		X
			130	Polypropylene		X
Medrad	Mark IV	Electromechanical	65	Polypropylene		X
			130	Polypropylene		X
			130	Polycarbonate	X	
			260	Polycarbonate	X	
Medrad	Mark V	Electromechanical	150	Polypropylene		X
Liebel-Flarsheim	Angiomat 3000		200	Polypropylene		X
			100	Molded polypropylene		X
			100	Polycarbonate	X	
			100	Stainless steel	X	
Liebel-Flarsheim	Angiomat 6000	Electromechanical	150	Polypropylene		X
			260	Polypropylene		X
Liebel-Flarsheim	Angiomat CT	Electromechanical	150	Polypropylene		X
			260	Polypropylene		X

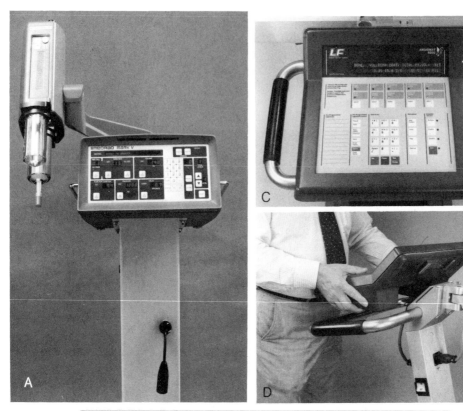

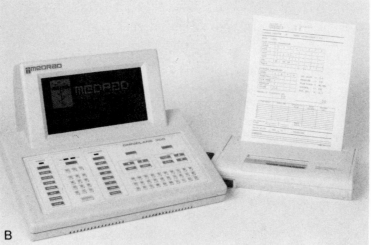

Figure 3–1. (A) Photograph of the Medrad Mark V injector system showing the control panel attached to the unit. (B) Photograph of the Medrad Omniplane 300 combination control panel and program selector, which is capable of controlling the automatic injection system as well as the Omniplane image recording system. Also shown is the printer attachment, which can produce a hard copy of the parameters of the study. (C) Photograph of the Liebel-Flarsheim Angiomat 6000 injector system control panel attached to the floor-mounted stand. (D) Photograph of the Liebel-Flarsheim Angiomat 6000 injector system control panel being removed from the stand. (A and B from Medrad Corporation; C and D from Liebel-Flarsheim Company.)

available in the special procedures suite so that if syringe failure or contamination occurs, a prolonged delay can be avoided. Figure 3–2 shows some syringes in use today.

HEATING DEVICE

The heating system is an electronic device that heats and maintains the contrast medium at or near body temperature and reduces the viscosity of certain contrast agents, thereby facilitating the setting of certain flow rates from the injector. It is usually located on the injector head close to the syringe. The syringe temperature is thermostatically controlled and is usually preset at the factory to a nominal 37° C (approximately 98° F). Heating time varies with the injector being used. Most injection device heaters can only maintain the temperature of the contrast agent. Therefore, the contrast agent should be prewarmed when using injection devices equipped with this type of heater.

HIGH-PRESSURE MECHANISM

The main type of high-pressure mechanism used on automatic injectors is the electromechanical system. This is simply an electric drive motor connected to a jackscrew that drives the piston into or out of the syringe. Figure 3–3 depicts a simplified version of an electromechanical high-pressure device.

Automatic injection devices using compressed air as the high-pressure mechanism are no longer manufactured for use during special procedures in the United States.

Cordis Corporation is marketing a device for use during hand injections that uses compressed air to assist the practitioner in making the injection. The system consists of a hand-held, three-ring–controlled, 10-ml syringe that connects to a supply of carbon dioxide. During the injection, the gas is released behind the syringe plunger to assist in maintaining a consistent pressure on the plunger and help the practitioner provide an accurate rate of delivery of the contrast agent through small diagnostic angiographic catheters.[1]

When using systems that operate with high-pressure gas cylinders it is important to check and double-check the pressure that is to be applied. These systems are equipped with reducer valves or pressure regulators that allow for the adjustment of the air pressure required for the procedure. The pressure is usually read from a manometer or pressure gauge located on the system. In the case of the Hercules syringe system, two gauges are present. One of these shows the pressure in the carbon dioxide cylinder (0 to 1000 psi), and the other shows the syringe pressure (0 to 450 psi). The bursting pressure of the catheter system being used must be considered when setting the amount of pressure needed to make the injection. The pressure should be checked against all of the parameters before initiating the study.

Optional Components

Electrocardiogram Triggering Device. One optional feature of some automatic injectors is the electrocardiogram (ECG) triggering device. With this option the injection can be synchronized with the R wave impulses received from the patient.

Electrical changes in the heart muscle taking place during systole can be led off from the surface of the body by electrodes to a recorder capable of producing an ECG. Standard locations on the body for these electrodes are the right and left arms, right arm and left leg, and left arm and left leg. Each segment of the ECG shows the electrical cycle of the heart (Fig. 3–4). The P wave initiates the cycle, and the excitation spreads from the sinoatrial node over the atrium to the atrioventricular node. Peaks

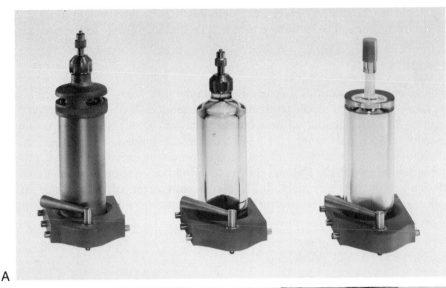

A

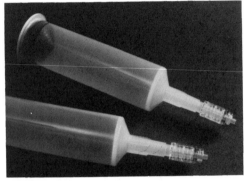

B

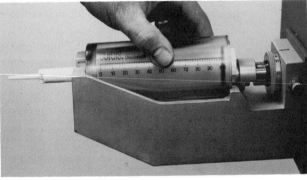

C

Figure 3–2. Automatic injection syringes. (*A*) Angiomat 3000 ClearVu disposable, plastic resterilizable, and stainless steel syringes; (*B*) Medrad polypropylene disposable syringes. (*C*) 100-ml plastic syringe for the Cordis Injector II. (*A* from Liebel-Flarsheim Company; *B* from Medrad, Inc.; *C* from Cordis Corporation.)

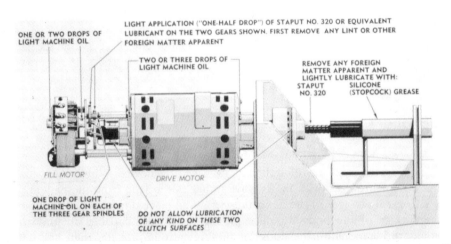

Figure 3–3. Schematic of a typical electromechanical drive mechanism of automatic injectors. (From Cordis Corporation.)

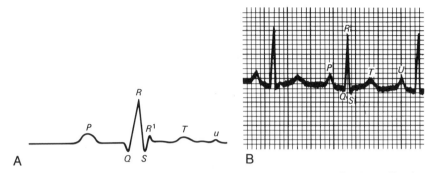

Figure 3–4. (A) Electrocardiogram showing the location of the major waves; (B) schematic of a segment of (A) showing excitation during one cycle. (From Hurst J. W., and Myerburg, R. J.: Introduction to Electrocardiography, 2nd ed. New York, McGraw-Hill, 1973.)

Q, R, and S follow as the impulse spreads throughout the atrioventricular bundle of His over the ventricles. At this time, the heart is in ventricular systole. Finally, as ventricular excitation subsides, the T peak is recorded.[2] The U wave is not usually attendant in the normal ECG; it is usually present when the serum potassium level is low and appears as a small upward wave.

A normal single heartbeat comprises five waves (P, Q, R, S, and T). The P wave causes the atria to contract. The presence of the QRS complex indicates that the ventricles are undergoing contraction. The T wave is the electrical recovery from the ventricular contraction phase.

The small and large blocks on the ECG paper and tracing illustrate the interval in seconds (horizontal blocks) and the measurement of electrical activity in millimeters (vertical blocks) of the wave. Each of the small horizontal blocks represents 0.04 s on the horizontal line and 1 mm on the vertical line (Fig. 3–5). Because each of the large blocks comprises five horizontal and five vertical blocks, its value can be stated as 0.2 s (0.04 s × 5 = 0.2 s) horizontal and 5 mm (1 mm × 5 = 5 mm) vertical. The vertical height is correlated to the electrical activity. Five millimeters of height (one large block) is equal to 0.5 mV of electrical activity.

Table 3–2 summarizes the normal ECG tracing and lists the wave, segment, or interval; the significant physiology; and how the normal pattern should be represented on the ECG paper.

Figure 3–5. Schematic showing time and voltage lines on ECG paper. Five large horizontal boxes (25 small squares) equals 1 s. Two large vertical boxes equals 1 mv or 10 mm.

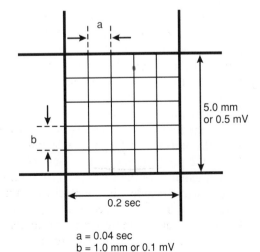

a = 0.04 sec
b = 1.0 mm or 0.1 mV

Table 3–2. SUMMARY OF THE NORMAL ELECTROCARDIOGRAM

Wave/Segment/ Interval	Significance	Normal Pattern
P wave	Upward deflection Begins with electrical discharge from sinus node Electrical current flows in the atria Depolarization of the atrial muscle produces the P wave	Less than 3 small blocks wide Less than 3 small blocks high

PR interval	Interval between the beginning of the P wave and the beginning of the QRS complex
	Electrical impulse spreads along the following route:
	    Atrium
	    Atrioventricular node
	    Bundle of His
	    Right and left bundle branches
		More than 3 and less than 5 small blocks wide

QRS complex	Three separate deflections:
	    Q—downstroke before the R wave (downward deflection)
	    R—first upward wave (upward deflection)
	    S—downstroke after the R wave (downward deflection)
	Represents a depolarization of the ventricles
	Electrical impulse travels along the following pathway:
	    Purkinje fibers
	    Ventricular muscle fibers
		Less than 2.5 small blocks wide

ST segment	Begins at the end of the S wave and ends at the beginning of the T wave Point at which the tracing "turns" following the S wave	The ST segment should not be elevated or depressed
T wave	Repolarization of the ventricular tissue	Normal wave less than 10 small blocks high in the chest leads and less than 5 small blocks high in the remaining leads
U wave	Small upward deflection that follows the T wave	Not normally present unless serum potassium level is low

ARRHYTHMIAS

The recognition of cardiac arrhythmias is a skill that is acquired through experience. Many of the abnormalities that appear on electrocardiographic (ECG) tracings can apply to more than one type of arrhythmia. A systematic analysis of the ECG tracing pattern can narrow the choices dramatically. The novice practitioner should be conversant with the normal ECG pattern and be able to recognize any deviation from the "normal" ECG pattern. During the procedure, any changes in the normal pattern should be noted, and the physician should be alerted.

Arrhythmias are basically changes in the ECG tracing and denote a change in the rate of the impulses (automaticity), the conduction of the impulses, or both. Variations from the normal ECG pattern should be immediately pointed out to the physician during the procedure; careful observation of the patient in conjunction with monitoring of the regularity of the ECG pattern is important during a special procedure. Symptoms to watch for include chest tightness, pain, palpitations, rapid or distressed breathing, restlessness, loss of consciousness, pallor, and cool, moist skin. The physician should be alerted if any of these symptoms appear in conjunction with an abnormal ECG trace pattern. These symptoms can be invaluable in determining the exact diagnosis and treatment protocol to be followed subsequent to the event.

The ECG tracing should be systematically evaluated in the following categories:

1. **Rate of rhythm**. The rate of the cardiac rhythm should be categorized into one of the following.
   a. No rate. No waves present or any sign of electrical activity.
   b. Slow rate. Rates less than 60 beats/min (bradycardia).
   c. Normal rate. Rates between 60 and 100 beats/min.
   d. Increased rate. Rates in excess of 100 beats/min (tachycardia)
2. **Regularity of the rhythm**. This is measured by the distance between the QRS complexes, which is sometimes referred to as the RR interval. This should vary by no more than three small squares (0.12 s).
3. **PR ratio**. This is the ratio of the number of P waves to QRS complexes. The normal PR ratio is 1:1.
4. **PR interval**. This is measured as the distance between the onset of the P wave and the onset of the QRS complex. It should not be any less than three small squares (0.12 s) or more than five small squares (0.20 s).
5. **QRS complex interval**. This is measured as the distance from the start of the QRS complex to the end of the same QRS complex. The normal QRS interval is about two and one-half small squares (0.10 s).

ECG tracing pattern changes in any of these areas should be noted on the patient's chart, and the information should immediately be transmitted to the physician performing the procedure. Any change from the normal ECG tracing pattern usually signifies the presence of an arrhythmia. Table 3–3 summarizes a variety of major arrhythmias and their general characteristics.

Table 3–3. SUMMARY OF MAJOR ARRHYTHMIAS AND THEIR GENERAL CHARACTERISTICS

Type of Arrhythmia	Heart Rate	Pattern Regularity	PR Ratio	PR Interval	QRS Complex
Asystole	None	Regular flat line wave	None	None	None
Ventricular fibrillation	None	Irregular wavy line	None	None	None
Junctional rhythm	Slow	Regular	1:1 or 0:1	None or shortened	Within limits
Sinus bradycardia	Slow	Regular	1:1	Within limits	Within limits
Idioventricular rhythm	Slow	Regular	0:1	None	Increased
First-degree heart block	Normal to slow	Regular	1:1	Increased with regular pattern	Within limits
Mobitz I heart block (second-degree)	Normal to slow	Irregular	Between 1:1 and 2:1	Increased with irregular pattern	Within limits
Mobitz II heart block (second-degree)	Normal to slow	Regular or irregular	1:1, 2:1, or greater	Constant for beats that are conducted	Within limits
Third-degree heart block	Normal to slow	Regular	1:1	Variable	Increased
Atrial fibrillation	Slow or fast	Irregular	0:1	None	Within limits
Atrial flutter	Ventricular rate, normal Atrial rate, 250 to 300 beats/min	Usually regular	2:1 or greater	Regular	Within limits
Sinus tachycardia	Fast (100 to 150 beats/min)	Regular	1:1	Within limits	Within limits
Atrial tachycardia	Fast (150 to 250 beats/min)	Regular	1:1	Within limits	Within limits
Ventricular tachycardia	Fast	Regular	0:1	None	Increased
Junctional tachycardia	Fast	Regular	1:1	None or shortened	Within limits

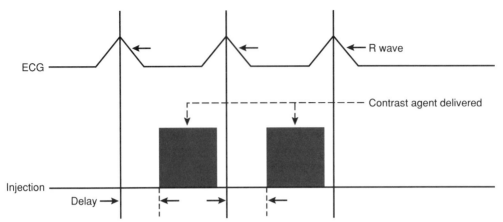

Figure 3–6. Schematic showing how multiple injections are accomplished using the R wave plus a prescribed delay. This allows the contrast agent to be delivered during a particular segment of the cardiac cycle.

The automatic injector can usually be adjusted to amplify the input to use the R wave as a triggering device for injection rather than any of the others present on the ECG. This adjustment should be made before the injector is armed. The injection can also be delayed after triggering by the R wave for as long as 0.8 to 0.9 s, depending on the particular injection device.

Some units, such as the Medrad Mark V, are equipped with an ECG triggering device that can deliver a single injection or a maximum of nine multiple boluses. Each of the boluses would be triggered by the R wave of the cardiac cycle plus a predetermined delay (Fig. 3–6). This unit makes it possible to control whether the injection continues through successive R waves. This means that the total selected volume would be delivered to the patient at the chosen flow rate even if it spanned more than one cardiac cycle (Fig. 3–7). In this situation, the total amount of contrast agent delivered would be the selected volume multiplied by the number of injections initiated.

The injector can also be set to terminate the injection at the next R wave regardless of the volume of contrast agent delivered (Fig. 3–8). The total amount of contrast agent delivered to the patient would be the bolus volume multiplied by the number of boluses delivered.[3]

Depending on the injector purchased and the options added, the ECG option may

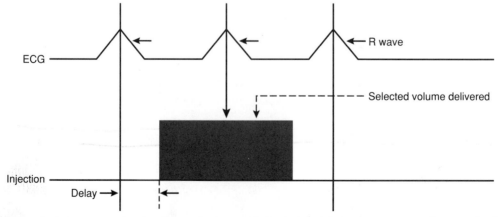

Figure 3–7. Schematic showing the contrast agent bolus being delivered across several successive R waves.

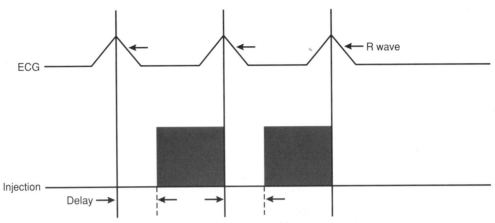

Figure 3–8. Schematic showing the termination of the injection at each successive R wave.

be a simple device whereby the entire injection is triggered by the R wave or it may be a more sophisticated system that permits many smaller injections, each initiated by an R wave received from the patient (Fig. 3–9). With some devices, such as the Medrad Mark V, the x-ray exposure can also be initiated automatically during this sequence of events.

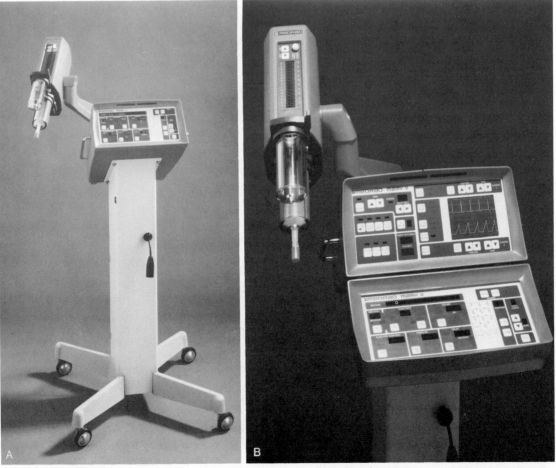

Figure 3–9. (*A*) Medrad Mark V automatic injector showing the ECG triggering device and optional oscilloscope module (*B*). (From Medrad, Inc.)

STRIP CHART RECORDERS AND/OR OSCILLOSCOPE MONITORS

Injectors can be equipped with equipment for strip chart recording and/or oscilloscope monitoring of the ECG. The Médrad Mark V oscilloscope module uses a two-channel, nonfading display that shows the patient's ECG on one channel and the injection profile on the other. This allows a review of the entire ECG-triggered injection without the necessity of a chart recorder.

DETACHABLE INJECTOR HEAD

Another interesting feature found on some injectors is the detachable injector head (Fig. 3–10). This feature is useful for procedures such as femoral arteriography when

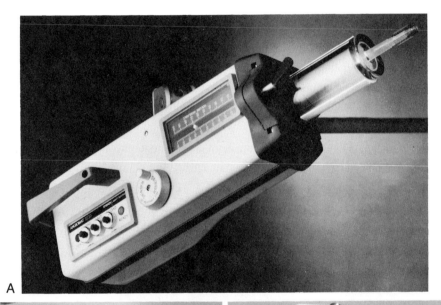

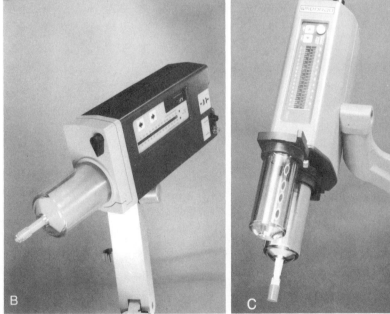

Figure 3–10. Detachable injector heads of two automatic injection devices. (*A*) Liebel-Flarsheim Angiomat 3000; (*B*) Liebel-Flarsheim Angiomat 6000; (*C*) Medrad Mark V injector head detached from the injector console, also showing the double-syringe assembly. (*A* and *B* from Liebel-Flarsheim Company; *C* from Medrad, Inc.)

done on the specialized arteriographic step-table. An attachment is available that permits the injector head to be monitored directly on the radiographic table, while the console portion is located in the control booth.

DOUBLE-SYRINGE ASSEMBLY

Also of interest is the double-syringe assembly of the Medrad injector, which allows preloading of two syringes. When one syringe has been emptied, the plunger is retracted and the assembly is turned 180° to position the second syringe with minimum resulting time loss.

SAFETY DEVICES

Acceleration regulators and pressure-limiting devices can add optional safety features to the automatic injection device. The acceleration regulator allows the drive motor to be accelerated over a specific period of time, which reduces the possibility of catheter whip (Fig. 3–11).

Available are simple devices, such as the rate rise control on the Angiomat 3000, and sophisticated systems by which the flow rate may be selected according to various parameters, such as the Medrad universal flow module. The latter not only can increase flow rate to a specific level and maintain this level for the duration of the injection but also achieve a final acceleration or deceleration of the flow rate after an initial level has been reached. With the Medrad Mark V injector, multiple-level injections can be programmed to allow for a wide variety of unusual flow patterns during the study. This is accomplished by having the flow rate change during the injection. The Medrad Mark V injector has the capability for nine flow rate changes per injection. Multiphasic and biphasic injection patterns as well as backflow studies and positive and negative accelerations are possible with this system. The rate rise is controlled in the Angiomat 6000 injector by digitally setting the transition time on the control panel.

Pressure-limiting devices set a maximum on the pressure permitted to be generated, thereby ensuring safe use of even low-pressure catheters (Fig. 3–12).

Volume-limiting devices are designed to set a maximum limit on the volume of contrast agent injected into the patient. The automatic safety stop device on the Medrad Mark V will reposition itself automatically for each injection, providing for a recurring volume-limiting action and preventing the plunger from moving past a certain point. The Angiomat 3000 and the Cordis injectors are equipped with mechanical volume-limiting devices. These are designed to be used only as a safety feature and not as injection volume regulators. Both these units must be set manually and checked before each injection.

Function-monitoring devices are available on all types of units. These may be simple, such as a ready light, or sophisticated, such as in the Medrad Mark V Sentinel, which monitors the key functions and operation sequences of the injector. This device will alert the operator to an arming procedure or control setting that was overlooked as well as indicate both primary and secondary circuit features.

Most automatic injectors are designed to be triggered with the head pointed toward the floor to allow air bubbles that may be present to collect at the far end of the syringe and not be injected into the patient.

Injector Operation

When programming the automatic injector, the radiographer must be concerned with one primary factor—the *flow rate*. Flow rate can be defined simply as the delivery rate

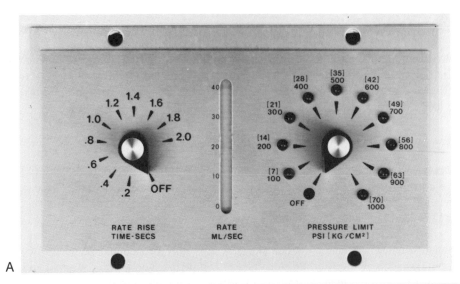

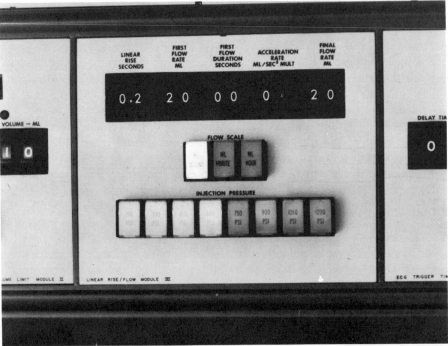

Figure 3–11. Acceleration-regulating mechanisms of two automatic injectors. (*A*) Rate-rise control of the Angiomat 3000. Also shown are the pressure-limiting control and the achieved rate indicator. The pressure-limiting control monitors pressure in 100-psi increments up to 1000 psi. The achieved rate indicator shows at a glance the rate of injection in 2-ml/s increments up to 40 ml/s. (*B*) The Medrad linear-rise flow module III provides for not only simple acceleration regulation but also secondary acceleration or deceleration of the injection rate. With this option, it is possible to program an accelerating flow rate followed by one that decelerates. This technique of providing two separate flow rates is called the biphasic injection technique. (*A* from Liebel-Flarsheim Company; *B* from Medrad, Inc.)

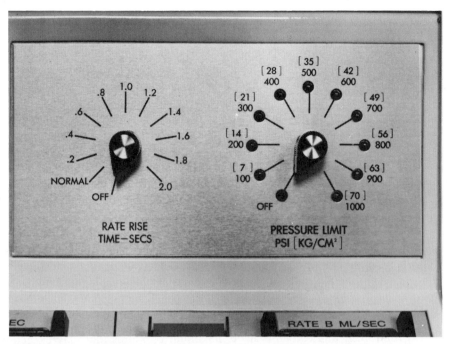

Figure 3–12. Close-up of the Angiomat 3000 pressure-limiting device. This permits a maximum amount of pressure to be generated by the automatic injector, thereby ensuring that low-pressure catheters may be used without the concern of rupture. (From Liebel-Flarsheim Company.)

(amount delivered per unit of time). It is dependent on the viscosity of the contrast agent, the length and diameter of the catheter, and the injection pressure. The flow rate chosen for a specific special procedure is governed by the procedure itself, the vessel entered, the patient, and the nature of the disease. Flow rates can vary from as low as 4 ml/s to as high as 30 to 40 ml/s, depending on these factors.

Automatic injectors can be divided into two basic types in regard to delivery of contrast material—those that automatically provide a constant flow rate, and those that give a constant pressure (W. L. Smith, Barber-Coleman Co., 1973; personal communication). The constant flow rate injector maintains a selected flow rate regardless of the variable parameters involved (e.g., catheter length, diameter, contrast viscosity, etc.). The constant pressure injector maintains a constant pressure but does not take into account the various parameters that determine the flow rate; these must be considered before the pressure is selected.

CONSTANT FLOW RATE

When constant flow injectors are used, the desired flow rate and injection time are set, and the selected volume in milliliters per second will be delivered regardless of the variables involved (Fig. 3–13). For example, if a flow rate of 50 ml/s and a volume of 100 ml are required, they are programmed on the injector as 50 ml/s injection rate for 2 s. This setting will deliver the specific volume at the desired flow rate regardless of the viscosity of the contrast medium or any other parameters involved. Care must be exercised when flow rates are set because too high a flow rate may injure the patient or damage the catheter.

Constant flow rate injectors provide adjustable pressure during the injection. The unit changes the pressure to adapt to the parameters involved in the study. These types of injection systems are usually equipped with pressure-limiting devices that prevent the injector from producing pressures beyond the safety limits of the catheter being

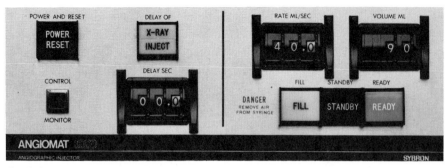

Figure 3–13. Close-up of the Angiomat 3000 console panel. This illustrates one method by which constant flow injectors are programmed to achieve a specific flow rate for an injection. If a total volume of 80 ml and a flow rate of 4.0 ml/s are desired, these parameters are set on the control panel. This will then provide a flow rate of 4.0 ml/s for an injection period of 20 s. On other flow rate injectors, it is necessary to set the rate of flow and the total injection period. In other words,it would be necessary to set 4.0 ml/s for an injection period of 20 s. Milliliters per second multiplied by the injection period yields the total volume injected, in this case, 80 ml. (From Liebel-Flarsheim Company.)

used. The radiographer is responsible for setting this factor on the injector before the study. It is important that the pressure limitations of the catheters being used are known. Some low flow catheters have a maximum bursting pressure of 500 psi, while higher flow, reinforced-wall catheters have maximum pressures that may exceed 1000 to 1200 psi. If the pressure-limiting device for a low flow catheter were set for a maximum of 800 psi, this would exceed the safe operating range and be potentially harmful to the patient.

Another consideration involves setting the pressure-limiting device too low for the parameters involved. Each combination of parameters used (catheter length, diameter, number of side holes, type and viscosity of the contrast agent, etc.) requires a minimum amount of pressure to maintain the selected flow rate. (This pressure should be below the maximum rating for the catheter involved.) If the pressure-limiting device was set below this minimum level, the injection would be made with a decreased flow rate. For example, assume that a particular set of parameters requires 450 psi to maintain a flow rate of 6 ml/s and the catheter is rated at 800 psi. If the radiographer sets the pressure-limiting device at 150 psi, the injector would not be able to produce the minimum pressure required for the desired flow rate; in this case, the flow rate would be reduced to 3 ml/s.

Varying the parameters used for a particular study can change the pressure required. If the maximum safe operating pressure is exceeded and the desired flow rate cannot be achieved with the selected parameters, other combinations should be considered. The types of changes that can be considered are summarized as follows.

1. Catheter diameter. The catheter with the larger overall internal diameter (ID) (lumen) will provide less resistance against the flow of contrast and require less pressure to maintain a selected flow rate.
2. Catheter length. The catheter with the overall greater length will provide more resistance to flow than one that is shorter.

If the major parameters cannot be varied, the removal of nonessential components in the system can decrease the resistance to flow and drastically reduce the pressure needed to maintain the flow rate; this refers to any tubes or fittings that would be in the path of the syringe and the catheter.

If the components of the system cannot be varied, a reduction in the resistance can be accomplished by warming the contrast agent or using a contrast medium with a lower viscosity (less iodine concentration). It should be remembered that the contrast agent must not be heated above the nominal 37° C (approximately 98° F).

CONSTANT PRESSURE

Constant pressure injectors usually require only one setting on the console—the pressure. However, the variable parameters that influence delivery rates must be taken into consideration by the radiographer before the pressure is dialed into the unit. A detailed analysis of the causes and effects of these factors is beyond the scope of this text, but an understanding of their influence on delivery rate is necessary to obtain optimum opacification of the anatomy with the least possible risk to the patient.

EFFECT OF CATHETER LENGTH. The delivery rate of contrast material is inversely proportional to catheter length (Fig. 3–14).[4] It is readily seen that delivery rates can be increased by using shorter catheters and decreased by using longer catheters.

EFFECT OF CATHETER DIAMETER. Increases in catheter ID result in increases in the delivery rate of contrast media. This relation is not is not a direct one, and delivery rates increase nonlinearly with increases in catheter diameter. Tapering the catheter tip effectively reduces the ID of the catheter. At lower pressures, there is a negligible decrease in flow rate; however, as pressure increases, there is a relatively greater decrease in flow rate. This is a result of the increased turbulence caused by the obstructive influence of the tapered end of the catheter.[5]

EFFECT OF VISCOSITY. Decreases in viscosity of the contrast agent with all other factors kept constant will result in an increase in delivery rate.

EFFECT OF CATHETER SIDE HOLES. Side holes in catheters result in delivery rates from 10 to 20% greater than those of catheters without side holes. The presence of side holes in catheters also adds stability to the catheter tip, which tends even at high

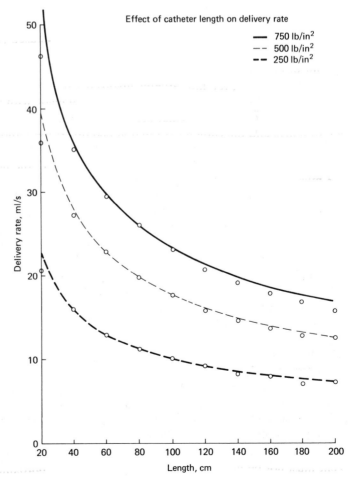

Figure 3–14. This graph shows the effect of varying catheter lengths on the delivery rate of distilled water. It can be readily seen that shorter catheter lengths provide greater flow of material. (From Krovetz, L. J., et al.: An analysis of factors determining delivery rates of liquids through cardiac catheters, Radiology, 86:124, 1966.)

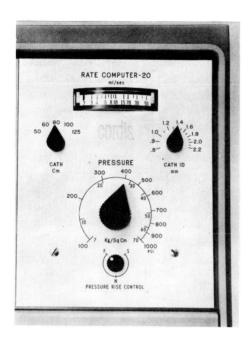

Figure 3–15. Close-up of the injection rate computer of the Cordis automatic injector. The computer meter indicates the injection rate resulting from the combination of the injection pressure with the parameters set on the module. (From Cordis Corporation.)

pressures to minimize the whiplash effect of the catheter. The greatest effect will be noted when the side holes are arranged symmetrically around the circumference of the catheter.[5]

Injection Pressure

Electromechanically powered injectors usually indicate the actual pressures used during the injection procedure. The pressure range available is from 100 to 1000 lb/in², which allows a wide range of flow rates when combined with the variable parameters discussed previously.

An optional feature of the Cordis 2 injector is an injection rate computer (Fig. 3–15). This enables the radiographer to preset variable parameters such as syringe size and catheter length, diameter, and wall thickness before adjusting the pressure to a setting that will indicate the desired flow rate in milliliters per second on the meter. This eliminates the necessity for predetermining flow rates for the combinations of variable parameters that can be used.

By following the operating instructions of the Cordis injector, a nomogram can be supplied that can be used to obtain the flow rate for various combinations of catheters (length and ID) and injector pressures (Fig. 3–16).

Tables 3–4 and 3–5 illustrate the typical parameters used for various angiographic procedures with the Angiomat 6000 and Medrad Mark V injectors.

CT INJECTORS

CT procedures require a high degree of control over the injection and its parameters to maximize the accuracy of the study. Injection systems used for CT have the same basic components as those used for angiography. The Angiomat CT is a microprocessor-based system equipped with a 260-ml polypropylene syringe (an optional 150-ml syringe is available). The injector head can be either floor mounted or track mounted on an

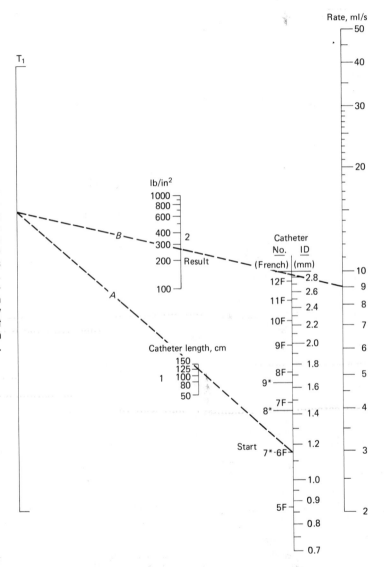

Figure 3–16. Nomogram supplied with the Cordis automatic injector. The nomogram applies only to contrast agents between 2 and 8 poise at 38° C. To use the nomogram, start by drawing a line from the chosen catheter number or ID through the length of the catheter. This line *(A)* should intersect the T scale. From the point at which the line intersects the T scale, draw a line *(B)* through the pressure (lb/in²) to indicate the flow rate. This indicates the flow rate that would result if the parameters through which the lines are drawn are used. (From Cordis Corporation.)

Table 3–4. SUMMARY OF PARAMETERS FOR VARIOUS ANGIOGRAPHIC PROCEDURES WITH THE ANGIOMAT 3000 INJECTOR†

Procedure	Contrast Medium Concentration (%)	Volume per Injection (ml)	Delivery (ml/s)*
Abdominal aortography	75–76	45–70	15–35
Adrenal arteriography			
Aortography	60–75–76	45–70	15–35
Selective injection of renal artery	60–75–76	6–10	4–6
Brachial arteriography	50–60	20	10–20
Brachiocephalic arteriography of the:			
Common carotid artery	50–60	12–14	10
Internal carotid artery	50–60	10	10
Vertebral artery	50–60	6	10
Innominate artery	50–60	30	10
Subclavian artery	50–60	25	10
Bronchial arteriography	75–76	6	2–4
Celiac angiography	75–76	40–70	10–15
Femoral arteriography	50–60	20–30	10–20
Gastroduodenal, dorsal pancreatic, intercostal, and lumbar arteriography	60–75–76	4–12	4–10
Hepatic arteriography	60–75–76	40	8–12
Hypogastric arteriography	60–75–76	15–20	5–10
Inferior mesenteric arteriography	75–76	15–30	8–12
Pulmonary angiography	75–76	60	15–25
Renal arteriography	60–75–76	8–10	4–10
Selective coronary angiography	60–75–76–85	6	4
Splenic arteriography	60–75–76	40–100	8–12
Superior mesenteric arteriography	75–76	20–40	8–12
Thoracic aortography via the femoral routes	75–76	50–70	15–30
Cardiac arteriography			
Left atrial angiography (transseptal or retrograde left ventricular route)	60–75–76–85	50–60	15–25
Left ventriculography	60–75–76–85	40–50	15–20
Right atrial angiography	75–76–85	60–80	30–40
Right ventriculography	60–75–76–85	40–50	15–20
Venography			
Adrenal venography	60–75–76	3–6	2–4
Ascending venography	50–60	50–100	5–15
Direct portography	60–75–76	35	20
Gonadal venography	60–75–76	15	5–10
Hepatic venography (wedged)	75–76	6–8	2
Inferior cavography	60–75–76	50	10–25
Pelvic venography	60–75–76	40–50	15–30
Renal venography	60–75–76	15–35	4–15
Splenoportography (direct)	75–76	60–80	4–8
Superior cavography	60–75–76	50	10–25

*Relative to catheter or needle flow rates and technique.
†These parameters are also valid for the Angiomat 6000.

Table 3–5. SUMMARY OF PARAMETERS FOR VARIOUS ANGIOGRAPHIC PROCEDURES WITH THE MEDRAD MARK IV AND MARK V INJECTOR SYSTEMS*

	Contrast Media Group†	Volume (ml)	Flow Rate (ml/s)	Comments
Selective Arteriography				
Brachiocephalic				
Common carotid artery	A	10	8	Pure meglumine medium
Internal carotid artery	A	8	6	Pure meglumine medium
External carotid artery	A	4	2	Pure meglumine medium
Vertebral artery	A	7	7	Pure meglumine medium
Innominate artery	A	25	15	Pure meglumine medium
Subclavian artery	A	16	8	Pure meglumine medium
Thyrocervical trunk	A	6	2	
Brachial artery	A	12	6	If hand study, inject 25 ml tolazoline intraarterially 1 min before study; increase volume to 18 ml
Abdominal and thoracic				
lumbar, intercostal, bronchial	B	6	2	May increase if supplying large tumor
Renal artery	B	8–12	4–6	Decrease if artery does not supply entire kidney
Celiac axis	B	40	10	
Splenic artery	B	30	8	Increase to 60 ml to show portal system
Hepatic artery	B	30	8	
Gastroduodenal artery	B	16	4	
Dorsal pancreatic artery	B	6	2	
Superior mesenteric artery	B	40	10	
Superior mesenteric artery	B	50	12	To enhance portal system, inject 50 mg
Inferior mesenteric artery	B	20	5	
Hypogastric artery	B	20	8	
Common femoral artery	A	24	8	Retrograde injection
Superficial femoral artery	A	18	6	Antegrade injection. If foot study, inject 25 ml tolazoline intraarterially 1 min before study
Angiocardiography				
Left coronary artery	B	8	3	Mixture of magnesium diatrizoate recommended (magnesium predominant); hand injection usually used
Right coronary artery	B	6	3	If not dominant, inject less
Saphenous-vein bypass graft	B	8	3	Decrease if graft supplies relatively small vascular bed
Internal mammary	B	6	2	
Left ventricle	B	40–50	10–12	For contractility and function. Increase volume to 50 ml if left ventricle is dilated
Left ventricle	B	45	15	To visualize septal defect
Left atrium	B	40	15	
Right atrium	B	60–80	30–40	To visualize left heart and aorta
Right ventricle	B	40	20	Increase if large right-to-left shunt
Main pulmonary artery	B	60	40	For pulmonary thromboembolism
Right or left				
Pulmonary artery	B	40	20	Vary to fit size of vascular bed
Branch pulmonary artery	B	20	10	
Pediatric studies				
Right heart		1–1.5/kg	2	
Left heart, aorta		0.5/kg	2	

Table continued on following page

Table 3–5. SUMMARY OF PARAMETERS FOR VARIOUS ANGIOGRAPHIC PROCEDURES WITH THE MEDRAD MARK IV AND MARK V INJECTOR SYSTEMS* *Continued*

	Contrast Media Group†	Volume (ml)	Flow Rate (ml/s)	Comments
Aortography				
Thoracic aorta	B	50	25	Increase if large aneurysm
Aortic arch	B	45–50	30–35	To visualize brachiocephalic vessels
Abdominal aorta	B	40	25	Open-end catheter
Abdominal aorta	B	30	20	Pigtail catheter
Abdominal aorta	B	60	20	For large aneurysm
Aortic-peripheral				
Suprarenal injection	B	60	15	Translumbar approach
Aortic bifurcation	A or B	50	12	Inject 50 mg tolazoline intra-arterially 1 min before study
Aortic bifurcation	A mixed with lidocaine (1 mg/ml)	70	8/5 and 6/5	Automatic variation of flow from 8 s^{-1} for 5 s to 6 s^{+1} for 5 s to prolong duration of injection when using moving table top; x-ray delay 3 to 4 s.
Venography				
Upper extremity	A	20	5	
Jugular vein	A	10	10	
Superior vena cava	B	40	20	Via catheter
Superior vena cava	B	40	10	Into each arm
Azygos vein	B	30	10	Selective azygos vein injection
Azygos vein	A	20	5	Intramedullary rib injection
Inferior vena cava	B	40	20	
Hepatic vein	B	8	2	Wedged
Hepatic vein	B	20	6	Unwedged
Adrenal vein	B	3–6	1–2	Determine flow volume fluoroscopically
Renal vein	B	20	10	
Gonadal vein	B	24	6	
Hypogastric vein	B	24	8	
Splenoportography	B	30	8	
Direct aortography	B	30	15	Umbilical approach

*Data compiled by J. H. Grollman, Jr., M.D., Clinical Professor of Radiology, UCLA Center for the Health Sciences, University of California, Los Angeles. This represents the typical parameters in use with the Medrad Mark IV Injector at UCLA. These settings can also be used with the Mark V system.
†Physical factors for contrast media given in Table 4–1.

overhead system (Fig. 3–17). In most cases, the console is mounted inside the control booth for maximum operator safety. The Angiomat CT allows a variable flow rate, from 10 ml/hr to 10 ml/s. This unit also allows programming injection delays from 0 to 255 s in 0.01-s intervals for use during multiphasic studies.

The Angiomat CT injector has the same safety systems as the Angiomat 6000, including pressure limitation and transition time. The unit is also equipped with a pause feature that permits a pause in the injection; the injection can then be resumed on command. The parameters of the pause, such as the phase number, pause mode, elapsed time, and volume remaining, are displayed on the console. The Angiomat CT is also capable of storing more than 60 programs that can be recalled when needed. Some typical parameters for use with the Angiomat CT can be found in Table 3–6. The Medrad Mark V injector allows multiple-level injections to be programmed, thereby allowing a wide variety of unusual flow patterns during the study. This is accomplished by having the flow rate change during the injection. The Medrad Mark V injector has the capability for nine flow rate changes per injection. Multiphasic and biphasic injection patterns as well as backflow studies and positive and negative accelerations are possible with this system.

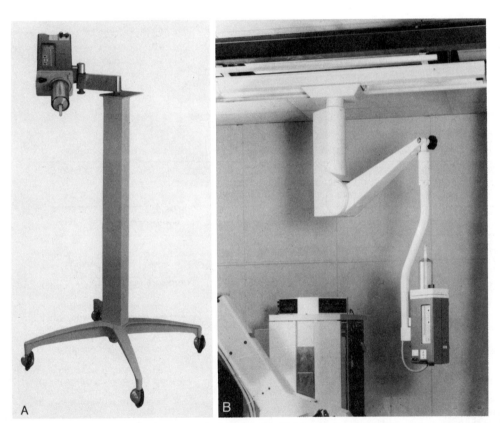

Figure 3–17. (*A*) Photograph of the floor-mounted Angiomat CT injector head. The stand is mobile and can be positioned conveniently during the procedure. (*B*) Photograph of the Angiomat CT injector head as attached to a ceiling mount. (From Liebel-Flarsheim Company.)

Table 3–6. SAMPLE CT INJECTION PARAMETERS FOR USE WITH THE ANGIOMAT CT INJECTION SYSTEM (From Liebel-Flarsheim Company)

GUIDELINE PARAMETERS IN USE AT THE MAYO CLINIC, ROCHESTER, MN, USING THE ANGIOMAT CT SYSTEM*
(Information supplied through the courtesy of Ms. Sherri Prescott, RN)

Region of Interest	Phase	Rate (ml/s)	Volume (ml)	Interphase Delay (s)	Comments†
Chest/abdomen	1/2	2	50	—	
	2/2	1	90	0	
Liver	1/2	3	45	—	
	2/2	2	95	0	
Abdomen–pelvis 1	1/3	3	50	—	Press *pause* during 120-s delay;
	2/3	1	60	0	restart at iliac crest
	3/3	3	50	120	
Abdomen–pelvis 2	1/3	2	50	—	Press *pause* during 120-s delay;
	2/3	1	70	0	restart at iliac crest
	3/3	1	60	120	
Abdomen–pelvis 3	1/4	2	50	—	Press *pause* during 120-s delay;
	2/4	1	25	0	restart at iliac crest
	3/4	2	50	120	
	4/4	1	75	0	
Abdomen–pelvis 4	1/3	3	60	—	Press *pause* during 120-s delay;
	2/3	2	50	0	restart at iliac crest
	3/3	1	75	120	
Abdomen 1	1/2	3	50	—	
	2/2	2	150	0	
Abdomen 2	1/2	2	45	—	
	2/2	1	95	0	
Lymphoma	1/1	1	140	—	

†Typical catheter used is Jelco 18 to 20 g. Contrast is 60%. Scanner is Picker 1200 SX. Scan delay is 20 to 30 s.

GUIDELINE PARAMETERS IN USE AT THE MARSHFIELD CLINIC, MARSHFIELD, WI, USING THE ANGIOMAT CT SYSTEM* (Information supplied through the courtesy of Thomas Hinke, M.D., and Debbie Arnt, CT Supervisor)

Region of Interest	Phase	Rate (ml/s)	Volume (ml)	Interphase Delay (s)	Comments†
Abdomen/chest					
50 to 75 lb	1/2	0.2	40	—	Press *pause* during delay; restart
	2/2	0.2	35	120	after patient is moved up and apex of lung is visualized
75 to 100 lb	1/2	0.28	50	—	Press *pause* during delay; restart
	2/2	0.28	50	120	after patient is moved up and apex of lung is visualized
100 to 150 lb	1/2	0.45	75	—	Press *pause* during delay; restart
	2/2	0.45	75	120	after patient is moved up and apex of lung is visualized
150 to 200 lb	1/2	0.55	100	—	Press *pause* during delay; restart
	2/2	0.55	100	120	after patient is moved up and apex of lung is visualized
>200 lb	1/2	0.62	112	—	Press *pause* during delay; restart
	2/2	0.62	112	120	after patient is moved up and apex of lung is visualized
Abdomen/pelvis					
50 to 75 lb	1/2	0.26	50	—	Press *pause* during delay; restart
	2/2	0.13	25	120	at iliac chest
75 to 100 lb	1/2	0.36	66	—	Press *pause* during delay; restart
	2/2	0.21	34	120	at iliac crest
100 to 150 lb	1/2	0.55	100	—	Press *pause* during delay; restart
	2/2	0.28	50	120	at iliac crest
150 to 200 lb	1/2	0.73	130	—	Press *pause* during delay; restart
	2/2	0.38	70	120	at iliac crest
>200 lb	1/2	0.82	150	—	Press *pause* during delay; restart
	2/2	0.47	50	120	at iliac crest
Single body area (chest/abdomen/pelvis)					
50 to 75 lb	1/1	0.28	62		
76 to 100 lb	1/1	0.48	87		
101 to 150 lb	1/1	0.68	125		
151 to 200 lb	1/1	0.97	175		
>200 lb	1/1	1.12	200		

†Typical catheter used is Jelco 18 g. Contrast is 60%. Scanner is Picker 1200 SX and GE 9800. Scan delay is 35 s.

GUIDELINE PARAMETERS IN USE AT THE FROEDTERT HOSPITAL, MILWAUKEE, WI, USING THE ANGIOMAT CT SYSTEM* (Information supplied through the courtesy of Dr. Dennis Foley, Radiologist, and Tom Roland, RT)

Region of Interest	Phase	Rate (ml/s)	Volume (ml)	Interphase Delay (s)	Comments†
Chest	1/2	3	50	—	
	2/2	1	130	15	
Abdomen	1/2	3	50	—	
	2/2	1	130	45	
Neck	1/2	3	30	—	
	2/2	0.3	150	20	
Abdomen/chest	1/3	3	50	45	Pause—Move patient back up
	2/3	1	100	—	to apex
	3/3	1.5	30	15	Restart at apex

†Typical catheter used is Deseret 20 g Insyte. Contrast is 60%. Scanner is GE9800 Quick Scanner.

GUIDELINE PARAMETERS IN USE AT ST. MICHAEL'S HOSPITAL, TORONTO, CANADA, USING THE ANGIOMAT CT SYSTEM* (Information supplied through the courtesy of Ann Marie Gaudet, CT Supervisor)

Region of Interest	Phase	Rate (ml/s)	Volume (ml)	Interphase Delay (s)	Comments†
Chest—hilum bolus	1/3	0.25	20 to 25	0	Infuse slowly from arch to hilum; bolus right at hilum
	2/3	2 to 3	50	0	
	3/3	0.8 to 1	65	0	Drip remaining contrast through lungs
Abdomen/pelvis	1/3	3	50	0	Press *pause* during 120-s delay; restart at iliac crest
	2/3	1	40	0	
	3/3	1.5	50	120	

†Typical catheter used is 20 g with nonionic contrast. All studies are dynamic. Scanner is Philips-Tomo. Scan LX. Scan delay is 10 to 15 s.

GUIDELINE PARAMETERS IN USE AT NEW YORK UNIVERSITY HOSPITAL, NEW YORK, NY, USING THE ANGIOMAT CT SYSTEM* (Information supplied through the courtesy of A. Birnbaum, M.D., Alec J. Megibow, M.D., and Edward Lubat, M.D.)

Region of Interest	Phase	Rate (ml/s)	Volume (ml)	Interphase Delay (s)	Comments†
Abdomen/pelvis	1/2	2.5	50	—	18- to 20-gauge Angiocath; 200 ml Conray 43%
	2/2	0.8	145	—	
Abdomen/pelvis	1/2	1.5	50	—	22-g Angiocath; 200 ml Conray 43%
	2/2	0.8	145	—	
Pancreas	1/2	3.0	50	—	18- to 20-g Angiocath; 150 ml Conray 60%
	2/2	1.0	95	—	
Pancreas	1/2	1.5	50	—	22-g Angiocath; 150 ml Conray 60%
	2/2	1.0	95	—	
Abdomen/pelvis for gynecologic or rectosigmoid pathology	1/3	2.5	50	—	20-g Angiocath; 200 ml Conray 43%
	2/3	0.8	95	—	
	3/3	1.0	50	240	Press *pause* during delay; restart at sacroiliac when patient re-scanned prone with rectal air
Abdomen/pelvis for gynecologic or rectosigmoid pathology	1/3	1.5	50	—	22-g Angiocath; 200 ml Conray 43%
	2/3	0.8	95	—	
	3/3	1.0	50	—	Press *pause* during delay; restart at sacroiliac when patient rescanned prone with rectal air
Routine chest	1/2	1.0	30	—	20- or 22-g Angiocath; 200 ml Conray 43%
	2/2	1.5	165	—	
Abdomen/pelvis/chest	1/3	2.5	50	—	20-g Angiocath; 250 ml Conray 43%
	2/3	0.8	135	—	
	3/3	1.0	60	240	Press *pause* during delay; restart before scanning chest
Abdomen/pelvis/chest	1/3	1.5	50	—	22-g Angiocath; 250 ml Conray 43%
	2/3	0.8	135	—	
	3/3	1.0	60	240	Press *pause* during delay; restart before scanning chest

†● Abdominal scanning should begin after the first phase of injection is completed. Chest scanning, however, may commence as the first phase begins.
● Pancreatic studies performed by scanning below the uncinate process superiorly to the level of the hepatic dome and commence as the first phase begins.
● Abdomen/pelvis three-phase studies initially are performed as a routine abdomen/pelvis examination. However, patients are scanned supine to the level of the sacroiliac joints. At this point, patients are repositioned prone and, after administration of rectal air, have their pelvis scanned as the third phase of the injection commences.

Table continued on following page

Table 3–6. SAMPLE CT INJECTION PARAMETERS FOR USE WITH THE ANGIOMAT CT INJECTION SYSTEM (From Liebel-Flarsheim Company) *Continued*

GUIDELINE PARAMETERS IN USE AT UNIVERSITY OF MINNESOTA, USING THE ANGIOMAT CT SYSTEM*
(Information supplied through the courtesy of Robert Halvorson, M.D., and Ms. Diane Tenney, RT, CT Department)

Region of Interest	Phase	Rate (ml/s)	Volume (ml)	Interphase Delay (s)	Comments†
Abdomen	1/2	2	75	—	
	2/2	1	65	0	
Chest	1/1	1	140	—	
Liver/chest	1/3	2	60	—	Press *pause* during 120-s delay;
	2/3	1	60	—	restart at apex of chest after
	3/3	1	60	120	patient is moved into gantry

†Typical catheter used is Jelco 22 g intercath. Contrast is 60% Hypaque. Scanner is Siemens Somatom DRH and DR. Scan delay is 20 s.

GUIDELINE PARAMETERS IN USE AT APPLETON MEMORIAL HOSPITAL, APPLETON, WI, USING THE ANGIOMAT CT SYSTEM* *(Information supplied through the courtesy of Mr. Mark Putzer, RTR Senior CT Technologist)*

Region of Interest	Phase	Rate (ml/s)	Volume (ml)	Interphase Delay (s)	Comments†
Chest	1/1	1	145	—	
Abdomen	1/2	2	60	—	
	2/2	1	85	0	
Serio (for vasculature)	1/1	2	30	—	Repeat scans of single-level; no table movement
Serio (for liver/organs)	1/1	2	40 to 60	—	Repeat scans of single-level; no table movement
Vascular (through chest)	1/1	1	145		
Upper abdomen	1/3	2	60	—	Press *pause* during delay; restart
(pancreas)	2/3	1	35	0	at tip of tail of pancreas
	3/3	2	50	120	

†Typical catheter used is Jelco 18 to 20 g. Contrast is 60%. Scanner is Siemens Somatom DR.

GUIDELINE PARAMETERS IN USE AT UNIVERSITY HOSPITAL, CINCINNATI, OH, USING THE ANGIOMAT CT SYSTEM* *(Information supplied through the courtesy of Jonathan S. Moulton, M.D., Director, Body CT Section; Dave Neidich, RT, Tech. Supervisor, CT Section; and Anthony Johnson, RT, Tech. Supervisor, CT Section)*

Region of Interest	Phase	Rate (ml/s)	Volume (ml)	Interphase Delay (s)	Comments†
Abdomen					
Liver/pancreas	1/2	1.5	30	—	
Renal, etc.	2/2	0.6 to 1	120	10	
Abdomen/pelvis	1/2	1.5	30	—	
pelvic primaries	2/2	0.5 to 1	120	10	Scan from bottom up; start at pelvis symphysis pubis and scan up
Abdomen/pelvis (other)	1/2	1.5	30	—	Start at diaphragm and scan
	2/2	0.6 to 1	120	0	down
Chest for bolus study of specific abnormality	1/1	1	50		Dynamic scan—delay scan 30 s—9 scans; Increase volume for 12 scans
Cerebral	1/2	1	50	—	
	2/2	0.4	100	60	
Abdominal (poor veins)	1/1	0.6 to 1	150	—	Used when patient has poor veins or nauseous and high rate bolus contraindicated; also use for neck studies; delay scan is 30 s
Liver photography	1/1	0.5	65	—	Patient catheterized in SMA. Delay scan is 30 s; dynamic scan with 3.5 s interscan delay; reduce mA to allow adequate number of scans

†Typical catheter used is Jelco 22 g. Contrast is 60%. Scanner is CT Scanner GE9800.

Table 3–6. SAMPLE CT INJECTION PARAMETERS FOR USE WITH THE ANGIOMAT CT INJECTION
SYSTEM (From Liebel-Flarsheim Company) *Continued*

*GUIDELINE PARAMETERS IN USE AT GENESIS COMMUNITY IMAGING CENTER, PHOENIX, AZ, USING THE
ANGIOMAT CT SYSTEM* (Information supplied through the courtesy of Claude S. Frey, M.D.)*

Region of Interest	Phase	Rate (ml/s)	Volume (ml)	Interphase Delay (s)	Comments†
Dynamic scans					
Chest	1/2	2	50	—	Scan delay, 20 s
	2/2	1	100	0	
Abdomen	1/2	2	50	—	Scan delay, 30 to 45 s*
	2/2	1	100	0	
Pelvis	1/2	2	50	—	Scan delay, 45 to 60 s*
	2/2	1	100	0	
Abdomen/pelvis	1/2	2	50	—	Scan delay, 30 to 45 s*
	2/2	0.7	100	0	
CT neck, face, and extremities (5 mm nondynamic)	1/1	1	150	—	Scan delay, 20 s
Head CT for aneurysm (single-level dynamic scan)	1/1	2	50	—	Scan delay, 20 s
Chest for aortic dissection (single level dynamic × 3)	1/1	2	50	—	Scan delay, 10 s

*Variable according to the age and cardiac output of the patient.
†Scanner is GE 9800.

*The above parameters are guidelines only. Actual parameters may vary based on experience, clinical indications,
intravenous access, contraindications, etc.

LYMPHANGIOGRAPHIC INJECTORS

The automatic injection devices previously discussed are designed for use with rapid serial film changers and are capable of delivering a large bolus of contrast medium in a matter of seconds. During lymphangiography, however, a slow, forced injection of contrast agent under steady pressure is necessary. The contrast agent must be delivered at a flow rate of 0.1 to 0.2 ml/min through a catheter with a very small ID. At times, this injection must be made simultaneously into both extremities (Fig. 3–18). This is difficult to accomplish manually, so a specialized injection device is used.

The lymphangiographic injector contains the same basic components of all automatic pressure injectors—the syringe, a heating device, and the pressure mechanism (Fig. 3–19).

Syringe

Syringes vary by manufacturer. Certain units will accept only specially constructed syringes, whereas others will accept standard glass syringes with Luer-Lok fittings. If specially designed syringes are required, additional units should be kept on hand in the department to replace broken or damaged syringes without creating serious delays.

Heating Device

As with pressure injectors, the contrast agent must be heated before instillation into the patient. This is essential to obtain a sufficient flow of the material through the catheters. Preheating of the contrast material to body temperature also minimizes discomfort to the patient. The temperature range of lymphangiographic injectors varies from 0° C to a maximum of 100° C on some units and from 55 to 80° C on other units. In general, temperatures of about 80° C should be used because heat loss occurs along

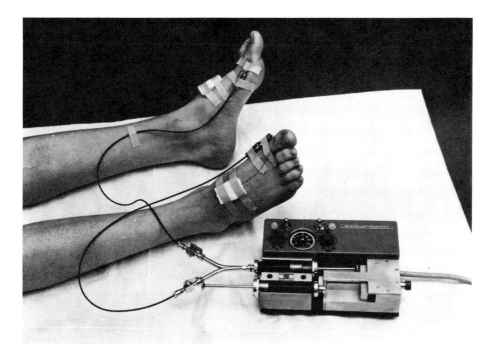

Figure 3–18. Automatic injection of contrast medium bilaterally during lymphangiography using the Elema-Schönander lymphography injector. (From Siemens Medical Systems, Inc.)

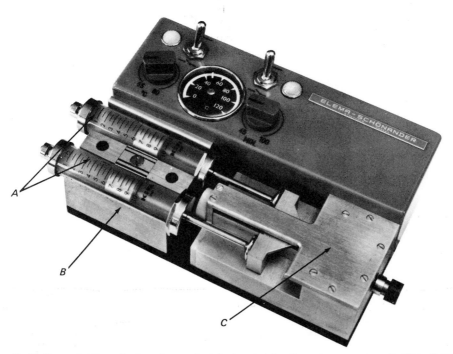

Figure 3–19. Elema-Schönander lymphography injector showing its major components: *(A)* syringes; *(B)* heating device; *(C)* pressure mechanism. (From Siemens Medical Systems, Inc.)

the length of the catheter during the slow injection. This will ensure that the contrast material is delivered to the patient at body temperature.

Pressure Mechanism

Lymphangiographic injectors are electromechanically powered. The pressure on the syringe is automatically controlled by the drive motor. Certain injectors are equipped with automatic rate controls that adjust the injection rate to compensate for variations of intralymphatic pressure. These injectors are also equipped for easy changeover to manual control, if necessary.

SUMMARY

Certain special procedures require the use of automatic injection devices. These devices vary by design but have certain features in common, including a syringe, a heating device, and a pressure mechanism. Automatic injection devices manufactured and in use today use an electromechanical high pressure device. The constant flow rate delivery of contrast media has become the standard. This implies that there will be a known amount of contrast agent delivered per unit of time regardless of the parameters of the system.

The delivery (flow rate) of the contrast agent to the patient is affected by any part of the system between the syringe and the patient that affects the resistance of the contrast medium to flow. Variables such as catheter ID, length, and side holes; contrast agent viscosity; and accessory items contribute to the resistance to flow. These factors should be considered when planning the study, and equipment choices should be made to optimize the delivery of the contrast agent.

Lymphangiographic injectors differ from other types of automatic injectors in that the delivery of the contrast agent is slow and constant and occurs over a long time period rather than in a large bolus that is delivered in a few seconds. Lymphangiographic injectors contain the same basic components as the other automatic injection devices.

REFERENCES

1. Personal communication from Latham, G., Cordis Corporation, 1991.
2. Kimber, D. C., et al: Anatomy and Physiology, 15th ed. New York, Macmillan, 1966.
3. Mark V Injector Operation Manual, Medrad, Inc., 1989, p. 1–94.
4. Krovetz, L. J., et al: An analysis of factors determining delivery rates of liquids through cardiac catheters, Radiology, 86:124, 1966.
5. Gonzalez, L. L., et al: A study of factors influencing delivery rates of contrast media during arteriography, Angiology, 15:284, 1964.

SUGGESTED READINGS

Abbot, J. A., Lipton, M. J., Hayashi, T., and Lee, F.: A quantitative method for determining angiographic jet energy forces and their dissipation: Theoretical and practical implications, Cathet. Cardiovasc. Diagn., 3:139, 1977.
Bjorno, L., and Pettersson, H.: Hydro- and hemodynamic effects of catheterization of vessels, Acta Radiol., 18(1):1–16, 1977.
Burchell, H., and Sturm, R. E.: Editorial: Electroshock hazards, Circulation, 35:227, 1967.
Gardiner, G. A., Jr., et al: Selective coronary angiography using a power injector, Am. J. Roentgenol., 146:831, 1986.
Hessel, S. J.: Complications of angiography, Radiology, 138:273, 1981.
Schad, N., Stucky, J., Brunner, H., Schad, H., and Wellauer, J.: The intermittent phased injection of contrast material into the heart, Am. J. Roentgenol., 2:464, 1968.
Williamson, D. E.: Experimental determination of flow equation in catheters for cardiology, Am. J. Roentgenol., 94:704, 1965.

four

Contrast Media

TYPES
Negative Contrast Agents
Positive Contrast Agents
REACTIONS
CHARACTERISTICS
Ionic Organic Iodine Compounds

Nonionic Contrast Agents
Low Osmolality Contrast Agents
Iodine Concentration
Miscibility
Persistence
Specialty Contrast Agents

All of the examinations designated as special procedures require the introduction of some type of material into the area of interest to provide contrast. This is necessary because the differences in density among the various tissues in the body are too small to provide adequate contrast for visualization of anatomic details. To compensate for this, it is necessary to increase or decrease the density of the organ to provide the desired contrast.

Contrast agents can be classified into one of two broad groups depending on their interaction with x-radiation—positive contrast agents (radiopaque) and negative contrast agents (radiolucent).

Some of the familiar, so-called routine special procedures (barium enemas, excretory urograms, etc.) increase organ density through the addition of a radiopaque substance, which renders the organ radiopaque. In some cases, however, it may be undesirable to increase the density of an organ. In these situations, the density of the organ can be decreased by the addition of a radiolucent substance.

TYPES

Negative Contrast Agents

The absorption of x-rays by a substance is dependent on its atomic weight. Substances with low atomic weights absorb less x-radiation and produce greater density on the finished radiograph. Some examples of negative contrast agents are air, oxygen, carbon dioxide, and nitrous oxide. Most available gases have been used as negative contrast agents with varying results; however, these four gases are commonly used as radiolucent contrast agents.

Some special procedures requiring the use of a negative contrast agent are pneumoarthrography and retroperitoneal pneumography. The use of these agents results in a silhouette of the anatomic structures against a radiolucent background.

Air or oxygen may be dangerous during certain procedures because they can cause gas emboli, but carbon dioxide and nitrogen do not pose the risk of gas emboli and can be used with relative safety. They are also able to be absorbed rapidly by the body. This factor can be advantageous when rapid absorption is desired, but in cases in which many radiographs are taken, it is a definite disadvantage.

Positive Contrast Agents

Positive contrast agents cause an increase in the absorption of x-rays, thus producing a positive image on the finished radiograph. These agents are made up of elements with high atomic weights, such as iodine, bromine, and barium. They can take the form of tablets, powders, and liquids and can be introduced into the body through a variety of routes. They are relatively nontoxic in most cases, but certain patients may exhibit reactions of varying severity, especially to agents containing iodine. In some cases, small doses of these agents may cause death.

Most of the positive contrast agents used during the special procedures discussed in this text will be organic iodine compounds. Table 4–1 presents the iodine content and other characteristics of various angiographic contrast media. The patient should be questioned before administration of the contrast medium about whether he or she is allergic to iodine. The possibility of a reaction should always be anticipated, and proper emergency medication should be available in the special procedure suite. The following is a list of typical emergency equipment:

Oxygen tank and masks
Airways (pediatric and adult)
Suction apparatus
Physiological saline
Emergency drugs (by physician preference)
    Diphenylhydramine hydrochloride
    Phenylephrine hydrochloride
    Metaraminol
    Hydrocortisone sodium succinate
    Epinephrine
Syringes and needles for drug injection
Aromatic spirits of ammonia
Blood pressure device and stethoscope

REACTIONS

The mechanism of patient reaction to contrast media is not fully understood. It is a complex issue because there is no accurate way to predict a reactive event, and the causative factors vary greatly. Reactions can occur in patients receiving contrast agents for the first time, yet patients receiving subsequent doses after experiencing a reaction may have fewer symptoms or no additional reactions.

Contrast agent reactions are considered adverse drug reactions. Some of the problems experienced by patients can be classified as allergic reactions. Some can be attributed to the hyperosmolality of the contrast agent administered, and some can be related to the chemotoxicity or specific, intrinsic chemical and pharmacological characteristics of the substance.

The reactions that occur during contrast examinations can be classified into one of five major groups; overdose, anaphylactic, cardiovascular, psychogenic, and activation system–triggering reactions. _Specials_

It should not be implied from these classifications that some patients are deliberately

Table 4–1. CHARACTERISTICS OF SOME INTRAVASCULAR CONTRAST MEDIA USED IN ANGIOCARDIOGRAPHY*

Group	Iodine Concentration	Agent	Iodine Content mg/ml	%	Chemical Components (% by weight/volume)† Anions	Cations	Viscosity (cP)‡ 25°C	37.5°C	Sodium Content mEq/ml	mg/ml	Vial Sizes (ml)	Manufacturer
A	28–31%	Hypaque 60%	282	28	Diatrizoate	Mg (60%)	6.22	4.18	0.001	0.02	20, 30, 50	Winthrop
		Conray 60%	282	28	Iothalamate	Mg (60%)	6.10	4.0	0.0014	0.03	20, 30, 50	Mallinckrodt
		Reno-M-60	282	28	Diatrizoate	Mg (60%)	6.7	4.0	0.04	0.91	10, 30, 50	Squibb
		Renografin 60	288	29	Diatrizoate	Mg (52%) Na (8%)	6.0	3.9	0.16	3.76	10, 30, 50, 100	Squibb
		Hypaque 50%	300	30	Diatrizoate	Na (50%)	3.25	2.5	0.8	18.1	20, 30, 50	Winthrop
		Renovist II	310	31	Diatrizoate	Mg (28.5%) Na (29.1%)	5.84		0.49	11.3	30, 60	Squibb
B	36–40%	Meglumine diatrizoate 76%	358	36	Diatrizoate	Mg (76%)	13.7	9.2	0.04	0.91	20, 50, 100, 200	Squibb
		Renografin 76	370	37	Diatrizoate	Mg (66%) Na (10%)	13.94	9.1	0.19	4.48	20, 50	Squibb
		Hypaque M75	385	39	Diatrizoate	Mg (50%) Na (25%)	13.4	8.35	0.39	9.0	20, 50	Winthrop
		Conray 400	400	40	Iothalamate	Na (66.8%)	6.7	4.4	1.05	24.1	25, 50	Mallinckrodt
		Vascoray	400	40	Iothalamate	Mg (52%) Na (26%)	14.5	9.0	0.408	9.38	25, 50, 200	Mallinckrodt
		Isopaque 440	440	44	Metrizoate	Mg (76%) Na (17%) Ca (0.8%) Mg (0.15%)	10.4	0.7		16.6	50	Winthrop

*Only the most popular contrast agents are listed; all data have been verified by the respective manufacturers.
†MG: meglumine; Na: sodium; Ca: calcium.
‡Where a combination salt of any contrast media product is used, the viscosity, whether measured at 25 or 37.5°C, is going to fall within a range rather than equal a specific number. Therefore, the numbers indicated are the average within each respective range.

overdosed with contrast agents. Under certain conditions, some patients may be predisposed to inadvertent contrast agent overdose. Infants, adults with acute renal failure, adults with incipient cardiac failure, or adults with hepatic failure with ascites are particularly at risk of receiving an osmotic load to the body that is excessive, and what is an overdose for these patients may have been considered to be within normal limits.

Anaphylactic reactions can occur and are usually considered to be of mild to medium severity; they are easily recognized and treated.

Cardiovascular reactions tend to cause a peripheral vasodilation and a decrease in systemic blood pressure, which in turn result in reflex tachycardia. They also affect myocardial contractility and cardiac electrophysiology and ultimately are cardiotoxic.

Psychogenic factors are described by Lalli[1] as important mediators of some major reactions. If patients are overanxious, they may respond to the subjective side effects produced by the introduction of the contrast agent with an autonomic response. This response becomes the basis for the adverse reaction. Substances less likely to cross the blood–brain barrier and enter the central nervous system reduce the reactions precipitated by this mechanism.

The triggering of a variety of activation systems (complement, coagulation, fibrinolysis, and histamine) can occur as a response to damage to the vascular endothelium at the injection site. These do not cause the same type of reaction in every patient because of the presence and action of inhibitors in the pathways of these systems. Histamine release, tissue damage, thrombus, and hemolysis are some possible manifestations of this category of reaction.

It is important that the radiographer become familiar with the signs and symptoms of these types of reactions and their treatment; a summary of some types of reactions, their signs, and their treatments is given in Table 4–2.

Table 4–2. SUMMARY OF MAJOR EMERGENCIES AND THEIR TREATMENT

Cause	Type	Complication	Treatment (in addition to oxygen in all cases)
Contrast media Anesthesia Local General	Cardiovascular system	Cardiac arrest Asystole	Cardiac massage, etc.
Cardiac catheterization		Ventricular fibrillation Hypotension, syncope	Defibrillation Posture vasopressor drugs
Pneumography		Pulmonary edema	Aminophylline IV Lasix IV, venesection, morphine, atropine, IV
Coronary disease Electric shock, etc.	Respiratory system	Respiratory arrest or obstruction	Maintain airway, natural tracheostomy Pulmonary ventilation nikethamide IV
Local anesthetic	Central nervous system	Toxic convulsions	Thiopentone IV
Contrast media		Coma	Corticosteroid IV
Contrast media and other drugs	Allergic	Angioneurotic edema Bronchospasm, iodism	Adrenaline SC Corticosteroid IV Aminophylline IV
		Pulmonary edema	Antihistamine IV Corticosteroid IV (see also "Cardiovascular system")
Pneumography		Gas embolism	Left lateral decubitus

From Ansell, G.: Notes on Radiological Emergencies. London, Churchill Livingstone, 1966, p. 1.

Table 4–3. SUMMARY OF SOME MAJOR SYMPTOMS OF REACTIONS TO CONTRAST AGENTS ADMINISTERED INTRAVENOUSLY

Mild to Moderate Symptoms		Severe Symptoms
Nausea*	Vomiting*	Dyspnea
Flushing	Hoarseness	Sudden drop in blood pressure
Sneezing	Coughing	Loss of consciousness
Shivering	Urticaria*	Paresthesias
Chest pain	Edema	Convulsions
Facial swelling	Warm feeling	Tissue necrosis
Abdominal pain		Cardiac arrest
Pain at injection site		Paralysis
Heat sensation*		
Vascular pain		
Itching*		

*These symptoms were found to be the most frequent by Katayama, H., et al.: Adverse reactions to ionic and nonionic contrast media, Radiology, *175*:622, 1990.

Because the reaction to the administration of a contrast agent is not predictable, all patients should be monitored closely during the procedure. The importance of assessing the patient before the procedure cannot be overemphasized. This will give the radiographer a baseline value from which to measure the patient's condition throughout the procedure. The radiographer should be familiar with the symptoms of the various reactions to contrast agents and note any changes in the patient during the procedure. If any of the symptoms appear, the physician should be notified and the incident documented. Table 4–3 lists some common symptoms of contrast-related reactions.

The onset of reactions is variable; approximately 70% of reactions occur within 5 min of the injection, whereas 16% occur more than 5 min after the injection.[2] Fourteen percent occur 15 min after the injection. It is advisable that the radiographer remain with the patient for at least 15 min after the injection.

When a particular contrast agent is being used, the radiographer should read the supplied product data sheet. Information provided about the contrast agent includes description, indications and contraindications, administration and dosage, warnings or precautions, and adverse reactions or complications. The section on adverse reactions or complications can prepare the radiographer for the possible types of reactions that the agent can produce. The following is a summary of some general precautions to be taken before and after the administration of contrast media:

Before injection
  Know the patient
    Check chart for history of allergy or hypersensitivity
    Check whether patient has other medical problems
      Hepatic or renal disease
      Pregnancy
      Multiple myeloma
      Homozygosity for sickle cell disease
      Known or suspected pheochromocytoma (solid tumors of neurogenic origin)
      Severe cardiovascular diseases
      Bronchial asthma
      Hyperthyroidism
  Know the procedure
    Contraindications and limitations to the specific special procedure
    Know the possible reactions that can occur with the contrast agent used
    Check emergency equipment

After injection
Know where physician may be reached
Evaluate patient's vital functions for abnormalities
   Respirations
   Pulse
   Blood pressure
   Presence of cyanosis
Remain with patient for at least 15 min after injection

CHARACTERISTICS

In the selection of a contrast agent, certain characteristics such as viscosity, toxicity, iodine content, miscibility, and persistence must be considered. The ultimate choice of a contrast agent is usually left to the physician performing the procedure, but the radiographer should understand the characteristics of contrast agents to be able to use them intelligently and efficiently during special procedures.

Contrast agents used for intravenous injection during special procedures fall into one of three major classes—ionic, low-osmolality, and nonionic contrast agents. All of these are organic iodine compounds that use iodine as the substance that provides the contrast.

It has been demonstrated that the nonionic contrast agents produce fewer adverse drug reactions. This has been attributed to the osmolality of the material. The ionic compounds have a greater tendency to pass the blood–brain barrier owing to their hyperosmolality. The *blood–brain barrier* is the anatomic/physiological aspect of the brain that separates the parenchyma (organ tissue) of the central nervous system from the blood. It is thought to prevent or slow the passage of various chemical compounds and other potentially harmful substances from the blood into the tissue of the central nervous system. The hyperosmolality of the ionic contrast agents has been thought to be the cause of many of the major reactions that occur during special procedures. Ionic contrast agents degrade into electrically charged particles within the body and can disrupt the heart's electrical activity and thereby increase the potential for arrhythmia.

The nonionic contrast agents have demonstrated clinically a marked reduction in adverse drug reactions relating to their use in special procedures. Another feature of this type of contrast agent is that patients are much more comfortable during the study. Also, there are fewer subjective side effects. This has the combined effect of producing less anxiety in the patient, and psychogenic responses, as described by Lalli,[1] are less likely to occur. Because the nonionics are less apt to damage the blood–brain barrier, they demonstrate a very low neurotoxicity. The nonionic agents also exhibit a high compatibility with other intravascular medications used during angiography and the treatment of allergic reactions.

This would lead one to think that it would be advantageous to use nonionic contrast agents exclusively in radiography. Adopting a policy of this nature would be easy from a medical standpoint, but there are economic considerations that make the decision difficult. The cost of the nonionic contrast agents can be as much as 20-fold to 25-fold that of ionic agents. A typical 50-ml vial of ionic contrast agent may cost from $4.00 to $7.00, whereas a similar-size vial of a nonionic substance could cost as much as $100.00. At the present time, the ionic contrast agents are still widely used. This may change as additional studies are completed, demonstrating the effectiveness and safety of the nonionic contrast agents. An increase in the use of the nonionics will probably occur if the cost of the material is reduced over time or there is a method by which the institutions can realize a reimbursement for the additional cost.

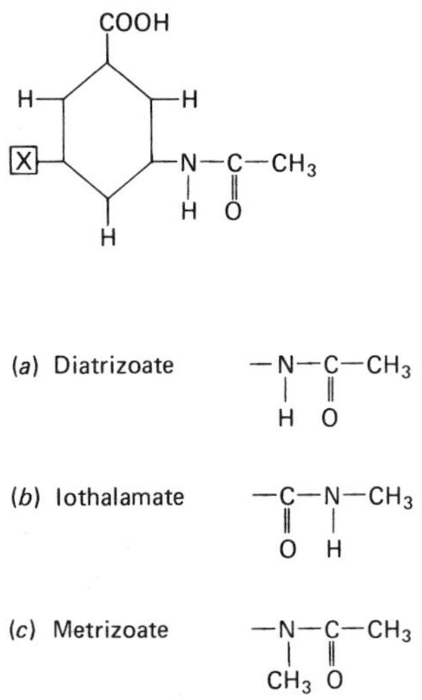

Figure 4–1. Basic structure of the anions of the organic iodine compounds used during angiography. The three side chains diatrizoate *(a)*, iothalamate *(b)* and metrizoate *(c)* can be substituted in the block marked X on the basic structure to form the different compounds.

Ionic Organic Iodine Compounds

The ionic contrast agents used for vascular studies are salts of organic iodine compounds. The compound is composed of an anion (negatively charged) and a cation (positively charged). The anions that have found common use in angiography have the same basic structure but differ in one side chain (Fig. 4–1). The cations that form the compound are either sodium or meglumine (*N*-methylglucamine).

The anions of the common angiographic contrast media begin as organic benzoic acids. These are iodinated and combined with a cation to form a salt (Fig. 4–2). Each of these salts has different characteristics and affects the patient differently.

Experimental results have shown that the meglumine salts are less toxic than the sodium salts of the organic iodine contrast agents (see Suggested Readings at the end of this chapter). However, the sodium salts are less viscous than solutions of the meglumine salts with the same iodine content.

The ionic contrast agents currently available for angiographic use are either meglumine salts or combinations of meglumine and sodium salts. The toxicity of the low-viscosity, sodium salt contrast agents can be reduced somewhat by the addition of calcium and magnesium to the solution.[3]

Nonionic Contrast Agents

Nonionic contrast agents are relatively new to special procedure radiography. These substances were developed because the high osmolality of the ionic contrast agents was thought to be responsible for the majority of the undesirable side effects. The basic structure of the nonionic compounds is the same as that of the conventional agents. However, the various side chains added to the basic building block create a substance

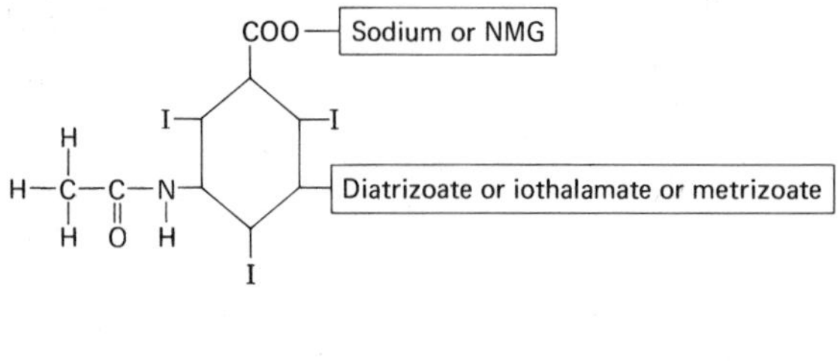

Figure 4–2. Schematic of the basic structure combined with the anionic side chains and cations to form an organic iodine compound.

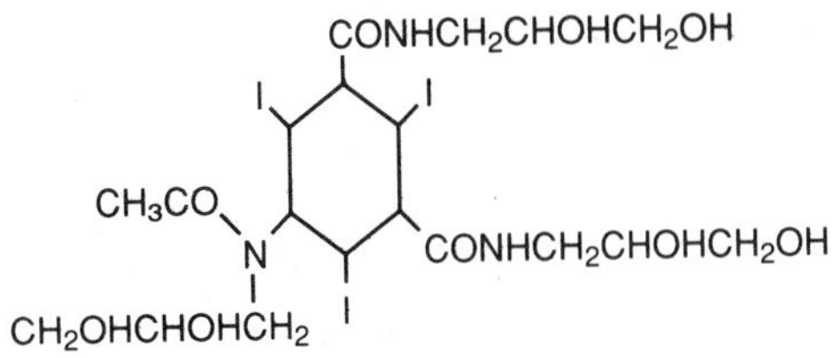

Figure 4–3. Schematic of chemical structure of "Omnipaque" (Iohexol) from Nycomed, an example of a nonionic contrast agent.

that does not ionize (i.e., separate into an anion and a cation) (Fig. 4–3). They are considered to be 3:1 compounds—they contribute three iodine particles in solution to provide contrast and only one particle to provide osmolality. The ionic compounds are 3:2 in that they also contribute three iodine particles for contrast and two particles for osmolality.

Osmolality depends on the number of particles in solution. The nonionic compounds exhibit less osmolality than conventional ionic contrast agents because they provide fewer osmotically active particles. This results in fewer patient reactions.

Although their chemical structure differs, nonionic contrast agents are as effective as ionic agents in providing the necessary contrast during special procedure radiography. Their main advantage is in the reduction of both subjective and objective side effects in the patient.

Low Osmolality Ionic Contrast Agents

This type of contrast agent overlaps characteristics of the two previously mentioned types of substances; the compound uses the same basic building block but forms what is called a monoacid dimer. This compound is an ionic contrast agent, but it has the same type of compound ratio as the nonionic substances. The contrast agent illustrated in Figure 4–4 (Hexabrix, Guerbet, Paris) is a 6:2 compound; that is, it provides six iodine particles for contrast and two particles for osmolality. This type of contrast agent lies between ionic and nonionic agents in the mediation of side effects. Its advantages are that it more closely mimics the nonionic compounds, but it is not as costly and thereby reduces the economic considerations for its use.

Iodine Concentration

As the iodine concentration of the contrast agent increases, the viscosity also increases. Compounds of the meglumine salts have a greater increase in viscosity than those of sodium salts. In considering the use of contrast agents during vascular procedures, the viscosity becomes an important factor when long, small-bore catheters are used. More viscous contrast agents require greater injection pressures to deliver the same amount of material, resulting in the possibility of patient trauma and catheter damage.

The iodine concentration itself is an important physical characteristic; it can be

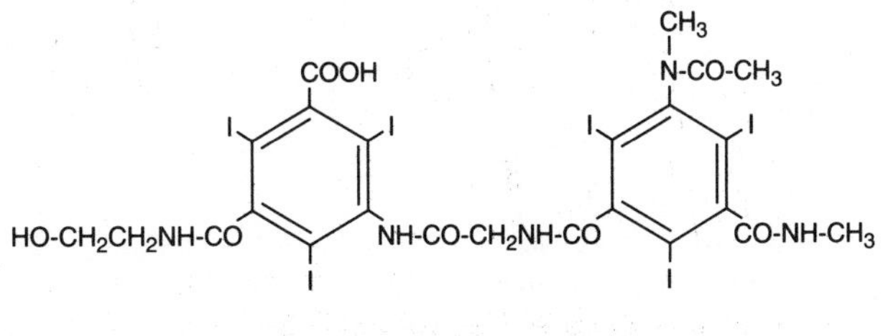

Figure 4–4. Schematic of sodium meglumine ioxaglate (Hexabrix), Guerbet, Paris, France. It is a monoacid dimer, a low osmolality compound with a 6:2 iodine atom–to–particle in solution ratio.

determined easily if the iodine content of the substance and the amount dissolved in its solvent are known. The iodine content is usually expressed in milligrams per milliliter or per cubic centimeter. Information relating to the physical characteristics of the contrast agents can be found in the product data sheet that is packaged with the contrast agent.

In comparing contrast agents, the amount of iodine delivered per second to the patient should be considered because contrast agents with a greater amount of meglumine salt usually have a lower iodine content as a result of the increased weight of the meglumine ion. Therefore, the amount of iodine delivered per second will be smaller. To illustrate this, if we compare the iodine content of Hypaque (sodium 50%) with that of both Conray (meglumine 60%) and Renografin 60% (meglumine 52%, sodium 8%) (see Table 4–1), it can be seen that the Hypaque has a greater iodine content. It should be noted that Hypaque 50% contains 100% sodium salt, whereas Renografin 60% is a mixture of sodium and meglumine salts, and Conray 60% contains 100% meglumine salt.

Miscibility

The miscibility or immiscibility of a contrast agent is an important factor in procedures in which the radiopaque material must be removed. For example, in myelography, the immiscibility of the contrast agent is of some concern. In this procedure, it is important that the radiopaque material remain unmixed with the cerebrospinal fluid to facilitate its collection and removal at the completion of the procedure. The angiographic contrast media, however, must be completely miscible with the blood to prevent any possibility of contrast media embolization. Certain procedures, such as bronchography, lymphography, and hysterosalpingography, can result in contrast agent persistence embolization due to the oily base of the radiopaque iodized compound.

Persistence

A final factor to consider regarding choice of contrast agent is the agent's persistence within the body. Because radiopaque agents instilled either directly or indirectly into body organs are foreign substances, it is important that they be excreted rapidly from the body. However, they should remain and concentrate in the body organs long enough to provide an adequate radiographic study. This is an important criterion in the design of a suitable contrast agent. Some contrast media are quite persistent and can remain in the body for months or even years without being excreted.

Specialty Contrast Agents

The organic iodine compounds have found widespread use in special procedure radiography and CT. However, they do not possess the characteristics necessary to function as contrast agents during MRI procedures. Iodinated contrast media function through absorption and subsequent attenuation of the x-ray beam. MRI does not use x-radiation to produce images; therefore, the usefulness of the iodinated compounds is limited. The substances used for contrast production in this specialty alter the micro-chemical environment to change the relaxation times (T1 and T2) and thereby increase the signal intensity.

The substance that has found favor as an intravenous contrast agent in MRI is gadolinium diethylenetriaminepenta-acetic acid (Gd-DTPA). This substance is a metal chelate. Metal ions tend to bind with certain body tissues, such as in the kidneys, liver, heart, brain, bone, spleen, and lungs. As a result, they can remain in the system for a long period of time and may cause undesirable side effects. If the metal ion can be linked with a substance that prevents such binding, it could be used safely. The process of chelation makes the metal ion available for use while eliminating the negative effects of tissue binding within the body. DTPA is the chelating agent used in the production of Gd-DTPA.

The side effects of this agent are minimal and include a slight transient increase in serum bilirubin (up to 15 mg/dl above normal), mild headache, rash, gastrointestinal upset, nausea, vomiting, and hypotension. This substance has not demonstrated toxicity to organ systems such as the heart, brain, kidney, or liver, which would be primary target organs if decomplexation of the substance occurred.

The primary excretory pathway is via the kidneys; approximately 80% of the Gd-DTPA is eliminated within 3 h. Approximately 98% is eliminated from the body through urination and defecation within 1 week of administration. It should be noted that because the primary method of excretion is via the urinary system, the use of the substance in patients who exhibit poor renal function or advanced renal disease is contraindicated.

The usual effective dose of Gd-DTPA is 0.1 ml/lb, not to exceed a total of 20 ml. This dose is sufficient for most MRI studies; however, doses approaching 0.2 ml/lb have been used to image some metastatic lesions. Increases above this level have demonstrated decreased signal intensity. Other chelated forms of Gd are being researched that would provide better contrast with smaller doses, but these have not emerged in clinical use.

SUMMARY

Contrast agents can be divided into negative and positive varieties. Negative contrast agents silhouette the anatomy against a radiolucent background, whereas positive contrast agents produce areas of decreased density on the finished radiograph. Commonly used negative contrast agents are air, carbon dioxide, oxygen, and nitrous oxide. The positive contrast agents are primarily substituted benzoic acid compounds. They differ in the types of side chains and the extent of carbon atom substitution. They all use iodine to provide the contrast in the organ, but they vary in the number of particles that provide the osmolality of the substance. They are divided into agents that are ionic, and those that are nonionic in nature. There is a category of iodinated compounds that are considered to have a lower osmolality than the purely ionic agents. Nonionic compounds have been proven to cause fewer reactions than other varieties, but the economic considerations have prevented these from gaining universal use. These compounds are usually used in high-risk cases.

The important physical characteristics of contrast agents—viscosity, toxicity, iodine content, miscibility, and persistence—are usually considered when a contrast agent is chosen for a specific special procedure. MRI has its own specific criteria for contrast agent selection. The iodinated contrast agents are not effective during these types of procedures. Gd-DTPA, a metal chelate, is the most widely used substance for MRI.

REFERENCES

1. Lalli, A. F.: Urographic contrast media reactions and anxiety, Radiology, *112*:267, 1974.
2. Katayama, H., et al.: Adverse reactions to ionic and nonionic contrast media, Radiology, *175*:621, 1990.
3. Fischer, H. W.: Viscosity, solubility, and toxicity in the choice of an angiographic contrast medium, Angiology, *16*:764, 1965.

SUGGESTED READINGS

Ansell, G.: Adverse reactions to contrast agents: scope of problem, Invest. Radiol., 5:374, 1970.

Appleby, A., and Gryspeerdt, G. L.: Controlled trial of certain contrast media in cerebral angiography, Acta Radiol., 5:91, 1966.

Assem, E. S. K., Bray, K., and Dawson, P.: Release of histamine from human basophils by radiological contrast agents, Br. J. Radiol., 56:647–652, 1983.

Bettmann, M. A., Holzer, J. F., and Trombly, S. T.: Risk management issues related to the use of contrast agents, Radiology, 175:629, 1990.

Burchell, H., and Sturm, R. E.: Editorial: Electroshock hazards, Circulation, 35:227, 1967.

Cattell, W. R.: Excretory pathways for contrast media, Invest. Radiol., 5:473, 1970.

Dawson, P., Grainger, R. G., and Pitfield, J.: The new osmolar contrast media: a simple guide, Clin. Radiol., 34:221, 1983.

Eaton, S., et al.: Assays for plasma complement activation by x-ray contrast media, Invest. Radiol., 25:789, 1990.

Eaton, S. M., Hagan, J. J., Tsay, H. M., et al.: A predictive test for adverse reactions to contrast media, Invest. Radiol., 23(Suppl 1):S206, 1988.

Fischer, H. W.: The toxicity of the sodium and methylglucamine salts of diatrizoate, iothalamate, and metrizoate, Radiology, 85:1013, 1965.

Gomes, A., et al.: Acute renal dysfunction after major arteriography, Am. J. Roentgenol., 145:1249, 1985.

Grainger, R. G.: The clinical and financial implications of the low osmolar radiological contrast media, Clin. Radiol., 35:251, 1984.

Hessel, S. J.: Complications of angiography, Radiology, 138:273, 1981.

Higgins, C. B.: Effects of contrast media on the conducting system of the heart: mechanism of action and identification of toxic component, Radiology, 124:599, 1977.

Jacobsen, P. D., Rosenquist, C. J.: The introduction of low osmolar contrast agents in radiology: medical, economic, legal and public policy issues, JAMA, 260:1588, 1988.

Kallehauge, H. E., et al.: Iopamidol, a new ionic contrast media in peripheral angiography, Cardiovasc. Intervent. Radiol., 5:325, 1982.

Lang, E. K.: Prevention and treatment of complications following arteriography, Radiology, 88:950, 1967.

Lasser, E. C., Lang, J. H., Hamblin, A. E., Lyon, S. G., and Howard, M.: Activation systems in contrast idiosyncrasy, Invest. Radiol., 15:S2, 1980.

Magill, H. L.: Iodinated contrast media in pediatric radiology, Radiol. Rep., 1:364, 1989.

Mannhire, A., Dawson, P., and Dennett, R.: Contrast agent induced emesis, Clin. Radiol., 35:369, 1984.

Palmer, F. G.: The RACR survey of intravenous contrast media reactions: final report, Australas. Radiol., 32:426, 1988.

Reuter, S. R.: The use of conventional vs low osmolar contrast agents: a legal analysis, Am. J. Roentgenol., 151:529, 1988.

Shehadi, W. H., and Toniolo, G.: Adverse reactions to contrast media, Radiology, 137:299, 1980.

Tirone, P., and Boldrini, E.: Effects of radiographic contrast media on the serum complement system, Arch. Toxicol., 6(Suppl):37, 1983.

Wolf, G. L., Arenson, R. L., and Cross, A. P.: A prospective trial of ionic vs nonionic contrast agents in routine clinical practice: comparison of adverse effects, Am. J. Roentgenol., 152:939, 1989.

five

Catheters and Accessories

CUSTOM-SHAPING
Preparation of Tip
Cutting of Tip
Cutting to Length
Custom-shaping Distal End
Placement of Side Holes
Forming Proximal End

SIZE
SHAPE AND UTILITY
GUIDE WIRES
NEEDLES AND ACCESSORIES
PROCEDURE TRAYS AND SETS
ACCESSORIES

Catheters used during diagnostic radiography act as pipelines for transporting the contrast agent from an external source to a location within the body. In special procedures, the instillation of contrast material by catheters allows the radiographer to selectively demonstrate specific anatomic areas. The most common use of catheterization is during vascular radiography (angiography), although catheters are also used in many other special radiographic procedures such as bronchography and sialography.

Catheterization offers some definite benefits in radiography. If selective angiographic procedures are performed, the amount of contrast agent delivered to the patient is reduced. In these cases, a smaller amount of contrast agent delivered to a specific area through a catheter will maintain the proper concentration for good radiographic visualization. Direct injection into a remote vessel with the bolus traveling through the circulatory system to a specific location requires that a large amount of contrast material be injected to offset the dilution that occurs. If less contrast media is used, the procedure is easier for the patient to tolerate; fewer subjective and objective symptoms are produced, and the patient is more relaxed and cooperative during the procedure. Other advantages of catheterization include the possibility of biopsy and the ability to measure pressures within the lumen of vessels or directly from the chambers of the heart.

Catheters are simply tubes of varying lengths and inside diameters (IDs) with holes in each end that allow the contrast agent to flow through. Originally, catheters were adaptations of ureteral catheters that were constructed of rubber, but this soon gave way to the various thermoplastic catheters manufactured today. One major advance in catheter manufacturing was the development of the radiopaque polyethylene catheter, which allowed the radiologist to follow the path of the catheter through the body to its destination. Radiopaque catheters usually have different characteristics than the nonopaque varieties.

There are a wide variety of catheters and catheter systems available for use during special procedure radiography. These range from the simple straight catheter with one end hole to complex catheter systems designed to perform more than one function.

The Paceport catheter system (Fig. 5–1), for example, is designed to provide sophisticated hemodynamic monitoring capabilities as well as the ability to deliver reliable temporary pacing of the heart on demand. A discussion of every type of catheter and catheter system is beyond the scope of this textbook. However, the companies that manufacture catheters and accessories will provide catalogs illustrating their product lines. In most cases, the catalogs include data sheets that usually illustrate and reference each product and provide a short description of each catheter or accessory (Fig. 5–2).

All catheters manufactured today are disposable; that is, they are designed to be used once and then discarded. Several of the accessory items are still manufactured as "reusable." These items are designed to be cleaned, repackaged, and sterilized after the procedure. These must be inspected carefully during the cleaning process for any visible flaws. If any are noted, the item should be discarded.

The choice of the catheter or catheter system is made by the physician performing the procedure and is usually designated in the special procedure or catheterization laboratory procedure protocols.

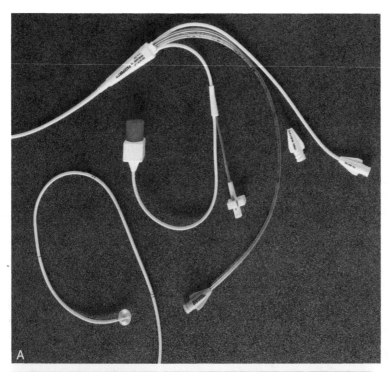

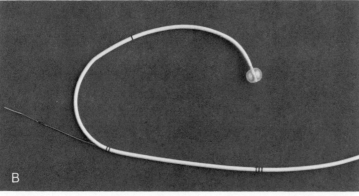

Figure 5–1. *(A)* Swan-Ganz Thermodilution Paceport catheter model 93A-931H-7.5F. Swan-Ganz is a registered trademark of Baxter International, Inc. Copyright 1988, Baxter Healthcare Corporation. *(B)* Paceport Catheter and Chandler V-Pacing Probe. (Reprinted with permission of Baxter Healthcare Corporation, Edwards Critical Care Division. Swan-Ganz® is a registered trademark of Baxter Corporation.)

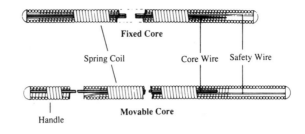

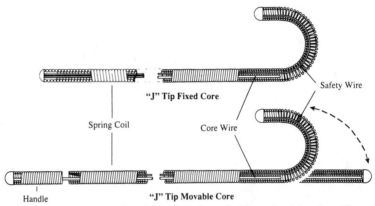

Figure 5–2. Sample catalog page describing the characteristics of guide wires. (From United States Catheter and Instruments Corporation, C. R. Bard, Inc.)

CUSTOM-SHAPING

Catheters supplied today are preshaped and molded. Becton Dickinson and Company offers a service that provides for the manufacture of custom specialty instrumentation. Many large institutions that perform research using newer techniques require catheters designed or shaped to specifications not usually available through product catalogs. Previously, it was possible to custom-shape catheters in the special procedures department. To some extent, this is still being done, although it is relatively infrequent. The process is simple; it requires the use of thermoplastic catheter tubing and is outlined as follows:

1. Prepare the catheter tip.
2. Cut the catheter tip.
3. Cut the catheter to the required length.
4. Custom shape the distal end of the catheter.
5. Place the catheter side holes.
6. Form the proximal end.

The equipment necessary for this process includes a guide wire matching the ID of the catheter tubing, an alcohol burner, a scalpel handle and blade, a hole-punching tool, a hot water bath, and a flanging tool. Figure 5–3*A–F* illustrates the process of the custom formation of catheters. The catheters made with this technique are used only for research purposes. If it was determined that a particular catheter design was viable for a particular procedure, it could be manufactured by one of the companies for general use.

Preparation of Tip

Insert the guide wire into the lumen of the catheter tubing approximately 20 cm. Heat the tubing over the alcohol burner while pulling the tubing in opposite directions

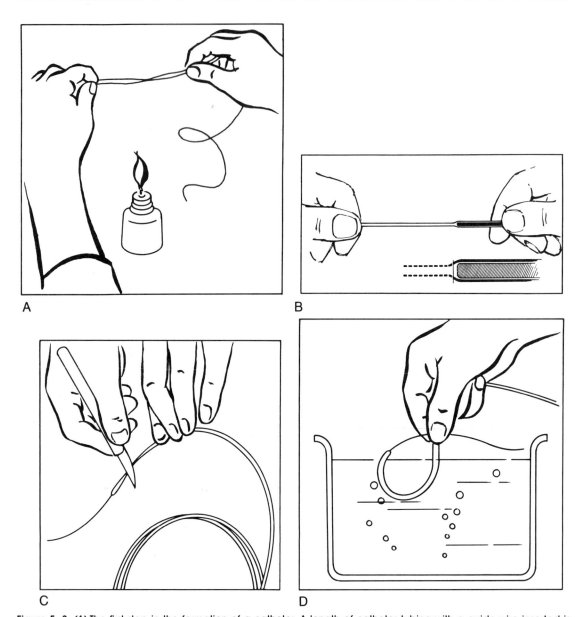

A

B

C

D

Figure 5–3. *(A)* The first step in the formation of a catheter. A length of catheter tubing with a guide wire inserted is heated over an alcohol burner. It is gently stretched to adapt to the diameter of the guide wire. The guide wire used in this procedure should not be used during a special procedure. *(B)* The cold formation used primarily with radiopaque Teflon, radioparent polyethylene, radioparent Teflon, and radiolucent vinyl tubings. After stretching, the catheter tubing will conform to the guide wire insert and should be cut off close to the insert. This will form a rounded catheter tip. *(C)* Cutting the catheter tip after stretching. The catheter should be rolled on a flat surface while applying gentle pressure on the knife blade. *(D)* Shaping the distal end of the catheter. The catheter-guide wire combination is placed in hot water. As the catheter softens, the desired shape can be formed. The combination is then transferred to a cold water bath to fix the position of the tip.

(see Fig. 5–3*A*). The tubing will soften, and the lumen will conform to the diameter of the guide wire and form an even taper. Immerse the catheter in cold water to fix the shape.

Another method of forming the distal end of the catheter is shown (see Fig. 5–3*B*). There is no need for heat because the tubing will stretch to conform to the tip of the guide wire in the lumen of the tubing. This method is used with catheter tubing other than radiopaque polyethylene tubing. When the tubing is sufficiently stretched around the guide wire, the unfilled portion should be cut off close to the tip of the guide wire. This procedure is used to form a rounded catheter tip.

Cutting of Tip

After the tip has been tapered and while the guide wire is still in the lumen of the tubing, the free end of the tubing should be cut with a sharp scalpel. The guide wire used to prepare the catheter tip should never be used in a procedure. The tubing should be cut at the point that best approximates the diameter of the guide wire used. The Kifa Catheter Manufacturing Company recommends rolling the tubing on a flat surface while applying slight pressure on the scalpel blade (see Fig. 5–3C).[1] It is essential that the cut tip be smooth to avoid trauma to the patient's vascular system.

Cutting to Length

When the tip of the catheter has been prepared, the tubing should be cut to the proper length for the procedure.

Custom-shaping Distal End

With the guide wire still in place, blend the catheter into the shape required for the procedure, and immerse it in hot water. It is important that the thinner walls of the tapered tip *not* be placed in the hot water because of possible deformation of the walls and end holes (see Fig. 5–3D). When the entire wall of the tubing has been heated and the catheter has softened, transfer the tubing to a cool water bath to fix the desired shape.

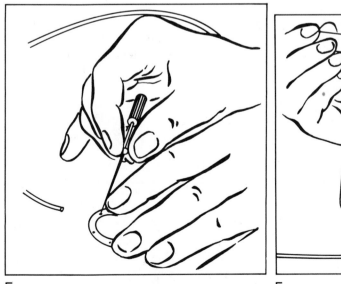
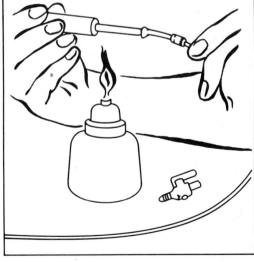

E

F

Figure 5–3 *Continued (E)* The procedure for punching holes in the distal tip of the catheter. *(F)* The formation of the proximal end of a catheter. The adapter cap is placed on the tubing, and the catheter tubing is heated over an alcohol burner. When it has softened, the flanging tool is used to form the cone-shaped proximal end. The shape is fixed under cold water with the flanging tool in place. (From Firma AB Kifa.)

Placement of Side Holes

Placing side holes in the distal end of the catheter reduces the whiplash effect created by injection of contrast media through a single end hole and increases the delivery rate of the catheter. Side holes should be placed so that the catheter wall is not weakened; they should not be placed in areas in which the guide wire could lodge as catheters are being exchanged. Therefore, holes should never be placed in the thin walls of the tapered tip or in direct opposition to each other.

Side holes are made with a punching tool that is a hollow cannula with a sharp cutting edge. Rotate the punching tool while applying slight pressure to it (see Fig. 5–3E). A stylet longer than the cannula is used to remove the plugs of tubing from inside the cannula. It is important that the piece of catheter wall not be left in the lumen of the catheter to avoid its introduction into the patient's vascular system.

Forming Proximal End

An adapter must be fitted to the proximal end of the catheter tubing to connect it to the injection device. A catheter flanging tool can be used to shape the proximal end of the tubing to fit the adapter cone (see Fig. 5–3F). Place the adapter cap on the tubing with the opening facing the proximal end. Heat the flanging tool, and then carefully press it to the end of the catheter tubing. With the tool in place, fix the flange under cold water. The connection should be tested for leakage before use.[1]

A second method of forming the flange in the end of the catheter tubing is to rotate it slowly over an alcohol burner while holding the tubing horizontally. Fix the shape in the usual manner under cool water.

SIZE

Catheter sizes are expressed in inches or millimeters or by French number.

The gauge scale known as the French scale was developed by Charrière, a French instrument maker (1803–1876). On Charrière's gauge scale, 1 Charrière [or 1 French (1F)[1]] is equal to a diameter of ⅓-mm, with each consecutive Charrière differing from the previous one by ⅓ mm. Table 5–1 lists the millimeter conversions for French numbers from 1 to 30.

If the diameter is expressed in inches, it is necessary to know that 1 in = 25.4 mm. To convert from inches to millimeters, simply multiply the number of inches by 25.4. For example, if the catheter diameter is 0.056 in, the conversion to millimeters is accomplished by multiplying 0.056 by 25.4 to give 1.42 mm as the catheter diameter.

Table 5–1. FRENCH GAUGE SCALE CONVERSIONS

Charrière	OD (mm)	Charrière	OD (mm)	Charrière	OD (mm)
1	⅓	11	3⅔	21	7
2	⅔	12	4	22	7⅓
3	1	13	4⅓	23	7⅔
4	1⅓	14	4⅔	24	8
5	1⅔	15	5	25	8⅓
6	2	16	5⅓	26	8⅔
7	2⅓	17	5⅔	27	9
8	2⅔	18	6	28	9⅓
9	3	19	6⅓	29	9⅔
10	3⅓	20	6⅔	30	10

From Firma AB Kifa: Instruments and Catheters for Radiography, Solna, Sweden, Firma AB Kifa.

A gauge scale is available that lists size specifications for cardiovascular catheters, facilitating the conversion from inches to millimeters or to French size (Fig. 5–4). Table 5–2 lists the size specifications for both standard and thin-walled cardiovascular catheters.

Some companies, such as Cordis Corporation, imprint sizing information on the hub, the proximal portion of the catheter that provides an attachment for the injector or syringes. Diagnostic catheters have the French size, length, and guide wire size imprinted on the hub. Interventional catheters show the same information on the injectate hub, whereas the inflation hub shows the inflated balloon size in millimeters and the usable balloon length in centimeters.

SHAPE AND UTILITY

The distal end of the catheter can be either straight or shaped. The shape of the catheter depends on the type of procedure being done and the anatomic part being

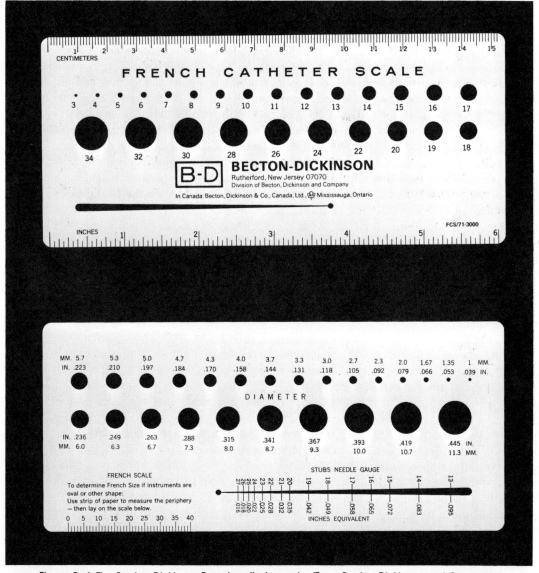

Figure 5–4. The Becton Dickinson French catheter scale. (From Becton Dickinson and Company.)

Table 5–2. SIZE SPECIFICATIONS FOR CARDIOVASCULAR CATHETERS

	Standard Wall							Thin Wall					
French Size	Inside Diameter		Outside Diameter		Needle Equivalent		French Size	Inside Diameter		Outside Diameter		Needle Equivalent	
	in	mm	in	mm	ID	OD		in	mm	in	mm	ID	OD
3	0.014	0.36	0.039	1.00	23+	20+							
4	0.018	0.46	0.052	1.33	22+	18+	4	0.023	0.58	0.052	1.33	20	18+
5	0.026	0.66	0.065	1.67	19	16	5	0.034	0.86	0.065	1.67	19+	16
6	0.036	0.91	0.078	2.00	18+	15+	6	0.046	1.17	0.078	2.00	17+	15+
7	0.046	1.17	0.091	2.33	17+	13–	7	0.058	1.47	0.091	2.33	15+	13–
8	0.056	1.42	0.104	2.67	15+	12–	8	0.068	1.73	0.104	2.67	14+	12–
9	0.064	1.63	0.118	3.00	14+		9	0.078	1.98	0.118	3.00	13+	
10	0.072	1.83	0.131	3.33	13+		10	0.088	2.24	0.131	3.33	12+	
11	0.083	2.11	0.144	3.67	12–		11	0.098	2.49	0.144	3.67		
12	0.094	2.39	0.157	4.00			12	0.108	2.74	0.157	4.00		
14	0.144	2.90	0.183	4.67			14	f0.128	3.25	0.183	4.67		

From United States Catheter and Instruments Corporation: Cardiovascular Catheters and Accessories, Glens Falls, NY, United States Catheter and Instruments Corporation.

imaged. Specialized shapes are used primarily for entry into smaller vessels during selective angiography (Fig. 5–5). There are a wide variety of catheter shapes available; some possible configurations of the distal ends of catheters are illustrated (Fig. 5–6).

Interventional radiology and cardiac catheterization have spawned the development of catheters that serve a variety of purposes. Catheters are available that contain attachments allowing various tests and measurements to be performed during the procedures (Fig. 5–7). Other catheters are equipped with small balloons that mechanically occlude vessels and allow hemodynamic studies to be performed as well as providing hemorrhage control, segmental isolation, and selective distribution of contrast media or therapeutic drugs. Catheters are also manufactured and equipped with baskets or forceps that allow the physician to remove foreign bodies or to perform biopsies. A variety of balloon catheters are also available. Figure 5–8 illustrates some of the types of interventional balloon catheters. Catheters that have permanently attached balloons have the capabilities of injecting contrast or therapeutic drugs either proximal or distal to the balloon depending on the design. In some catheters, the design permits the balloon to be detached in situ and left in place to provide a permanent occlusion. (A more in-depth discussion of the interventional catheters is given in Chapter 20.)

GUIDE WIRES

Catheters inserted by the percutaneous catheterization method are threaded over a stainless-steel guide wire. The guide wire is basically composed of an outer case of tightly wound stainless-steel wire enclosing a wire core that may be either fixed or movable. The inner core is a straight piece of stainless-steel wire. If the inner core is fixed, it is usually secured a short distance from the distal tip of the guide. This provides a flexible spring-wire tip that facilitates passage of the guide through sclerotic or tortuous vessels. The length of the standard length flexible guide tip is 3 cm, but 7.5-cm flexible distal-tipped guides are also available.

The movable-core spring guide has a movable inner core that can be used to vary the length of the flexible tip. When fully inserted, the inner core is used to straighten guides that have a precurved distal tip. When the inner core is withdrawn, the curve returns.

The length of spring guide wires ranges from 45 to 260 cm; guide wires used for exchanging catheters are usually more than twice the normal catheter length to prevent the loss of the guide while the catheter is being removed. Other lengths of guide wires

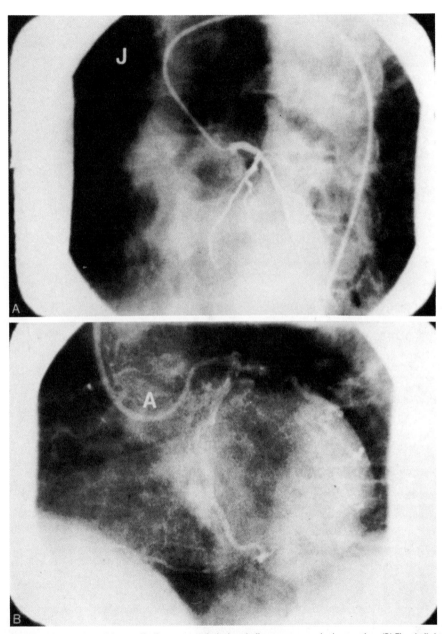

Figure 5–5. *(A)* The left Judkins catheter as used during left coronary arteriography. *(B)* The left Amplatz catheter as used during left coronary arteriography. These catheters are shaped to facilitate entrance into the desired coronary vessel during arteriography. (From Putman C., and Ravin, C.: Textbook of Diagnostic Imaging, vol. 3, Philadelphia, W. B. Saunders, 1988, p 1714).

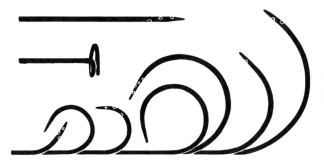

Figure 5–6. Illustration of possible shapes for the distal end of vascular catheters used in special procedures.

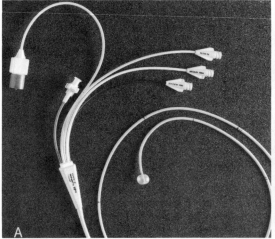

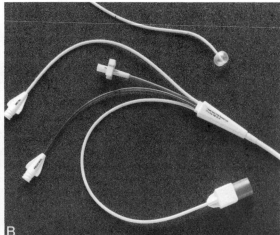

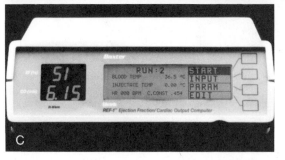

Figure 5–7. Catheters with multiple purposes. When used with the Edwards cardiac output computer, changes in the patient's hemodynamic status can be monitored. *(A)* Swan-Ganz VIP (Venous Infusion Port) catheter model 93A-831H-7.5F. Swan-Ganz® is a registered trademark of Baxter International, Inc. Copyright 1988, Baxter Healthcare Corporation. *(B)* Swan-Ganz S-Tip femoral catheter model 93A-151H-7F. Swan-Ganz is a registered trademark of Baxter International, Inc. Copyright 1988, Baxter Healthcare Corporation. *(C)* REF-1 Ejection Fraction/Cardiac Output Computer. Copyright 1990, Baxter Healthcare Corporation. All rights reserved.

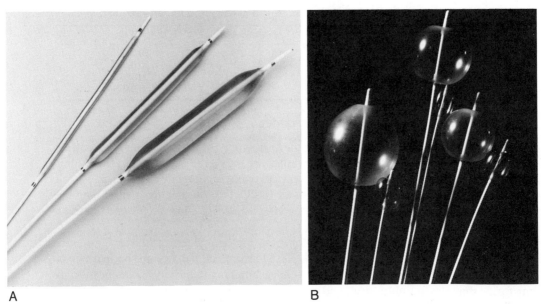

A   B

Figure 5–8. *(A)* Balloon dilation catheters; *(B)* balloon occlusion catheters. (From Medi-tech div. of Boston Scientific Corporation.)

can be made to order. The size of the guide chosen should be a minimum of 10 cm longer than the catheter.

Spring guide wires are very delicate instruments and should be handled with care. Spring guide holders serve as protective devices for the guide during sterilization and storage (Fig. 5–9). These holders can also be used as dispensers during the procedure, facilitating the handling of the guide wire and aiding in maintaining the distal end of the guide wire within the sterile field. It is generally recommended that spring guides be used only once and then discarded. If used more than once, a thorough inspection of the guide both before sterilization and during the procedure is recommended to prevent complications resulting from the use of a damaged guide.

NEEDLES AND ACCESSORIES

Needles are used extensively during procedures. The most frequently used needles are venipuncture needles. This type of needle is used for percutaneous vein punctures. These are usually disposable and are available in a wide range of gauges. Venipuncture

Figure 5–9. An example of a spring guide wire holder.

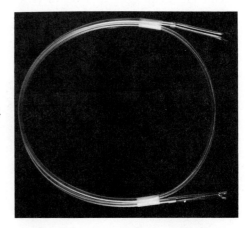

Table 5–3. EXAMPLES OF NEEDLE SIZING USING THE STUBBS NEEDLE GAUGE SYSTEM

Needle Gauge	OD (in)	Needle Gauge	OD (in)
27	0.016	21	0.032
26	0.018	20	0.0355
25	0.020	18	0.050
22	0.028	16	0.065

needles are relatively inexpensive, and a generous supply in various gauges should be kept in the special procedure suite. These needles are measured according to the Stubbs needle gauge, which, like the French system for catheters, relates needle size to a whole number. The Stubbs number represents the OD of the needle—the larger the Stubbs number, the smaller the OD of the needle. Table 5–3 illustrates some common needle sizes.

Arterial puncture needles are necessary for most angiographic procedures. These are manufactured under a wide variety of eponyms. Most arterial needles are basically two- or three-piece sets. Each set consists of an outer cannula with either a short bevel or a blunt tip, a sharp metal obturator, and a matching blunt-tip metal obturator (Fig. 5–10). These arterial puncture needles are equipped with a specialized flange that facilitates holding the needle during the puncture. The sharp inner obturator has either a regular bevel or a trocar point.

Certain angiographic procedures require the use of specially designed needles; these include a transthoracic catheter needle for left heart catheterization by the transthoracic route (Fig. 5–11D), various transseptal needles for left heart catheterization (Fig. 5–11C), transaxillary needles for catheterization of the descending aorta (Fig. 5–11B), and aortography needles for translumbar aortography (Fig. 5–11A). Table 5–4 summarizes some common needle types used during angiography. Procedures such as myelography, discography, sialography, and even bronchography also require specialized needles for the injection of contrast media. (Detailed descriptions of the various needles are available from the companies listed in Table A–1 of the "Appendix.")

PROCEDURE TRAYS AND SETS

Prepackaged, sterile procedure trays are available for many special procedures. These contain all of the accessory items necessary to prepare the patient and perform the percutaneous puncture. Becton Dickinson and Company manufactures general procedure trays for those performing direct puncture and for those using the Seldinger technique for arterial catheter insertion. These sets are divided into two sections; the top section contains the materials necessary for patient preparation, and the bottom

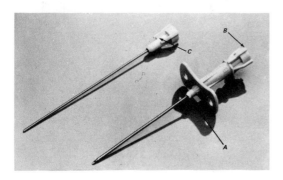

Figure 5–10. The Becton Dickinson sterile disposable arterial needle. The three-part set consists of an outer cannula (A), a sharp metal obturator (B), and a matching blunt tip obturator (C). (From Becton Dickinson and Company.)

Table 5–4. SOME COMMON NEEDLES AND THEIR APPLICATIONS

Needle Type	Description	Application
Angiocath	Needle with a beveled metal cannula and a Teflon sheath; the angiocath comes in various sizes.	Used for cubital vein puncture for DSA, peripheral venography, and pediatric angiography.
Amplatz	A three-part needle with a beveled cannula, stylet, and fitted radiopaque Teflon outer sheath. The Amplatz needle comes in 16-, 18-, and 20-gauge sizes.	Used for femoral, brachial, and axillary artery puncture; for the femoral vein, and for vascular grafts.
PTCA needle (Chiba Needles)	These are long, thin needles that usually are available in two sizes (22- and 23-gauge).	Used for percutaneous transhepatic cholangiography and splenoportography, and as a percutaneous biopsy needle.
Potts-Cournand needle	A two-part needle with a beveled outer cannula and a hollow, beveled stylet. This type of needle is also available with a blunt obturator. It is available in 16-, 17-, and 19-gauge sizes.	Used for arterial and venous puncture.
Seldinger needle	A two-part needle that has a thin-walled outer cannula with an inner stylet that can be beveled, diamond shaped, or pointed. It is available in 16-, 18-, and 20-gauge sizes.	Used for arterial or venous puncture.
Translumbar aortography needle	A long three-part needle having a Teflon outer sheath, metal cannula, and stylet with a diamond-shaped tip. It is available in 18 gauge.	Used for performing translumbar aortography.
Butterfly needles	These are available in various gauges. They have small "ears" attached to the hub portion of the needle to facilitate entering the vessel.	These needles are generally used to enter smaller veins. They can be used during a wide variety of procedures.

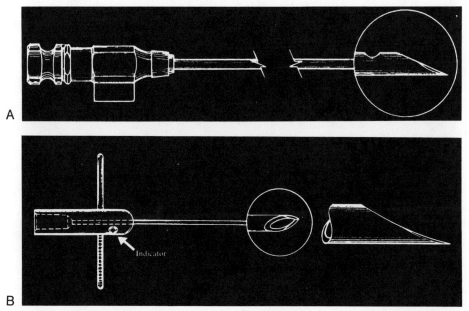

Figure 5–11. Some specialized needles available for use during special procedures radiography. *(A)* Aortography needle; *(B)* transaxillary needle.

Illustration continued on following page

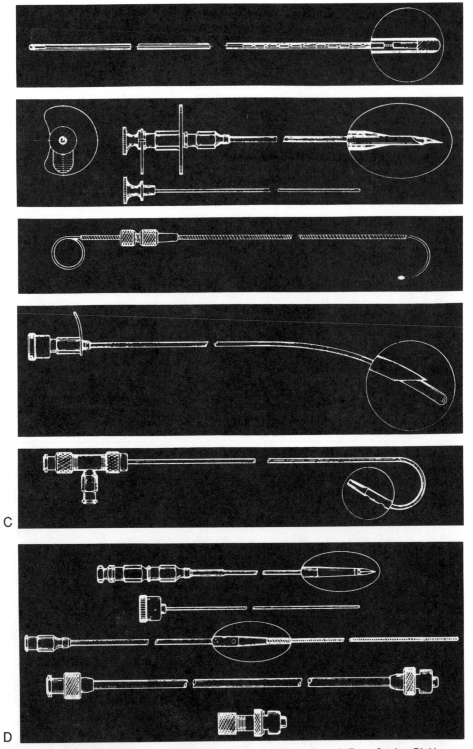

Figure 5–11 *Continued (C)* Cope outfit; *(D)* Levy-Amplatz transthoracic set. (From Becton Dickinson and Company.)

section contains the components for the particular procedural technique being performed.

Two common prepackaged sets that are available are the arthrography and myelography sets (Fig. 5–12*B*). The arthrography set, for example, contains the following items (Fig. 5–12*A*):

One 5-ml Luer-Lok syringe
One 10-ml Luer-Lok syringe
One 30-ml Luer-Lok syringe
One 18-g × 1½-in transfer needle
One 20-g × 1½-in short bevel needle
One 25-g × ⅝-in needle

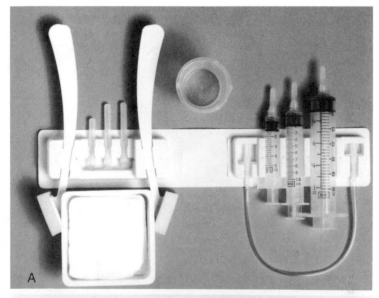

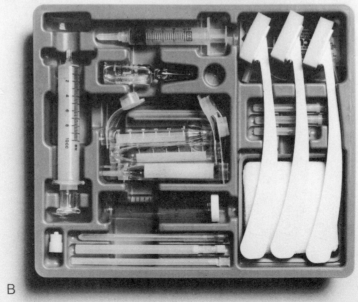

Figure 5–12. *(A)* Sample prepackaged arthrography tray. *(B)* Sample myelography tray for aspiration procedures using oil-based contrast media. (From Becton Dickinson and Company.)

Five 3 × 3-in gauze pads
One absorbent fenestrated drape
Two small basins
Two absorbent towels
One 2-oz medicine cup
One 10-in connecting tube
One adhesive bandage
Two prep sponges

The myelography tray comes supplied with different accessories depending on whether an oil-based or a water-soluble contrast agent is used. Each tray contains a variety of items from each of three basic groups of equipment (see Fig. 5–12*B*): (1) prep group (fenestrated absorbent drape, prep applicators, absorbent towels, 3 × 3-in gauze

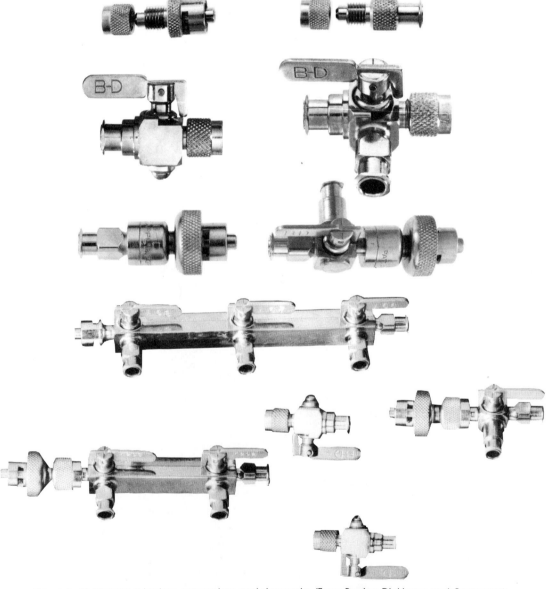

Figure 5–13. Various adapters, connectors, and stopcocks. (From Becton Dickinson and Company.)

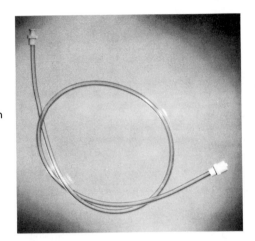

Figure 5–14. The sterile, disposable, flexible connector set with Luer-Lok fittings. (From Becton Dickinson and Company.)

sponges, and removable antiseptic basin), (2) anesthetic group (5 ml lidocaine, 5-ml syringe, 25-g × ⅝-in needle, 21-g × 1 to 1½-in needle, 18-g × 1½-in transfer needle, 16-g × 3-in transfer needle, and 18-g × 3-in transfer needle), and (3) insertion and contrast removal group (10-ml glass syringe, 20-ml glass syringe, 20-ml plastic syringe, 10-in extension tubing, 20-in extension tubing, 20-ml collection container, 3 × ¾-in adhesive bandage, male Luer-Lok cap, and specimen tubes). The trays are also supplied with different myelography needles that match a variety of different clinical requirements.

ACCESSORIES

Accessory items that should be kept in the special procedure suite include adapters, connectors, and stopcocks (Fig. 5–13). These are usually constructed of stainless steel and are reusable. They can be sterilized by autoclaving and should be thoroughly inspected and cleaned after each use. Connectors are usually supplied as sets containing vinyl tubing with male and female metal Luer-Lok adapters securely fastened. These are available in various lengths ranging from 10 in (25 cm) to 6 ft (180 cm) (Fig. 5–14). These are also sterilized by autoclaving and should be thoroughly cleaned and rinsed after each use.

REFERENCE

1. Adapted from: Instruments and Catheters for Radiography, Solna, Sweden, Firma AB Kifa, 1970.

SUGGESTED READINGS

Amplatz, K.: Techniques of coronary arteriography, Circulation, *27*:101, 1963.

Amplatz, K., Formanek, G., Stranger, P., and Wilson, W.: Mechanics of selective coronary artery catheterization via femoral approach, Radiology, *89*:1040, 1967.

Andrews, R., et al.: Catheter end-hole dilating guide wire, Am. J. Roentgenol., *139*:402, 1982.

Arani, D. T.: A new catheter for angioplasty of the right coronary artery and auto-coronary bypass grafts, Cathet. Cardiovasc. Diagn., *11*:647, 1985.

Baur, H. R., Mruz, G. L., Erickson, D. L., and Van Tassel, R. A.: New technique for retrograde left heart catheterization in aortic stenosis, Cathet. Cardiovasc. Diagn., *8*:299, 1982.

El Gamal, M., et al.: Selective coronary arteriography with a preformed single catheter: percutaneous femoral technique, Am. J. Roentgenol., *135*:630, 1980.

El Gamal, M., Bonnier, J., Michels, H. R., and Van Gelder, L.: Improved success rate of percutaneous transluminal coronary angioplasty with the El Gamal guiding catheter, Cathet. Cardiovasc. Diagn., *11*:89, 1985.

Hildner, F. J., et al.: New principles for optimum left ventriculography, Cathet. Cardiovasc. Diagn., *12*:266, 1986.

Hunter, T. B., et al.: Breakage of percutaneous catheters [Letter], Invest. Radiol., *17*:193, 1982.

Judkins, M. P.: Percutaneous transfemoral selective coronary arteriography, Radiol. Clin. North Am., 6:467, 1968.

Judkins, M. P., and Judkins, E.: Coronary arteriography and left ventriculography. *In* Coronary Arteriography and Angioplasty. New York, McGraw-Hill, 1985.

Kensey, K. R., Nash, J. E., Abrahams, C., and Zarins, C. K.: Recanalization of obstructed arteries with a flexible rotating tip catheter, Radiology, *165*:387, 1987.

Saxton, H. M., and Strickland, B.: Practical Procedures in Diagnostic Radiology. New York, Grune & Stratton, 1972.

Schoonmaker, F. W., and King, S. B.: Coronary arteriography by the single catheter percutaneous femoral technique, Circulation, *50*:735, 1974.

Sharma, G. V. R. K., Cella, G., Parisi, A. F., and Sasahara, A. A.: Thrombolytic therapy, N. Engl. J. Med., *306*:1268, 1982.

Sones, F. M., and Shirey, E. K.: Cine coronary arteriography, Mod. Concepts Cardiovasc. Dis., *31*:735, 1962.

Wells, D. E., Befeler, B., Winkler, J. B., Meyerburg, R., Castellanos, A., and Castillo, C. A.: A simplified method for left heart catheterization, including coronary arteriography, Chest, *63*:959, 1973.

White, R. I., French, R. S., and Amplatz, K.: An improved technique for right coronary artery catheterization, Am. J. Roentgen. Radium. Ther. Nucl. Med., *113*:562, 1971.

Zucker, R., Rothfeld, E. L., and Bernstein, A.: A new multipurpose cardiac catheter, Am. J. Cardiol., *15*:45, 1965.

2

Special Modalities

six

Digital Subtraction Angiography

MEDICAL ASPECTS

BASIC PRINCIPLES

Procedure

Image Processing

Image Storage

EQUIPMENT

IMAGING CAPABILITIES

Computer-assisted (digital) radiography differs from conventional radiography and fluoroscopy in the manner of data collection and/or processing. In conventional radiography, the data (remnant radiation that passes through the patient) is collected as a latent image on a film-based material that is subsequently processed via chemical means to produce an image. This image is usually viewed by passing light through the processed film.

Conventional fluoroscopy collects the data with an electronic image receptor, intensifies the image, and displays it as a television image. The image can then be stored on a variety of devices for future retrieval and study.

Computer-assisted (digital) radiography also collects the data via an electronic image receptor. Data collected in this manner is referred to as *analog data.** It is converted into *digital data*, processed, and stored in a computer system. It can be retrieved at a later time, reconverted to analog data, and viewed by means of an electronic device that displays the image. Digital radiography has several advantages over conventional radiography and fluoroscopy; these are summarized in Table 6–1.

Digital radiography has the same type of limitation as conventional radiography when it comes to the image. Because tomographic principles are not applied to digital

---

*Analog refers to signals that vary continuously with time, such as voltage.

Table 6–1. ADVANTAGES OF DIGITAL SUBTRACTION ANGIOGRAPHY

Imaging of low contrast structures is improved.
Data can be stored for analysis.
Information is processed quickly and reviewed without delay.
Diluted contrast agents (1:1 with saline) can be used.
Stored images can be electronically manipulated.
  Image contrast can be changed.
  Vessel edges can be enhanced.
  Portions of the image can be magnified.
  Remasking of images can be performed easily.

radiography in general, there is some superimposition of details in the image. As in conventional radiography, the superimposition can obscure details and compromise the diagnostic value of the procedure. In conventional radiography, a technique called subtraction removes the superimposition by eliminating the nonessential structures from the film (see Chapter 26). Digital radiography uses the principle of subtraction to achieve an image without superimposition. Digital radiography is usually referred to as digital subtraction angiography (DSA) when applied to special procedure radiography.

DSA is a diagnostic imaging method that uses a computer to convert the attenuated x-ray beam (analog information) into binary numbers (digital information), which can be manipulated and/or stored as required by the physician. DSA is more than just a technical method of producing a diagnostic film; it is a computer-assisted diagnostic procedure.

MEDICAL ASPECTS

DSA can be accomplished by both the intravenous and intra-arterial methods of introducing the contrast agent into the patient. Originally, a somewhat modified technique of the basic intravenous method for contrast injection was used exclusively. The use of the intravenous injection presented several advantages over catheter angiography—the procedure could be performed on an outpatient basis, thus avoiding the cost of a hospital stay, and complications and pain that can result from the placement of catheters could be avoided. The procedure promised to be less of a risk and much less expensive than catheter angiography.

The intravenous digital subtraction method had several disadvantages. Among these were the constant problem of both voluntary and involuntary motion artifacts, super-imposition of vessels caused by the generalized opacification from the intravenous injection, limitations on the study imposed by diminished cardiac output in certain patients, and the disadvantages of the large volume of contrast agent required for intravenous injection.

Modifications of the injection procedure and the ability of the system components to detect lower levels of contrast made intravenous DSA a relatively safe and cost-effective technique for vascular visualization.

Intra-arterial concentrations of 40 to 50% are required to produce satisfactory contrast images during standard angiographic procedures. Generally speaking, concentrations of less than 5% are not visible, even when routine subtraction techniques are used. Digital subtraction enables contrast agent concentrations as low as 1 to 3% to be visualized when they are administered intravenously. The amount of contrast agent that will produce satisfactory digital subtraction angiograms is generally about 0.70 ml/kg body weight. For example, a person weighing 150 lb (68.04 kg) would require approximately 48 ml of contrast agent to provide the necessary arterial contrast. An automatic injection device is required to deliver the contrast agent bolus. The intravenous injection procedure can be modified by first loading approximately 40 ml of saline solution into the syringe and then loading the appropriate amount of contrast agent. This "layering" of saline solution and contrast agent allows the contrast medium to be pushed through the venous system as a bolus to allow the maximum concentration to be delivered to the arterial system. Intravenous injections can also be made with a catheter placed in the superior vena cava. Another modification to the injection method is the use of the "intracath" type of venous catheter, which reduces the possibility of contrast agent extravasation.

A variety of advances in intra-arterial catheter techniques have changed the approach to DSA. Intra-arterial catheter insertion is now being done on a "same-day" basis. After the procedure, the patient is returned to the ambulatory surgery department for recovery and is usually released the same day. The primary reason, however, for the change to intra-arterial injection was the consistency of the results and the dramatic increase in the quality of the images produced.

The improved image quality resulted from the reduction and/or elimination of many of the disadvantages of the intravenous injection method. Motion artifacts were limited because the contrast agent was delivered to the site under study and imaging could proceed without delay. Lower doses of the contrast agent (15 to 20 ml for arterial DSA versus 40 to 50 ml for intravenous DSA) coupled with use of the nonionic contrast agents reduced the incidence of many of the symptoms experienced by the patient. This made the study more comfortable, which further reduced involuntary motion. The smaller doses and direct delivery also diminished the dependence on cardiac output to deliver a sufficient bolus for opacification of the anatomy. The arterial injections are also made with smaller catheters (usually 4F or 5F), which diminishes the incidence of postcatheterization bleeding. One added advantage of the intra-arterial method was that conventional angiography could be used interchangeably with DSA. This allowed the performance of the conventional procedure without the need for a return visit or additional catheterization if the study could not be performed using the DSA method.

Most DSA performed today is accomplished via the intra-arterial injection technique. In cases in which there is not a suitable arterial catheterization location, intravenous DSA is the method of choice.

BASIC PRINCIPLES

DSA depends on the use of image acquisition system components for successful results. The major components include a high-performance generator system (with capabilities in the 1000 to 1300-mA range), a high-quality image intensifier, a high-quality video camera, and an electronic computer system capable of processing and storing data. Figure 6–1 illustrates how these components can be integrated to provide the information flow in a DSA system. These components are usually matched to provide the highest-quality image possible. DSA may be described in terms of the procedure, image processing, and image storage.

Procedure

The medical aspects of the procedure have been discussed. The specific methodology varies, depending on the anatomy being examined. The physical principles of radiography that are used during this phase are the same as those that would be used during conventional radiography. In this phase, the radiation passes through the patient and is attenuated, and the resultant radiation is picked up by the image intensifier. The light image from the intensifier tube is focused and strikes the plumbicon tube of the video camera. At this point, the image is displayed on the television monitor.

The output from the video camera is also transferred to the second component, the image processing center, as a timed sequence of electrical pulses (the analog data). To understand this process, it is important to realize that the analog data (image) are measured in a point-by-point fashion in the image processing center. A radiographic image consists of many different density levels. The image processor "looks" at the image as if a rectangular grid (matrix) were placed over it. This grid divides the image into many squares, which represent discrete "picture elements" (pixels). Some common image matrix sizes are 256 × 256, 512 × 512, and 1024 × 1024 pixels. Given a standard field size, the larger the number of pixels in the matrix, the greater the resolution and the smaller the size of each pixel, yielding a greater spatial resolution.

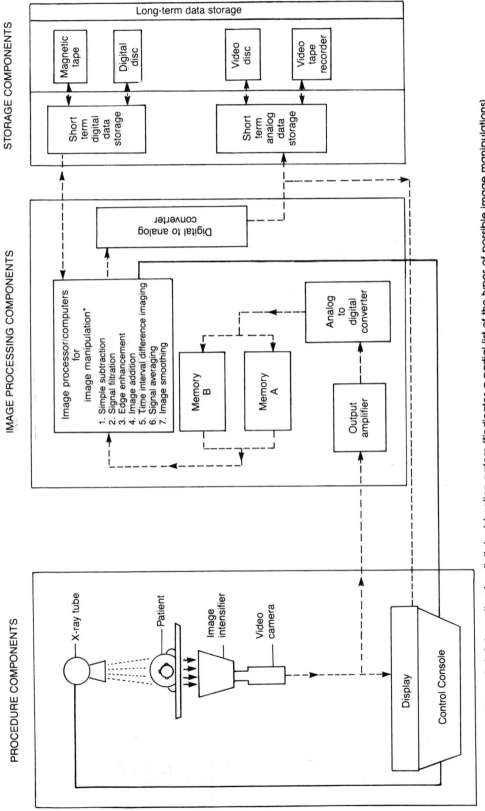

STORAGE COMPONENTS

IMAGE PROCESSING COMPONENTS

PROCEDURE COMPONENTS

Long-term data storage

Magnetic tape

Digital disc

Video disc

Video tape recorder

Short term digital data storage

Short term analog data storage

Digital to analog converter

Image processor/computers for image manipulation*

1. Simple subtraction
2. Signal filtration
3. Edge enhancement
4. Image addition
5. Time interval difference imaging
6. Signal averaging
7. Image smoothing

Memory B

Memory A

Analog to digital converter

Output amplifier

X-ray tube

Patient

Image intensifier

Video camera

Display

Control Console

Figure 6–1. Schematic of a digital subtraction system (*indicates a partial list of the types of possible image manipulations).

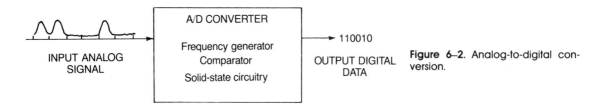

Figure 6–2. Analog-to-digital conversion.

Image Processing

When the video output (analog data) reaches this stage, the signal may be amplified. There are two methods available for the amplification of the output signal—logarithmic amplification and linear amplification. The former method is used most often with amplification of the data being proportional to the strength of the signal itself. It is usually used for carotid and vertebral studies. Linear amplification is used when the anatomy under study is of a uniform tissue density. This type of amplification is most often used for studies of the abdominal area.

In the next step of the process, the analog data signals are passed through an analog-to-digital (A/D) converter (Fig. 6–2). The intensity of the analog signal of each pixel is measured, and a numerical value is then assigned. This number represents the average density (analog signal) within the individual pixel areas. The A/D converter "digitizes" the analog information, that is, it transfers the analog signal into a digital number (Fig. 6–3). The digital data (numerical values) are represented by binary numbers.

Currently available A/D converters allow from 256 (2^8, or 8 bits) to 1024 (2^{10}, or 10 bits) gray levels for each image point (pixel). A bit is the contraction for the term *binary digit*. The human eye can distinguish only 16 shades (gray levels) at one time. The gray levels can be manipulated for optimal demonstration of different structures

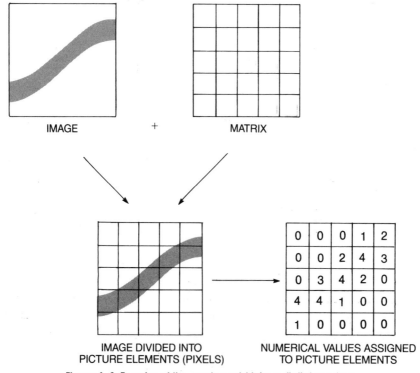

Figure 6–3. Transfer of the analog grid into a digital number.

in the image. Displaying a grouping of 16 shades at a time is termed *windowing*. The window level corresponds to the midpoint of the chosen gray scale as represented on the master scale.

The binary number system is made up of only 0s and 1s. It differs from the decimal system in that its base is 2. The decimal system has a base of 10 and is represented by the numbers 0, 1, 2, 3, 4, 5, 6, 7, 8, and 9. In the decimal system, numbers are formed using these digits multiplied by a power of 10.

Table 6–2 illustrates the differences between the binary number and decimal systems. It can be seen from the examples in Table 6–2 that binary numbers can be very long. To facilitate reading these numbers, other systems were developed based on the binary system—the octal system and the hexadecimal system. Each of these is a variation of the binary system using groups of binary numbers to represent larger numbers.

Table 6–3 illustrates the relationship between the binary number system and the other systems available for computer use. Each binary digit is called a *bit*. The term *byte* is used to describe a group of one or more bits. However, it is normally used to identify a group of eight bits, which is also known as an eight-bit code. For this information to be useful to the computer, it must be represented by a binary number system code.

After the A/D conversion (digitization) has taken place, the information is entered into the memory system. In most digital subtraction units, two memory systems are used, with the digitized image stored in one of the two memories. The second memory holds the images taken during the passage of the contrast medium. The information from the memories can then be integrated, and the images are manipulated in the computer. The resulting images can be stored in a short-term storage system as either digital or analog data. If the images are to be kept for any length of time, long-term storage capabilities are essential.

Before the digitized subtracted image can be displayed on a cathode ray tube screen or stored as analog data, it must be passed through a digital-to-analog (D/A) converter. This process is similar to that occurring in the A/D converter, but in this case the solid-state electronics generate an output voltage proportional to the digital number. The

Table 6–2. RELATIONSHIP BETWEEN THE DECIMAL AND BINARY SYSTEMS*

Decimal System			Binary System							
100	10	1	128	64	32	16	8	4	2	1
		1	0	0	0	0	0	0	0	1
		2	0	0	0	0	0	0	1	0
		3	0	0	0	0	0	0	1	1
		4	0	0	0	0	0	1	0	0
		5	0	0	0	0	0	1	0	1
		6	0	0	0	0	0	1	1	0
		7	0	0	0	0	0	1	1	1
		8	0	0	0	0	1	0	0	0
		9	0	0	0	0	1	0	0	1
	1	0	0	0	0	0	1	0	1	0
	1	1	0	0	0	0	1	0	1	1
	1	5	0	0	0	0	1	1	1	1
	2	0	0	0	0	1	0	1	0	0
	3	0	0	0	0	1	1	1	1	0
	4	0	0	0	1	0	1	0	0	0
	5	0	0	0	1	1	0	0	1	0
	7	5	0	1	0	0	1	0	1	1
1	0	0	0	1	1	0	0	1	0	0
1	5	0	1	0	0	1	0	1	1	0
2	0	0	1	1	0	0	1	0	0	0
2	5	0	1	1	1	1	1	0	1	0
2	5	5	1	1	1	1	1	1	1	1

*Base 10 in the decimal system uses the digits 0, 1, 2, 3, 4, 5, 6, 7, 8, and 9; base 2 in the binary system uses the digits 0 and 1.

Table 6–3. RELATIONSHIPS BETWEEN THE VARIOUS NUMBER SYSTEMS USED FOR COMPUTERS

Decimal	Binary	Octal	Hexadecimal
150	10010110 150	001, 101, 000 1 5 0 150	1111, 000 F 0 15 0 150
Base 10	Base 2	Groups of three digits are represented by one octal digit	Groups of four binary digits are represented by one hexadecimal digit
Ten digits are represented: 0, 1, 2, 3, 4, 5, 6, 7, 8, 9	Two digits are represented: 0, 1	Eight digits are represented: 0, 1, 2, 3, 4, 5, 6, 7	Sixteen digits are represented: 0, 1, 2, 3, 4, 5, 6, 7, 8, 9, 10 (A), 11 (B), 12 (C), 13 (D), 14 (E), 15 (F)

resultant electrical pulses are then converted into the light and dark patterns of the image on the television monitor.

Image Storage

The images resulting from the subtraction process can be stored in a short-term storage system as either digital or analog information. This type of storage can be considered primary storage, which occurs in the memory unit of the computer. If another procedure is performed, the short-term stored information is replaced by the newly generated data.

The long-term storage of data requires that secondary storage systems be available. Long-term data storage can be done using either analog or digital data. The analog data are stored on videodiscs or, more often, videotape. The digital data are stored on magnetic tape or digital discs.

EQUIPMENT

The computer hardware and system designs used for DSA vary with the individual manufacturers of the components. Figure 6–4 *A* and *B* shows an image acquisition and processing system.

The x-ray tube should be specifically designed for digital subtraction, especially in a dedicated DSA suite; however, standard angiographic tubes will function adequately during DSA under normal use.

The tube should have a high thermal capacity anode as well as dual focal spot capabilities. The larger focal spot will be used during DSA, because this is a low-resolution procedure. The small focal spot can be used for fluoroscopy, cineangiography, and some magnification work. Figure 6–5 illustrates one type of tube available for use during DSA, and Table 6–4 presents some design factors for a tube specifically designed for DSA.

The x-ray generator used should be a three-phase system. It should be linked with the computer to provide test exposures that are then computer adjusted to optimize the final exposure factors and provide the correct amount of light output from the image intensifier. The generator should be able to provide pulsed as well as continuous fluorography. If possible, the generator should be able to control the radiation dose (photon flux) according to the amount of contrast agent used. This is useful when DSA is performed on a patient whose tolerance to large doses of contrast agent is low. In

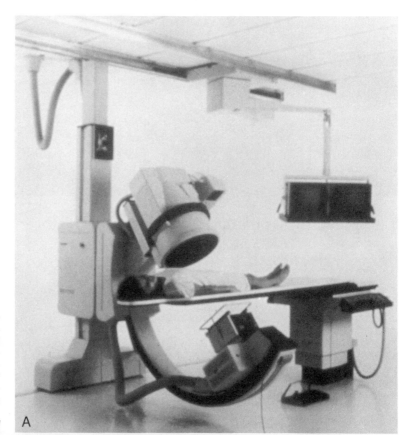

Figure 6–4. *(A)* Siemens Multiskop DSA x-ray imaging system showing the 85 cm radius C-arm and a large-format (40-cm) image intensifier. *(B)* Siemens Angiostar incorporates digital subtraction for both angiography and radiography and is equipped with a Puck CM film changer.

Illustration continued on following page

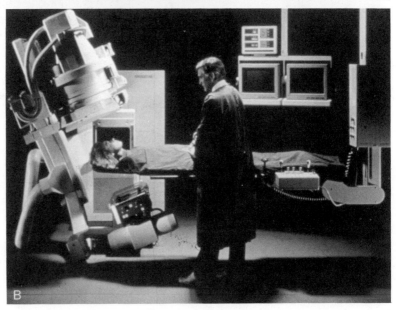

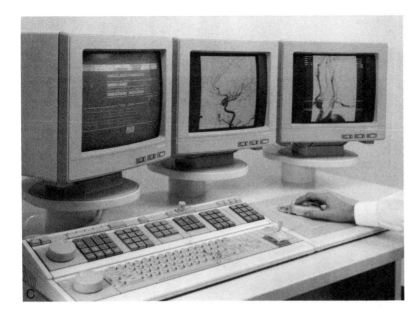

Figure 6–4 Continued (C) Siemens Polytron image acquisition and processing system for digital radiography. (From Siemens Corporation.)

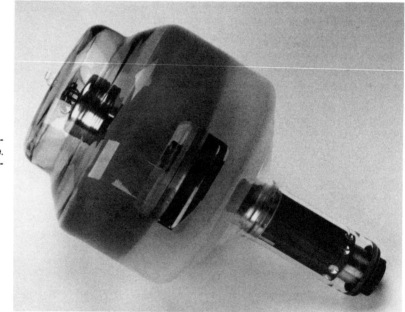

Figure 6–5. An 80° digital subtraction angiography x-ray tube. (From Varian Power Grid and X-ray Tube Products.)

Table 6–4. DIGITAL SUBTRACTION ANGIOGRAPHY X-RAY TUBE DESIGN FACTORS*

Specific Design Factor	Specification
Anode thermal characteristics:	
Heat unit storage	HU (maximum) 800,000
Heat unit dissipation	2,000–4,000 HU/s
Anode material	Rhenium-tungsten alloy-faced target on a molybdenum alloy anode disc
Anode size	125 mm (5 in)
Effective target angle	10°
Cathode	Dual focus: 0.6 mm/1.0 mm
X-ray field size/distance	35 × 35 cm (14 × 14 in)/100 cm (40 in) SID

*A800 series x-ray tube, Varian.

Table 6–5. SUMMARY OF SIGNAL-TO-NOISE RATIOS OF VARIOUS RADIOGRAPHIC SYSTEMS

System	Signal-to-Noise Ratio
Standard radiography	100:1
Standard fluoroscopy	200:1
Dedicated digital fluoroscopy	1000:1

such cases, the x-ray exposure could be increased and a smaller amount of contrast agent used, with satisfactory results.

The image intensifier should be of the cesium iodide variety for DSA. It should operate without loss of contrast at an exposure rate of 1 to 2 mR per image. The image intensifier must also have some type of filtration or aperture system to control the light level striking the television camera and to allow for the change of photon flux provided by the generator.

The television camera is the next link in the digital subtraction system. In this component, the signal-to-noise ratio (SNR) is a critical factor. Generally, noise as it applies electronically refers to anything that serves to hide the signal to be measured. The SNR is the ratio of the signal voltage to the noise voltage. Table 6–5 illustrates the SNRs of different radiographic systems currently in use. A television system should be chosen that provides the highest SNR possible to control the intrinsic system noise.

Another component in the television link is the monitor itself. Conventional television monitors have a format of 525 lines (rasters) for a single frame of video information. There are two methods by which the video information is displayed on the television monitor—the interlaced scan and the progressive scan. The interlaced scan mode reads out the video information in two separate scanning fields, with each containing half of the total 525 raster lines of the television tube. The completed video picture, also called a frame, is read out onto two separate scanning fields, with each containing 262½ raster lines. When the two 262½ raster line fields are interlaced, they form one complete frame comprising 525 raster lines.

The progressive scan reads out the entire frame of video information on the single 525-line field. Using the progressive system decreases the possibilities of motion artifacts occurring and allows for what is called the "snapshot" mode in digital fluoroscopy. The snapshot mode separates the x-ray exposure from the camera readout. The exposure is made with the television system blanked out, and the resultant image is stored on the face of the pickup tube. The information is read and then can be digitized. The advantage of using this type of mode is that the exposure time can be very short, which has the effect of stopping any motion. It is disadvantageous in that the rapid acquisition of information is compromised. In considering the components for this segment of the system, it would be useful to have both scan modes available—the progressive scan mode for snapshot digital fluorography and the interlaced mode for regular fluoroscopic applications.

IMAGING CAPABILITIES

All digital subtraction units available today provide for real-time subtraction. This means that the subtracted images can be displayed for viewing while the procedure is still being performed. The images can be produced by pulsed digital fluorography (serial imaging) or continuous digital fluorography (dynamic imaging). Figure 6–6 A and B provides typical examples of digital subtraction images.

Pulsed digital fluorography is similar to conventional serial radiography. It is often used when image acquisition rates range from one to eight images per second.

Continuous digital fluorography is similar to cineradiography, with image acquisition occurring at a rate of 30 frames per second. This type of imaging is used for visualizing

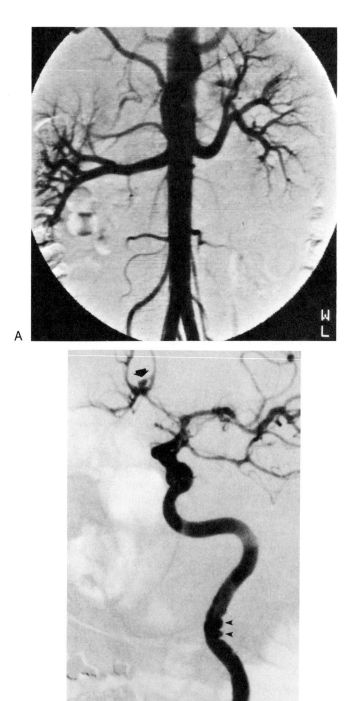

Figure 6–6. *(A)* Normal abdominal aorta and renal arteries as demonstrated by intra-arterial digital subtraction angiography. *(B)* Left internal carotid angiogram in the right posterior oblique projection using intra-arterial digital subtraction angiography. (From Putman, C., and Ravin, C.: Textbook of Diagnostic Imaging, Philadelphia, W. B. Saunders Company, 1988; vol 3, p. 1725; vol 1, p. 295.)

dynamic or rapidly changing processes. A disadvantage of the continuous digital fluorography method is the decrease in resolution of the image compared with images produced by the pulsed digital method. There also is a decrease in exposure times when this type of imaging is used.

There are three methods of performing subtraction in digital radiography—temporal (mask mode) subtraction, energy subtraction, and hybrid subtraction.

Temporal subtraction requires that an image be recorded before the introduction of the contrast agent. This image is referred to as the *mask*. Images recorded after the introduction of the contrast agent are then "subtracted" from the mask, that is, all of the information that was present on the mask is eliminated from subsequent images, leaving only the images of the opacified vessels. Temporal subtraction can be performed in different modes depending on how the images are collected. The various modes of temporal subtraction are serial mask mode, continuous mode, time interval difference, and postprocessing subtraction. Table 6–6 lists the differences among these methods.

Energy subtraction is based on the attenuation differences of the various types of tissue and the iodine in the contrast agent and on their relationship to the energy (kVp) of the x-ray beam. This method of subtraction requires equipment that differs from that used for temporal subtraction. The generator must be capable of switching kilovoltage during the exposures; there must also be a changing filtration system because this type of subtraction requires that images be recorded at two different energy levels (a low energy level and a high energy level). The two images can then be subtracted, and either bone or soft tissue can be removed from the subsequent images. One advantage to this type of subtraction is that motion artifacts can be reduced.[1]

Hybrid subtraction combines the best characteristics of temporal and energy subtraction methods. Images can be produced with the motion artifacts eliminated or reduced by subtracting the soft tissue via energy subtraction while the bone is eliminated via temporal subtraction.[2]

Temporal subtraction is by far the most common method of digital subtraction.

Table 6–6. COMPARISON OF THE VARIOUS MODES OF TEMPORAL SUBTRACTION

Mode	Method of Acquisition	Use
Serial mask	1. X-ray beam is pulsed. 2. Preinjection mask image is recorded. 3. Contrast is injected. 4. Postinjection images are subtracted from mask at a rate of about one or two per second. 5. Images are stored.	Carotid arteriography Peripheral arteriography Visceral arteriography Renal arteriography
Continuous	1. X-ray beam is continuous, similar to conventional fluoroscopy but with higher mA values. 2. Preinjection mask image is recorded. 3. Contrast is injected. 4. Fluoroscopic images are continually subtracted from the mask. 5. Images are stored.	Pulmonary arteriography Assessment of heart wall motion Coronary arteriography for bypass patency
Time-interval	1. Image acquisition occurs at a rate of 30 frames per second. 2. Preinjection mask image is recorded. 3. Contrast is injected. 4. Subtraction is performed at specified time interval. 5. Subtracted image becomes new mask. 6. New mask is subtracted from subsequent images at the predetermined interval. 7. Each new subtracted image becomes the new mask for the next interval subtraction. 8. Images are stored.	Cardiac angiography Imaging of moving structures
Postprocedure	1. Stored images are retrieved. 2. Images are manipulated or reviewed.	Stored image manipulation

Once the digital subtraction images are produced, they can be either stored or manipulated. A useful component is the array processor, which can perform a series of image manipulations very rapidly. One such manipulation is *image reregistration* (remasking). We have already seen that motion of any sort between the production of the images can interfere with the subtraction process by causing misregistration. The array processor shifts the contrast agent image up or down in relation to the precontrast agent mask image to compensate for any motion between the two images, a process known as image reregistration. This can be an extremely important option when performing digital subtraction in areas in which motion cannot be avoided, such as during cardiac imaging.

A variety of other manipulations can be performed on the stored images to aid the physician in arriving at a diagnosis.

Image magnification, sometimes referred to as *image zoom*, is the process of enlarging a portion of the image. This process cannot increase the amount of detail present; it can only make what is already present more easily visible.

Because DSA is often done as a presurgical procedure, the technique of *surgical landmarking*, or providing some visible landmarks for the surgeon to follow, can be beneficial during surgery. This is easily accomplished by returning a small part of the original image to the subtracted image.

Edge enhancement is a computer technique that makes the edges of the vessels more apparent, which facilitates visualization of the smaller details of the subtracted image.

State-of-the-art units are currently performing various quantitative evaluation functions, such as producing time–density curves, point measurements, and segment measurements; adding annotations to the image to identify items of interest; analyzing wall motion in left ventricular imaging; and performing statistical analysis in a specific area of interest.

SUMMARY

Digital radiography combines a computer system with a radiographic/fluoroscopic system that can provide a quick and accurate imaging method. It also allows for the manipulation of stored images of the study to aid in the diagnosis. Special procedures use this technology in conjunction with the basic principles of subtraction in DSA. This modality is equipment dependent and usually can be accomplished only in a dedicated DSA suite.

DSA collects the attenuated x-ray beam that passes through the patient, passes the beam through an image intensification system, converts the analog data into digital data, processes it in a computer, and then either stores or displays the information.

DSA was previously accomplished via intravenous injection; however, newer advances in arterial catheterization coupled with better image quality have changed how DSA is performed. The most common method used today is the intra-arterial method. DSA has several advantages over conventional angiography, including imaging of low-contrast structures, manipulation of the image, and use of a lower volume of contrast.

Digital subtraction can be accomplished by various means such as serial mask mode, continuous mode, time interval, postprocedure, and energy subtraction as well as a hybrid of energy and temporal subtraction.

REFERENCES

1. Brody, W. R., and Macovski, A.: Dual energy digital radiography, Diagn. Imag., *3*:18, 1981.
2. Guthaner, D., Brody, W. R., et al.: Clinical application of hybrid subtraction digital angiography: Preliminary results, Cardiovasc. Intervent. Radiol., *6*:290, 1983.

SUGGESTED READINGS

Crummy, A. B., et al.: Computerized fluoroscopy: Digital subtraction for intravenous angiocardiography and arteriography, Am. J. Radio., *135*:1131, 1980.

Foster, C. J., Butler, P., and Freer, C. E.: Digital subtraction angiography of the left ventricle, Br. J. Radiol., *61*:1009–1013, 1988.

Kruger, R. A., et al.: Digital K-edge subtraction radiography, Radiology, *125*:243, 1977.

Kume, Y., et al.: Investigation of basic imaging properties in digital radiography, Med. Phys., *13*:843–849, 1986.

McDermott, J. C., Babel, S. G., Crummy, A. B., et al.: Review of the uses of digital "road map" techniques in interventional radiology, Ann. Radiol., *32*:11–13, 1989.

Ovitt, T. W., et al.: Intravenous angiography using digital video subtraction: X-ray imaging system, Am. J. Neuroradiol., *1*:387, 1980.

Strother, C. M., et al.: Clinical applications of computerized fluoroscopy: The extracranial carotid artery, Radiology, *136*:781, 1981.

seven

Computed Tomography

STANDARD COMPUTED TOMOGRAPHY
Historical Perspective
Physical Principles
Room Design
Equipment
Technical Considerations

Patient Preparation
ULTRAFAST COMPUTED TOMOGRAPHY
Physical Principles
Room Design
Equipment
Technical Considerations

Computed tomography (CT) is a specialized modality that links the basic theory of body section radiography with a computer system to produce the anatomic images. The fundamentals of computer technology as it applies to radiography are presented in Chapter 6. The basic principles and terminology are similar for all computer-enhanced techniques, with minor variations applicable for CT and magnetic resonance imaging (MR). The physical principles of CT are presented, but a detailed discussion is beyond the scope of this book.

STANDARD COMPUTED TOMOGRAPHY

Historical Perspective

CT appears to be a very recent innovation, but the theoretic principles of CT were presented by Radon in 1917.[1] This Austrian mathematician proved that it was possible to reconstruct a three-dimensional object from the infinite set of all of its projections. The actual breakthrough in making CT a useful diagnostic tool was made by Hounsfield in 1967.[2] It was not until 1971, however, that the first working model was installed and ready for clinical trials. The transition from Radon's hypothesis to Hounsfield's breakthrough was aided by the experimental work of many researchers, including Oldendorf and Cormack.[3, 4] The use of CT has expanded since 1971, and new developments are occurring rapidly. Each major innovation heralds a new "generation," or category, of CT scanners. These generations are identified primarily on the basis of the geometry of the mechanical scanning motions. Each successive generation has shown improvement in scanning mode, detection system, and rotational movement (degrees of rotation). One common result of these changes has been the reduction in time required by the unit to produce a scan; this has been reduced from approximately 5 min for the first-generation CT units to from 2 to 10 s for the fourth-generation CT units. Figure 7–1 shows the four generations of CT scanners.

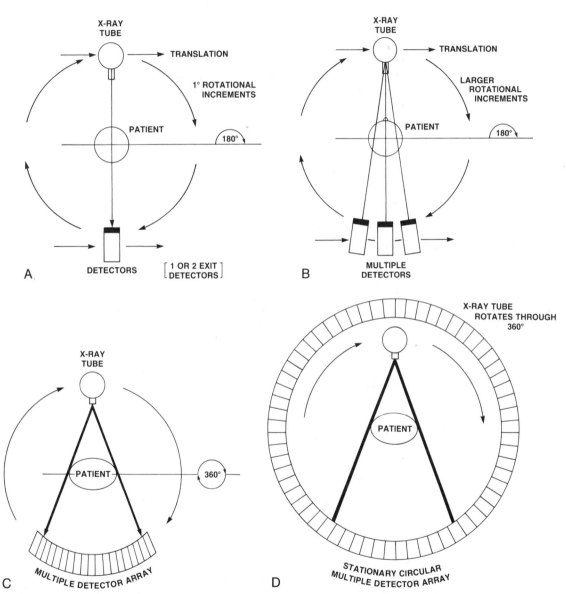

Figure 7–1. *(A)* Rectilinear pencil beam scanning typical of first-generation CT scanners, based on the rotate-translate principle; *(B)* rectilinear multiple pencil beam scanning used in second-generation CT scanners, based on the rotate-translate principle; *(C)* continuously rotating pulsed fan beam scanning typical of third-generation CT scanners; and *(D)* fourth-generation CT scanning scheme. (From Seeram, E.: Computed Tomography Technology. Philadelphia, W. B. Saunders, 1982.)

Physical Principles

"Tomography" is the term used to describe body section radiography. The procedure produces a sectional image, or "slice," of the body part being examined. Traditional tomography uses the principle of blurring to remove unwanted superimposed structures while keeping the selected layer in focus. This can be accomplished by moving the x-ray beam and film through mechanical linkages or similar devices. Blurring can also be achieved by moving the patient and the film, the x-ray beam and the patient, or only the patient (automography). All of these methods use conventional radiographic principles to produce the image, that is, to acquire diagnostic data. Conventional radiography and tomography, however, have several disadvantages. Superimposition of structures is one encountered problem. Conventional tomography can remedy this problem to some degree but not without a trade-off. With conventional tomographic methods, the blurring procedure can be somewhat distracting, and it cannot be completely eliminated from the final image produced by the scattered radiation.

CT is accomplished in three steps—scanning the patient, processing data, and displaying the image. The first step, scanning the patient, is the radiographic portion of the study. The method used to scan depends on the equipment.

CT equipment has undergone many changes since it was first available for diagnostic imaging. It has gone through four generations of geometrical design—rotate-translate using a pencil beam and a single detector, rotate-translate using multiple pencil beams and from three to 60 detectors, rotate-rotate using a narrow fan beam and an array of 128 to 600 detectors with a pulsed x-ray beam, and rotate-stationary using a wide fan beam and a circular array of 600 to 2000 detectors with a continuous x-ray beam (see Fig. 7–1). Most of the units in use today are third- or fourth-generation devices. The major disadvantage of the first- and second-generation units is the long scan time required for the study. Third- and fourth-generation scanners have scan times ranging from 2 to 10 s depending on the equipment design and the type of scan being performed.

In the fourth-generation scanning process, the x-ray tube rotates around a stationary circular set of multiple detectors (rotate-stationary). These detectors completely encircle the patient. Unlike third-generation units (rotate-rotate), the detectors do not move when the x-ray tube is rotated. A wide fan beam enters the patient around the edge of the slice being imaged. The scanning process consists of the x-ray tube's making a 360° rotation around the patient; one rotation of the x-ray tube creates one image. A typical CT study comprises many images at different slice locations. The slice scans can be made with the rotation smaller or larger than the standard 360° movement. This parameter can be adjusted and is usually set by the radiographer performing the study. During the rotation, a continuous x-ray beam projects information to the array of detectors, which has the result of seeming to produce the image from many x-ray tube locations using one detector.

CT produces the image by the attenuation of the x-ray beam; the patient absorbs the radiation in varying amounts depending on its interaction with the various tissues. The remnant radiation is collected by the detectors and transmitted to the computer for processing.

The measurements acquired from the scan are recorded in digital form by the computer. From this information, the computer reconstructs the image.[5] The data are processed by the computer software that runs the image reconstruction process. The algorithm sorts and manipulates the digital information to reconstruct the image. The radiographer can alter the processing procedure in two ways that affect both the quality and the appearance of the image—through selection of matrix size and selection of the reconstruction algorithm. In general, the larger the matrix size (128×128, 256×256, or 512×512), the greater the resolution (and quality). Many different algorithms are used for processing the data; algorithms are specific for the type of equipment and software options used.

Three methods used for image reconstruction are back projection, iterative reconstruction, and analytic reconstruction. The back projection method is the simplest one, but the image reconstruction is not very sophisticated or popular. The image produced lacks clarity and can produce an artifact commonly known as the "star pattern."

Iterative reconstruction can be accomplished in several ways:

1. Algebraic reconstruction technique (ART)
2. Simultaneous iterative reconstruction technique (SIRT)
3. Least-squares technique (LST)

All of these methods use the iterative mathematical technique to arrive at a reconstructed image. "Iterative" can be defined as a method of using successive approximations, starting with an arbitrary image, and applying calculated correction factors. This correction-comparison process continues until there is agreement between the calculated ray projection and the measured ray projection. Iterative methods can be applied by the use of additive and multiplicative mechanisms. Additive iterative reconstruction divides the correction factor among the elements of the matrix in proportion to their weighting factors. Multiplicative iterative reconstruction applies the correction factor in proportion to the present density of the matrix element. The most often used mechanism is that of additive iterative reconstruction.[6]

Analytic reconstruction methods are also based on mathematical principles and include the filtered back projection, or convolution, method and the two-dimensional Fourier reconstruction. These methods produce very accurate reconstruction images in less time than the iterative methods. The filtered back projection algorithm is used most often.

CT is the production of reconstructed images from information received from the remnant radiation through one of the techniques discussed above. Remnant radiation is the portion of the x-ray beam transmitted through the patient. These transmitted x-ray photons represent some amount of attenuation within the patient. These are compared with the intensity of the radiation from the x-ray tube, which is measured by a special "reference" detector, to give relative transmission values after digitization. The attenuation values of various tissues are related to the attenuation value of water and may be arranged as a scale (Fig. 7–2). These scale values are called EMI, or Hounsfield, numbers and represent the various CT digital numbers used to reconstruct the image. When the image is produced, the scale (CT digital) numbers represent a certain brightness level. Figure 7–3 illustrates how the scale numbers and brightness level are related. The brightness level (gray scale) can be manipulated to demonstrate different structures in the image. This manipulation, or variation in the relation between the scale numbers and level of brightness, is often called *windowing,* or *setting a window*.

The window is controlled by the operator of the CT unit and usually set as a window width and window level. The window width represents the range of scale numbers used for the gray scale. Adjusting the window width is equal to adjusting the contrast of the image. The window level represents the midpoint of the gray scale and can be considered a density adjustment. When viewing an image, these values can be adjusted, usually by the radiographer, to enhance certain anatomic structures. The effect of varying window width and window level is illustrated in Figure 7–4. Completed scans are stored (archived) as hard copy or on magnetic tape or digital discs.

Room Design

As in special procedure radiography, CT requires specialized construction specifications. The nature of the equipment requires that there be three separate and distinct

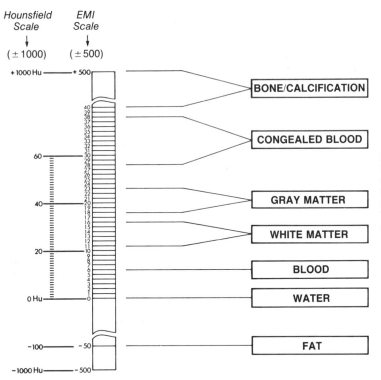

Figure 7–2. Absorption values common to clinical radiology. The values shown are for the EMI (±500) and Hounsfield (± 1000) scales. (From Seeram, E.: Computed Tomography Technology. Philadelphia, W. B. Saunders, 1982.)

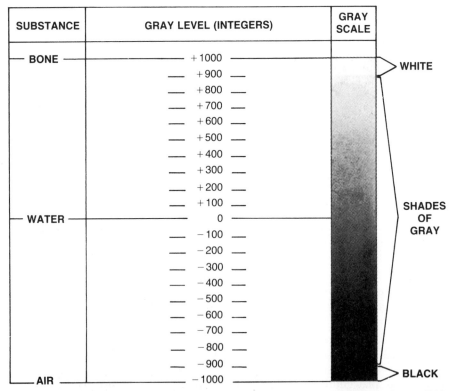

Figure 7–3. The relation between CT numbers and the brightness level (gray scale) for the ± 1000 scale. (From Seeram, E.: Computed Tomography Technology. Philadelphia, W. B. Saunders, 1982.)

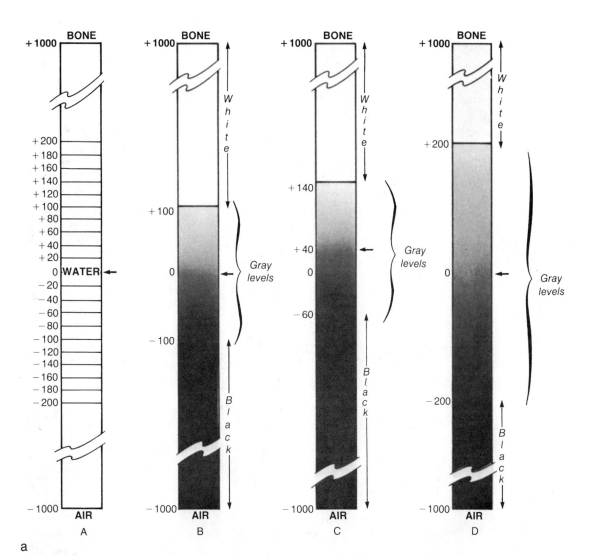

a

Figure 7–4. *(a)* Graphic illustration of the effect of different WW and WL settings on the CT image.

Illustration continued on following page

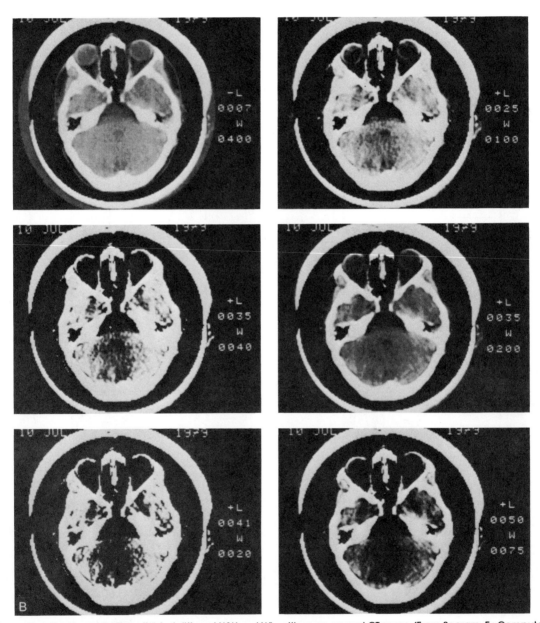

Figure 7–4 *Continued (b)* The effect of different WW and WL settings on several CT scans. (From Seeram, E.: Computed Tomography Technology. Philadelphia, W. B. Saunders, 1982.)

areas—the scanning area, the control area, and the computer hardware area. The ultimate size and configuration of the CT suite are determined by the manufacturer's representative, the radiographer, the radiography administrator, and the architect. In general, a suite size of 600 ft² (55.74 m²) is necessary to house the CT components. About half of this space, or 300 ft² (27.87 m²), must be devoted to the scanning area, in which the imaging equipment is housed. There should be sufficient room around the scanning unit for stretchers or beds to be easily maneuvered. The doorway to the scanning area should be a minimum of 4 ft (1.2 m) wide to provide unobstructed access to the area.

The control area should have approximately 150 ft² (13.935 m²) of floor space. The control console, x-ray control unit, viewing equipment, and hard copy imaging recording devices are located in this room. Each manufacturer has different system configurations that may alter the room design. Some system designs provide for remote viewing stations in addition to the operating-viewing console station located in the main CT control area. The control area should allow a direct view of the scanning area so the radiographer can monitor the patient throughout the course of the procedure.

The computer area should be approximately 100 to 150 ft² (9.29 to 13.935 m²). The final room size depends on the type of computer hardware installed and the amount of peripheral equipment purchased.

The entire CT suite should follow the same basic design and construction requirements as those for a special procedures suite in regard to radiation protection standards, concealed wiring, emergency equipment, and air conditioning. All equipment should be explosion-proof and should meet the requirements specified by the National Fire Code.[7]

Equipment

CT systems can be broken down into three main groups—the imaging group, the computer group, and the control group. A fourth group takes into consideration image reproduction and storage.

The imaging group contains all of the elements necessary to produce an image, including the x-ray generator, x-ray tube, and detector system. The x-ray tube(s) and detector(s) are located in housing called a *gantry* (Fig. 7–5), which also contains the mechanics that provide the motion used in the CT unit. The gantry housing conceals the motion of the x-ray tube and/or detectors. The equipment will vary depending on the generation of CT equipment. (See "Suggested Readings" at the end of the chapter for references on the mechanics of the gantry.) Each CT gantry comes with a patient table or couch that is styled according to the individual manufacturer's specifications. The purpose of the table or couch is to support and move the patient through the central opening in the gantry (Fig. 7–6). Movement of the patient couch can be controlled either by the computer or manually in a horizontal plane. The gantry can be angled with respect to the body axis before the scanning procedure. With the images collected from a series of axial scans, it is possible for the computer to combine segments of the images to create a new image in an orthogonal plane.

The x-ray tubes used in CT units can be of either the stationary or rotating anode variety. These tubes should be relatively heavy duty to tolerate the production of many images in a short period of time. The focal spot size is usually determined by the type of tube used in the manufacture of the system; fixed anode x-ray tubes have larger focal spot sizes. The third- and fourth-generation scanners use the rotating anode x-ray tube, which can provide more intensity and power output for short exposure times than stationary anode tubes. These tubes have small focal spots and extremely high heat loading capacities.

Another component housed in the gantry is the detector system. There are two types of detectors in use today—the gas ionization and the scintillation detector. Each has

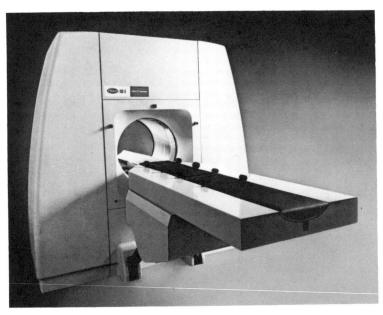

A

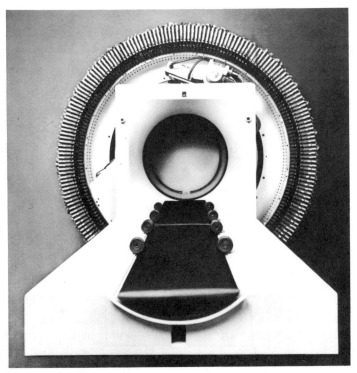

B

Figure 7–5. *(A)* One type of gantry system with a patient couch; *(B)* gantry system with cover removed showing how flow detectors *(outer circle)* and x-ray tube *(partially shown)* are mounted (fourth-generation). (Courtesy of Pfizer/American Science and Engineering.)

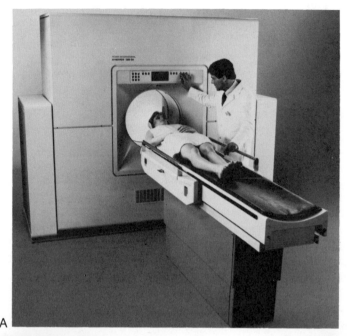

A

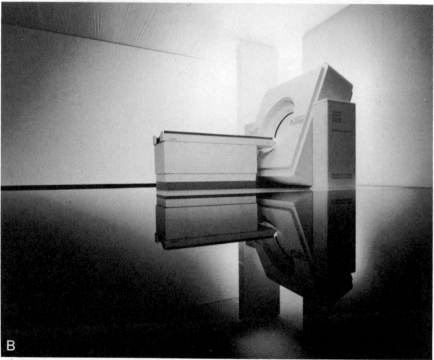

B

Figure 7–6. *(A)* Gantry and patient couch of the Picker Synerview 1200 SX. (From Picker International.) *(B)* Siemens HI Q/CT System. (From Siemens Corporation.)

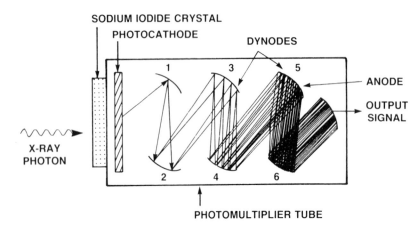

Figure 7–7. Schematic of a scintillation detector. (From Seeram, E.: Computed Tomography Technology. Philadelphia, W. B. Saunders, 1982.)

advantages and disadvantages. Scintillation detectors are usually more expensive than gas ionization detectors. They have the advantage of offering a high current amplification. The scintillation detector is basically a crystal of sodium iodide (NaI), cesium iodide (CsI), or calcium fluoride (CaF_2) connected to a photomultiplier tube (Fig. 7–7). These types of detectors produce an output signal that is dependent on the energy of the remnant radiation striking the crystal. Gas ionization detectors rely on the ionization of pressured xenon gas. The remnant radiation impinges on the detector cell and ionizes the xenon. The positively charged ions move toward the negatively charged side of the detector and the negative ions move to the positive side of the detector; this creates a weak electrical signal that is directed through an amplification system. The output signal of the detector is proportional to the number of x-ray photons

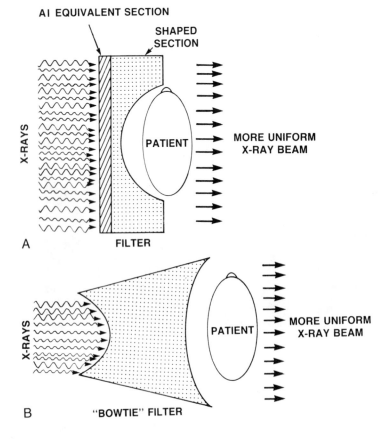

Figure 7–8. *(A, B)* Filters may be placed between the x-ray tube and object to reduce the dynamic range of the electronics (analog-to-digital converters) by shaping the beam to produce uniform beam hardening. (From Seeram, E.: Computed Tomography Technology. Philadelphia, W. B. Saunders, 1982.)

involved in the ionization. One problem with the gas ionization detector is its low absorption efficiency; many of the x-ray photons can pass through the detector cell without being ionized. The choice of detector depends on the manufacturer and equipment design specifications. The information produced by the detector system is transferred to the computer group for processing.

Filtration and collimation are two conventional radiographic principles that are also applied to CT. Filtration is used primarily to harden the x-ray beam, which, as in conventional filtration, is accomplished by absorption of the "softer," or less-penetrating, photons. Filtration also provides a uniform hardening effect across the entire x-ray beam (Fig. 7–8). In earlier head scanning units, water boxes were used to do this. Manufacturers supply different filtration systems with their units. Some units include selectable filtration modes, which have several different types of filters.

Collimation in CT is used to limit the patient dose and improve image quality. The collimation is accomplished at the x-ray source as well as at the detector. This type of system effectively limits the x-ray beam and reduces the scattered radiation that could reach the detector. Collimation in CT also determines the thickness of the scan section. Each generation of CT scanners has its own collimation design. (Many other factors are related to collimation, but they are beyond the scope of this discussion.)

The computer group is usually located in a room separate from the room that houses the gantry or scanner. The heart of the computer group is the central processing unit, which collects, reconstructs, and prepares the data for display. The central processing unit usually directs the movement of the patient table during the examination. It is equipped with short-term storage capabilities, which allow it to reconstruct and display an image in a relatively short period of time. This storage system is in the form of a digital disc. The Picker Synerview 1200 SX uses a 160-megabyte Winchester-type disc system for program and image storage. These digital disc systems are very costly and are not used for long-term storage. Most units currently in use are equipped with magnetic tape storage devices. However, some use the "floppy" disc system for storage, which is relatively inexpensive and can be used to store a small number of images per disc. Figure 7–9 shows a typical computer group with a magnetic tape storage system and a central processing unit. The computer group can also contain peripheral system components, including the interface connection between the imaging group and the computer group, a line printer, and the magnetic tape or disc storage system.

The control group contains the display control console and keyboard. The display

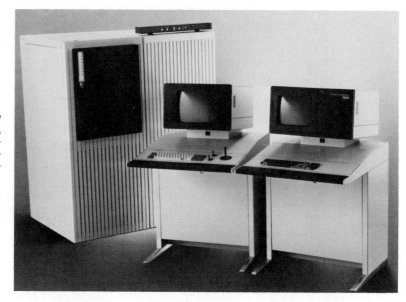

Figure 7–9. The Picker Synerview computer is shown on the left, along with a typical control console (center) and a viewing console (right). (From Picker International.)

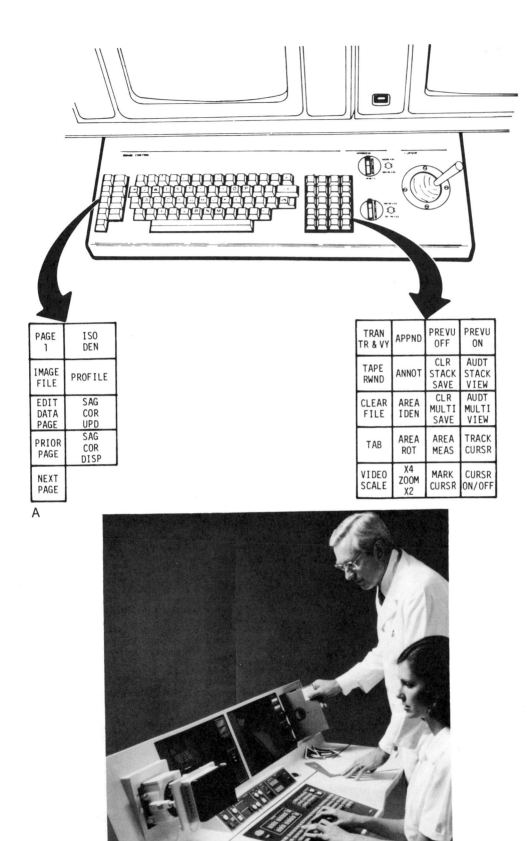

A

PAGE 1	ISO DEN
IMAGE FILE	PROFILE
EDIT DATA PAGE	SAG COR UPD
PRIOR PAGE	SAG COR DISP
NEXT PAGE	

TRAN TR & VY	APPND	PREVU OFF	PREVU ON
TAPE RWND	ANNOT	CLR STACK SAVE	AUDT STACK VIEW
CLEAR FILE	AREA IDEN	CLR MULTI SAVE	AUDT MULTI VIEW
TAB	AREA ROT	AREA MEAS	TRACK CURSR
VIDEO SCALE	X4 ZOOM X2	MARK CURSR	CURSR ON/OFF

B

Figure 7–10. *(A)* Interactive function keys on console of the Picker Synerview CT system. (From Picker International.) *(B)* EMI CT control console. (From Seeram, E.: Computed Tomography Technology. Philadelphia, W. B. Saunders, 1982.)

control console is similar to other x-ray machine consoles in that it has an on-off switch and a means of selecting the technical factors and section level. The scanning gantry is also energized from this point. In most CT room designs, the control group is stationed separate from the computer and imaging groups. The scanning gantry and patient should be visible from the display control console. Information is introduced into the system by the keyboard, which resembles a typewriter keyboard and consists of letters and numbers. There are also a number of keys devoted to various functions specific to the type of CT unit purchased. A console and keyboard are shown in Figure 7–10. Note the Polaroid camera on the left side of the unit used to make hard copy photographs of the scan and the floppy disc being inserted into the console on the right side for long-term storage of individual scans (Fig. 7–10*B*).

Image reproduction devices can have many different forms. In some CT designs, photographic capabilities are built into the control console. These are usually Polaroid-type cameras, which are mounted on the control console. Multiformat imaging devices (such as those produced by International Imaging Electronics), which can produce hard copy images on x-ray film or 35-mm slide film, are also available. These units can be equipped with character generators to insert patient identification information onto the hard copy print.

Technical Considerations

CT can be performed on any portion of the anatomy, and it is rapidly becoming the procedure of choice for the diagnosis of many disorders. There are many reasons for its popularity; the major advantages of performing CT examinations may be summarized as follows:

1. Precise demonstration of abnormalities, with minimal error
2. Ease of performance
3. Elimination of patient discomfort
4. Noninvasive procedure
5. Reduction in hospitalization cost
6. May be performed on an outpatient basis

The head region has been extensively studied with CT. The position and angulation of the patient are relatively standard. Positioning for scans in this area requires that the patient's head be adjusted so that Reid's baseline is perpendicular to the patient couch. The scan is then performed in relation to this plane. It can be done parallel to the infraorbital meatal line (Reid's baseline) or at an angle to the baseline. The determining factor for the scan angulation is the specific anatomy to be demonstrated. The specific protocol for the scan is given by the physician performing the procedure. The usual angulation for the head region is summarized in Table 7–1. CT is used to image anatomic structures throughout the body for both diagnostic and interventional purposes. Areas imaged include the chest, abdomen, mediastinum, kidneys, gastrointestinal tract, hepatobiliary system, and retroperitoneum. Scans can be taken in both a precontrast and a postcontrast stage. Some practitioners believe that all patients should have scans performed without the use of contrast media, and if the need arises, a second scan using contrast enhancement can then be performed.

Table 7–1. SUMMARY OF POSITIONING ANGULATION FOR CT HEAD SCANS

Structures Demonstrated	Angulation
Orbits; anterior portion of temporal lobe; sella turcica	Parallel to Reid's baseline, 0° angulation
Supratentorial cranial contents	20 to 30° angulation with Reid's baseline

Patient Preparation

Patient preparation for CT varies with the type of study. If the computed tomography study involves the administration of a contrast agent, the guidelines are similar to those of most contrast examinations.

For most head studies, the patient is instructed to consume no food and water for 2 to 4 h before the examination. CT of the body, including the abdomen and gastrointestinal system, requires food and water to be withheld from the patient from midnight before the examination. No special preparation is required for CT studies of the chest or extremities.

The procedure should be explained to the patient before the study begins. If iodinated contrast agents are to be used, a baseline of vital signs should be taken, and the patient should be questioned for a history of allergies and/or previous contrast reactions. If the patient is extremely agitated or nervous, a sedative may be prescribed; this should be administered by the special procedure nurse or the physician responsible for the procedure. If contrast agents are to be used or the procedure involves an interventional technique, the patient is usually required to complete a consent form.

Postprocedural care depends on the type of study and medication, if any, received by the patient. If a sedative is administered, the patient should have someone drive him or her home. Iodinated contrast agent studies require that the patient increase fluid intake for 24 to 36 h after the procedure. The patient should be monitored for 20 to 30 min after the procedure, especially if contrast agents are administered. If studies do not require the administration of a contrast agent, the patient will not need special care before discharge.

ULTRAFAST COMPUTED TOMOGRAPHY

One disadvantage of the current generation of CT systems has been the inability to perform real-time motion studies, three-dimensional volume imaging, and blood flow analysis. Scan times have to be dramatically reduced in conventional CT to make most studies feasible. Dynamic CT has been made possible by the C-100 Ultrafast CT system, a system manufactured by Imatron, Inc. This system design effectively reduces the scan time to between 50 and 100 ms, allowing scan rates of 17 scans/s without decrease in spatial and contrast resolution. The original application of Ultrafast CT (UFCT) was in cardiac imaging, but this modality can also be used for motion studies in other areas as well as all conventional CT applications.[8] CT arthrography is one example of an orthopedic application. In this type of study, many images can be taken in a short period of time, and they can be averaged to improve contrast resolution. The system can also be used for high throughput examination of areas in which involuntary or voluntary motion is not a problem. Scans can be performed rapidly and provide excellent artifact-free images in the head or body.

Physical Principles

The component parts of the Ultrafast CT System are similar to those of a standard CT system. The control and computer groups are similar in design to those of conventional CT and do not require a detailed discussion. The imaging group, however, is considerably different. The UFCT imaging system is made possible by the innovative design of the x-ray tube. In conventional CT units, the x-ray tube is a functional part of the gantry. In a matter of speaking, the UFCT unit actually is the x-ray tube. It consists of an electron gun that accelerates an electron beam along the length of the

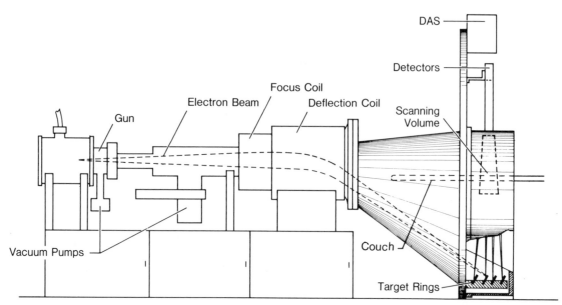

Figure 7–11. Schematic of a cine CT system, showing the components of the imaging group. (From Imatron, Inc.)

CT scanner (Fig. 7–11). The electron beam is focused with a magnetic lens and deflected toward the target rings. There are four target rings housed at the lower portion of the conical section of the gantry; these are fixed tungsten rings, and they envelop 210° of the gantry. The electron beam is magnetically rotated along the 330-cm target area at a speed of 66 m/s. The focal spot, less than 4 × 2 mm, sweeps around each target ring. These are usually scanned serially to provide rapid multislice volume studies.

The unique design of the x-ray tube allows the heat generated by the production of x-rays to be dissipated quickly into the target structure. Because of the mass of the cone that supports the target rings, x-ray production can be increased to provide the high-output, short-term exposures necessary for UFCT. When the electron beam strikes the target ring, an x-ray fan beam is produced. This is collimated to a 2-cm-thick fan-shaped beam, which is then used to produce the imaging information through attenuation. The remnant radiation strikes the detectors, which are arranged in two 216° arcs around the upper portion of the gantry. These are arranged as two contiguous rings to provide a pair of 8-mm-thick tomographic slices for each single scan.

The detector arrays are two stationary rings of crystals that convert the remnant radiation to a light signal. Ring 1 contains 864 detectors, and ring 2 contains 432 detectors. These crystals convert the x-rays to light and are linked to photodiodes, which convert the light signal into an electrical current that is proportional to the incident quantity of radiation. The electrical current is fed through an amplification system and directed to the computer group, which digitizes the signal in much the same way as in conventional CT systems.

The UFCT system is designed to operate in three different modes of operation—continuous, triggered, and volume—that can be used individually or together during a particular study. In the continuous mode, there can be as many as 17 dual-slice scans/s. These can be presented in a cine display to demonstrate cardiac function, any moving organ, or a bolus of contrast medium as it appears in real time. In the triggered mode, scans are initiated by a time signal, typically derived from electrocardiographic input. The rate of filming is less than in the continuous mode but provides a diagnostic flow study with much better temporal resolution than conventional or gated CT (Fig. 7–12). This type of scan can demonstrate selected phases of the heart cycle by producing a dynamic sequence of images at a particular cardiac phase. Blood flow analysis can be performed using the information produced during this operational mode. Volume mode

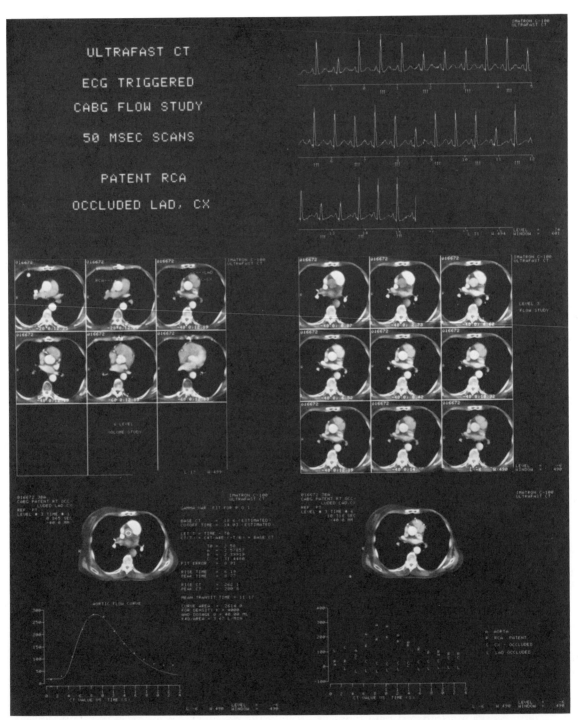

Figure 7–12. Sample cardiac flow study imaged with the Imatron Ultrafast CT system. (From Imatron, Inc.)

Table 7–2. SUMMARY OF CLINICAL APPLICATION OF THE C-100 ULTRAFAST CT SCANNER

Scanner Mode	Type of Scan Single-slice (100 ms)	Multislice (50 ms)	Scan Features	Examples
Continuous			Function study	Left and right ventricular functions
				Valve motion
		■	17 scans/s	Left and right systolic volumes
			Acquired in rapid sequence	Left and right diastolic volumes
				Ejection fraction
				Wall motion
	■		9 scans/s	Cardiac wall thickening
			Acquired in rapid sequence	Orthopedic joint motion
				Respiratory airway
Triggered	■	■	Flow study	Myocardial perfusion
			Cardiac R wave, timed trigger, or manual trigger	Coronary arteries
				Carotid arteries
				Cardiac output
				Valvular regurgitation
				Arterial grafts, shunts
				Blood flow in liver, kidneys, and brain
				Aortic dissection
				Coronary artery bypass graft patency
Volume			Anatomy	Myocardial infarct sizing
		■	Small volume	Aneurysm
			Eight 8-mm-thick slices cover 8 cm	Myocardial mass
				Pericardial disease
				Head
	■		Large volume	Chest
			Contiguous 3-, 6-, or 10-mm-thick slices with table incrementation	Pulmonary modules
				Spine
				Abdomen
				Neck
				Pediatric studies
				Trauma studies

From Imatron, Inc.

operation involves the production of scans using the multiple target rings. This mode produces scans over a span of as much as 8 cm that provide anatomic information as well as volume computations for specific cardiac chambers. The volume mode can also be used by moving the patient couch in selected increments, up to 17 cm/s, while performing a scan. The use of these three operational modes either individually or in combination provides a wide range of applications for cine CT. Table 7–2 is a summary of some of the basic applications of UFCT available with the C-100 Ultrafast CT scanner from Imatron, Inc.

Room Design

The basic room design considerations are similar to those required for conventional CT. The room should be large enough to house the scanner, control equipment, and computer hardware. The scanning area is divided into an examination and an equipment section. The examination area houses the gantry and patient couch, whereas the remainder of the scanner, high-voltage, couch control, and deflection systems are located in the equipment area.

The computer equipment should be placed in an environmentally controlled room, as in conventional CT. The room size and specifications are determined by the type of hardware to be housed (Fig. 7–13).

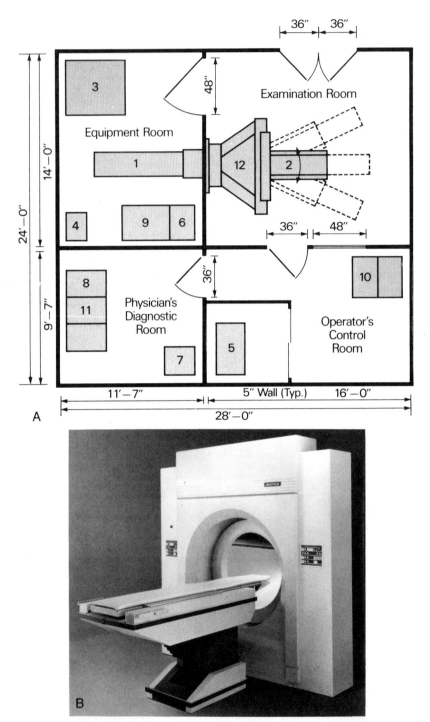

Figure 7–13. *(A)* Typical room layout (schematic) for an Imatron cine CT system; *(B)* Ultrafast CT system. (From Imatron, Inc.)

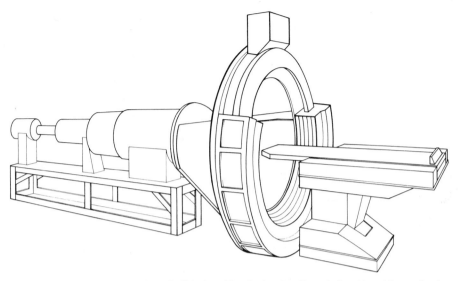

Figure 7–14. Schematic of the Imatron C-100 cine CT unit, showing the relationship of the patient couch to the imaging system. (From Imatron, Inc.)

Equipment

The UFCT system contains the same basic components as conventional CT. The imaging components' unique design has already been discussed. The gantry is similar in design to that of a conventional CT unit. The patient couch can support a weight of 136 kg (300 lb) and is designed to provide a wide range of positioning flexibility (Fig. 7–14). The couch can be moved in longitudinal (forward and backward), vertical (up and down), and horizontal swivel (side to side) planes, up to 25° in each direction. The couch can also be tilted at angles of up to 25° from the horizontal. A bicycle ergometer can be attached to the couch to stress the patient during a study to reveal abnormalities. The patient couch can be controlled from the table side as well as from the operator's console in the control room.

The computer component digitizes and stores the data from the detectors. It has a short-term memory capability that retains as many as 80 slices in the multislice mode of operation or up to 2 s of continuous scan data before transfer to a long-term storage system. The image storage system contains a laser camera that can provide images on 14 × 17-in film in a wide range of formats. A magnetic tape storage or optical disc capability is also integrated into the system for long-term data storage.

The scanner console is designed to permit display of the images produced by the UFCT scanner. It has an alpha-numeric keyboard for functional and operational control of the scanner and computer system. The system consists of the high-resolution display monitor, an alpha-numeric monitor, a trackball, window and level control knobs, and function keys for data processing.

Technical Considerations

UFCT can be used to image all areas of the body, and it is especially useful for imaging areas in which involuntary motion is present. The primary region of interest involves cardiac scanning, where it has capabilities for demonstrating flow studies as well as volume measurements (Fig. 7–15). One advantage of the UFCT system is that contrast agent studies can be performed using a bolus injection or drip infusion of the

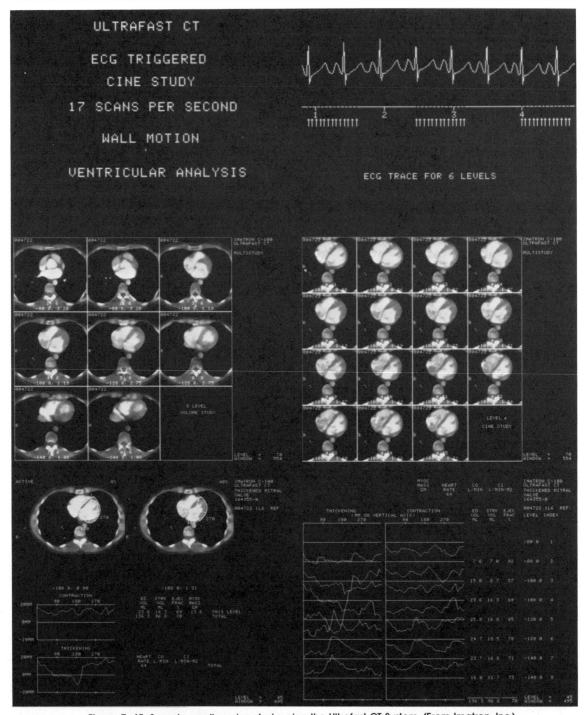

Figure 7–15. Sample cardiac cine study using the Ultrafast CT System. (From Imatron, Inc.)

radiopaque material. The following is a summary of the image display and range of image analysis of UFCT:

1. Real-time movie display
   a) Fixed level
   b) Fixed time
2. Measurement of blood flow and tissue perfusion with time–density graphs
   a) Heart
   b) Other organs

3. Quantitative measurement
   a) Motion of heart
   b) Thickening of heart wall
4. Quantitative volume measurements of any region of interest
5. Image enhancement
   a) Subtraction
   b) Averaging
6. Functional imaging
   a) Static
   b) Dynamic
7. Image reformation
   a) Movies
   b) Flow studies
   c) Oblique views
   d) Sagittal views
   e) Coronal views
   f) Parasagittal views
8. Region of interest
   a) Ellipse
   b) Rectangle
   c) Irregular
   d) Mean CT number
   e) Standard deviation
   f) Area
   g) Base value
9. Zoom function
10. Pan function
11. Identify
12. Save screen
13. Print screen

SUMMARY

CT uses the basic fundamentals of radiography to produce the diagnostic image. When performing these procedures, it is necessary to adhere to radiation safety practices identical to those for any radiographic examination to provide maximum protection for the patient and staff. Knowledge and proficiency come from observation and practical experience; the protocol for performing CT differs by institution. In addition, the radiographer must have a working knowledge of cross-sectional anatomy to position the patient properly and critique the images for diagnostic quality.

REFERENCES

1. Radon, J.: On the determination of functions from their integrals along certain manifolds, Berichte Sachische Akadamie der Wissenschafter, Liepzig Mathematische—Physische Klasse, 67:262, 1917.
2. Hounsfield, G. N.: Computerized transverse axial scanning (tomography). Part 1. Description of the system, Br. J. Radiol., 46:1016, 1973.
3. Oldendorf, W. H.: Isolated flying spot detection of radiodensity discontinuities—displaying the internal structure of a complex object, I.E.E.E. Trans. Biomed. Electron., 8:68, 1961.
4. Cormack, A. M.: Representation of function by its line integrals with some radiological applications, J. Appl. Phys., 234:2722, 1963.
5. Seeram, E.: Computed Tomography Technology. Philadelphia, W. B. Saunders, 1982, Chap. 2.

6. Brooks, R. A., and Di Chiro, G.: Theory of image reconstruction in computed tomography, Radiology, *117*:561, 1975.
7. National Fire Code: A Compilation of N.F.P.A. Codes, Standards, Recommended Practices and Manuals. Boston, The National Fire Prevention Association, 1978.
8. Brody, A. S.: Ultrafast CT scanning: Advantages and new developments, Clin. Update, *2*:3–4, 1989.

SUGGESTED READINGS

Arrington, J. A., Murtaugh, F. R., Martinex, C. R., and Schnitzlein, H. N.: CT of multiple intracranial cryptococcoma, Am. J. Nucl. Reson., *5*:472, 1984.

Berninger, W. H.: Physical aspects of dynamic computed tomography, Adv. Neurol., *30*:55, 1981.

Blumenfeld, M.: C. T.—The future in focus, Australas. Radiol., *25*:181, 1981.

Braunstein, E. M., et al.: Double-contrast arthrotomography of the shoulder, J. Bone Joint Surg. (Am.), *64*:192, 1982.

Breiman, R. S., et al.: Volume determinations using computed tomography, Am. J. Radiol., *138*:329, 1982.

Brooks, R. A., and Di Chiro, G.: Theory of image reconstruction in computed tomography, Radiology, *117*:561, 1975.

Brooks, R. A., and Di Chiro, G.: Principles of computer-assisted tomography (CAT) in radiographic and radioisotopic imaging, Phys. Med. Biol., *21*:689, 1976.

Caputo, G. R., and Higgins, C. B.: Advances in cardiac imaging modalities: Fast computed tomography, magnetic resonance imaging, and positron emission tomography, Invest. Radiol., *25*:838–854, 1990.

Gross, G., and McCullough, E. C.: Exposure values around an x-ray scanning transaxial tomograph, Med. Phys., *2*:282, 1975.

Jose, B., et al.: Computed tomography and radiotherapy in the treatment of cancer, J. Surg. Oncol., *23*:83, 1983.

Kirkpatrick, R. H., et al.: Scanning techniques in computed body tomography, Am. J. Roentgenol. Radium Ther. Nucl. Med., *130*:1069, 1978.

Marshall, C. H.: Principles of computed tomography, Postgrad. Med., *59*:105, 1976.

McCullough, E. C., and Payne, J. T.: X-ray transmission computed tomography, Med. Phys., *4*:85, 1978.

Nahamoo, D., et al.: Design constraints and reconstruction algorithms for transverse-continuous-rotate C. T. scanners, I.E.E.E. Trans. Biomed. Eng., *28*:79, 1981.

Parker, D. L., et al.: Design constraints in computed tomography: A theoretical review, Med. Phys., *9*:531, 1982.

Redington, R. W.: Possible direction in C. T. scanner design, Adv. Neurol., *30*:63, 1981.

Sagel, S. S., et al.: Gated computed tomography of the human heart, Invest. Radiol., *12*:563, 1977.

Seijo, C. A.: A C. T. scanning protocol for a quality assurance program, Radiol. Technol., *52*:497, 1981.

Suchato, C., et al.: A simplified multiformat film holder, Radiology, *143*:270, 1982.

Thiriet, M., et al.: Transverse images of the human thoracic trachea during forced expiration, J. Appl. Physiol., *67*:1032–1040, 1989.

Young, S. W., et al.: Computed tomography: Beam hardening and environmental density artefact, Radiology, *148*:279, 1983.

eight

Magnetic Resonance Imaging

PHYSICAL PRINCIPLES
GRADIENT SYSTEM
Spatial Encoding
Frequency Encoding
Phase Encoding
Three-Dimensional Imaging

ROOM DESIGN
EQUIPMENT
TECHNICAL CONSIDERATIONS
MAGNETIC RESONANCE ANGIOGRAPHY

Magnetic resonance imaging (MRI), formerly called nuclear magnetic resonance (NMR), is not a new concept. The basic principles were proposed in the early 1920s. Investigations continued throughout the 1930s and 1940s, during which the application of the technique was relegated primarily to investigating the principles of physics. In 1950, it was discovered that chemical shifts could be detected. This discovery led to the use of this technique in chemistry and biochemistry. Investigations were made into the properties of biological fluids as well as a variety of chemical compounds. The technique was commercialized in 1953 and marketed as NMR spectroscopy. By the middle of the 1960s, there was widespread application of NMR spectroscopy by the chemical and pharmaceutical industries in analyzing the structure of compounds.

In 1973, it was suggested by P. Lauterbur that the technique could be applied to imaging. However, it was not until 1977 that images of human anatomy were produced; this was accomplished almost simultaneously by W. S. Hinshaw, P. A. Bottomley, and G. N. Holland[1] and R. Damadian, M. Goldsmith, and L. Minkoff.[2]

By 1981, MRI began clinical trials as an imaging modality. Various advances in equipment and techniques have made the modality a viable diagnostic tool that not only yields anatomic information but also distinguishes between healthy and diseased tissue. Unlike computed tomography (CT), MRI can provide information about the functional and physiological conditions as well as the anatomic structure of the body's tissue without the use of x-irradiation. This chapter presents an overview of the basic theory behind MRI, the state-of-the-art hardware, and the potentials for its use in medical diagnosis.

PHYSICAL PRINCIPLES

It is important to first understand that MRI does not involve the use of radioisotopes or x-radiation to secure diagnostic information. The theory of MRI is based on the magnetic properties of certain atomic nuclei. The nucleus of an atom is composed of two types of particles—protons and neutrons. Atomic nuclei that contain either an even or an odd number of protons and an even number of neutrons or those with an even number of protons and an odd number of neutrons can be analyzed with MRI. It is well known that the atomic nucleus spins on its axis, similar to the planet earth. The nucleons (protons and neutrons) each possess a *spin*, or angular momentum. In atomic nuclei in which protons and neutrons are evenly paired, the individual spins tend to cancel each other out to produce a net spin of zero. In nuclei in which an unpaired proton or neutron exists, a net spin is produced, and because there is an associated net electrical charge, a magnetic field is generated that acts like a bar magnet with a north and a south magnetic pole, or a magnetic dipole.

A result of this phenomenon is that the nucleus will also act like a small magnet, and it can interact with magnetic fields. Some examples of elements with nuclei exhibiting these properties are ^{1}H, ^{31}P, ^{23}Na, and ^{43}Ca. If we looked at a sample of these small "nuclear magnets," we would see that they are equally oriented in a number of random directions, resulting in a total magnetization of zero. When an external magnetic field is applied around the sample of "magnetic nuclei," they would be expected to line up in the direction of this external magnetic field to produce some sort of net magnetization. In the case of the proton, there are only two possible states—the spin-up state, which parallels the external magnetic field (longitudinal component, z axis), and the spin-down state, which is antiparallel (parallel but in the opposite direction) to the external field. Each nuclear magnet can assume either state, and when an external static magnetic field is applied, some of the nuclear magnets line up in opposition to the externally applied magnetic field. Because it takes more energy to line up antiparallel with the external magnetic field, these nuclear magnets are considered to be at a higher energy level than those lined up parallel to the external field (Fig. 8–1). In general, the nuclei prefer to be in the lower energy level state parallel with the external magnetic field, and there are usually more nuclear magnets in this spin state.

When these nuclei are oriented either with or opposed to an external magnetic field, they can be made to undergo a transition from one energy level to another. This transition is actually a change in the orientation of the net magnetization vector (Mv), that is, the vector can be tipped from its longitudinal (parallel) orientation with the external magnetic field to another plane. To do this, the nuclei must either absorb a definite amount (quantum) of energy to move to a higher energy level or release a definite amount (quantum) of energy to return to a lower energy level. This *transition* energy is supplied by a pulse of radiofrequency (RF) energy from the low end of the magnetic spectrum. Figure 8–2 shows the electromagnetic spectrum and location of the

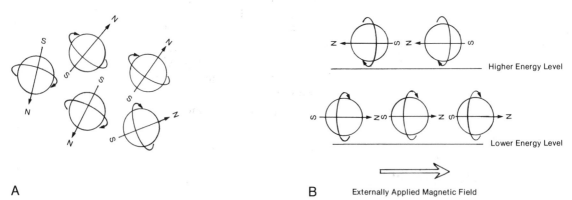

Figure 8–1. *(A)* Schematic of a sample of nucleons with net spins, showing the random orientation of the dipoles; *(B)* schematic of the same sample of nucleons placed in a magnetic field. Some of the nuclei line up in opposition to the direction of the external magnetic field; these represent nucleons with a higher energy level.

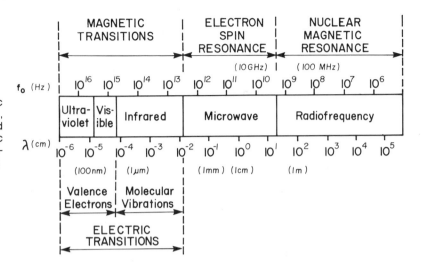

Figure 8–2. Electromagnetic spectrum. (From Partain, C. L., James A. E., Jr., Rollo, F. D., and Price, R. R.: Nuclear Magnetic Resonance (NMR) Imaging. Philadelphia, W. B. Saunders, 1983.)

transition RF energies used to change the energy levels of the nucleons. The RF pulse must have a specific frequency to accomplish transition. This frequency is dependent on the strength of the external magnetic field. For a 1.0-tesla (T) field, the RF should be 42.6 MHz. The gauss and the tesla are commonly used units that denote magnetic field strength. 1 T is equal to 10,000 gauss (G). A 1.5-T external magnetic field would require an RF of 63.9 MHz. This represents the amount of energy required to produce a transition, or it can be considered the difference between the spin-up (parallel) and spin-down (antiparallel) states. The RF pulse can tip the MV by an amount determined by its amplitude and duration. The transition from one energy state to another is called *resonance*.

The resonance caused by the RF pulse tips the MV from its longitudinal component. The amount of tipping caused by the RF pulse is described in degrees; if the vector were tipped halfway between the spin-up and spin-down states, the RF applied would be referred to as a 90° RF pulse. This has the effect of converting the longitudinal component (z axis) into a transverse component (xy axis). If the vector were already in the transverse component when the 90° RF pulse was applied, it would return to the longitudinal component.

This is an oversimplified explanation of the magnetic properties of the magnetic nucleus. When the external magnetic field is applied to the nuclei, their dipoles (north and south poles) do not line up exactly with it (Fig. 8–3). This causes a torque, which

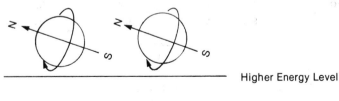

Higher Energy Level

Figure 8–3. When an external magnetic field is applied, the magnetic dipoles of the nucleons are not exactly lined up in the same direction.

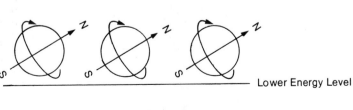

Lower Energy Level

Externally Applied Magnetic Field

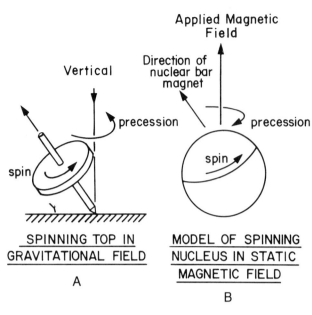

Figure 8–4. *(A)* A spinning top is precessing around the vertical field of gravity; *(B)* a spinning nucleus with the direction of its magnetization: its precession around the direction of the applied magnetic field is shown. (From Partain, C. L., James, A. E., Jr., Rollo, F. D., and Price, R. R.: Nuclear Magnetic Resonance (NMR) Imaging. Philadelphia, W. B. Saunders, 1983.)

creates a motion similar to that produced on the axis of a spinning top when it begins to slow down. The spinning top rotates and wobbles about the former vertical axis in a motion similar to that of a cone (Fig. 8–4). This motion is called *precession*. When the nuclei in a sample are exposed to an external magnetic field, their magnetic moments precess together in the direction of their spin state. The result can be visualized as two cones placed tip to tip (Fig. 8–5).

In the above example of magnetic nuclei in an externally applied magnetic field, the rate of frequency of the precession is proportional to the strength of the externally applied magnetic field and is related to the type of atomic nucleus. Hydrogen protons, for example, will have a natural resonance frequency of approximately 4.3 MHz in an externally applied magnetic field of 1000 G (0.1 T). The precessional frequency given above for the hydrogen proton is also known as the Larmor frequency.

Thus, when an external magnetic field is applied to a group of nuclei, there are two resultant energy states—spin up, following the direction of the field, and spin down, opposing the direction of the field. The overall magnetic effect of these energy states is usually a weak net magnetic moment in the direction of the externally applied magnetic field. The direction of this net Mv is usually considered to be the axis. This axis tends to be aligned parallel with the magnetic field and can be considered the longitudinal component (z axis). Figure 8–6 is a schematic representation of a group of nuclei precessing to create a net magnetic moment, or Mv.

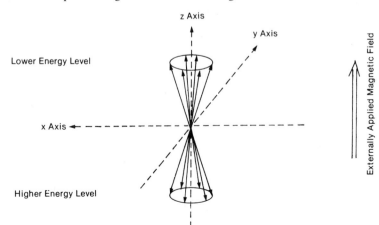

Figure 8–5. Schematic of the configuration of a sample of nuclei precessing in both spin states.

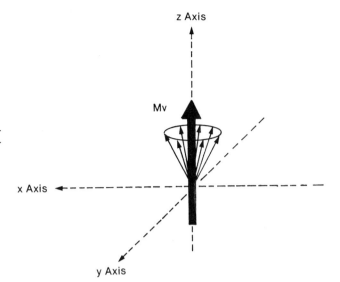

Figure 8–6. Schematic of the individual precessions of the nuclei and their net magnetic moment (Mv).

The net magnetic moment created by the magnetic nuclei can be precessed when a resonant magnetic field is applied to the transverse plane (*xy* axis) (Fig. 8–7). The amount of precession varies with the strength (amplitude) of the resonant magnetic field as well as with its duration. The resonant magnetic field is actually electromagnetic energy that has the same frequency as the precession of the nuclei. This frequency is in the RF band of the electromagnetic spectrum and is commonly known as the RF field. When this resonant (RF) magnetic field is applied, the nuclei actually absorb some energy, which puts them into a higher-level spin state. This has the effect of changing their relation with the originally applied external magnetic field, forcing them to approach the antiparallel spin state. When the resonant RF magnetic field is removed, the nuclei lose energy and ultimately return to their original spin state. The surplus energy is radiated from each nucleus, which allows it to return to the lower-level spin state; this process is called *relaxation*. This loss of energy can be detected and the sample can be analyzed, depending on the energy loss process. In general, the same unit used to produce the resonant RF magnetic field can act as the detector of the energy loss because the resonant RF field is usually applied as a pulse. These pulses affect the angle at which the magnetic nuclei are shifted. RF pulses are usually classified as 90° or 180° pulses; the change in angle depends on the length and amplitude of the pulse.

When the pulse is terminated, the precessional motion of the net Mv decays and a transient signal can be monitored; this is called the free induction or free induction decay (FID) signal. This signal decays to zero with a characteristic time constant.

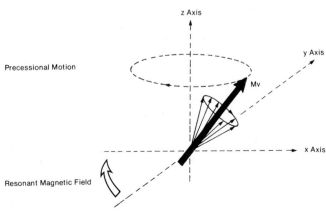

Figure 8–7. Schematic of the result of applying a resonant magnetic field in the transverse (xy) plane. The net magnetic moment of the nucleons will precess.

Immediately after the RF pulse, the magnitude of the FID signal can indicate the number of protons that are affected, thus yielding information about the proton density. This represents quantitative information about the overall concentration of specific nuclei in a sample of a certain type of tissue or about the numbers of specific nuclei in a sample of different types of tissue. In general, the greater the proton density, the stronger the MRI signal and the greater the image intensity. This does not have much effect in imaging most tissues because there is not much difference between proton density. In brain imaging, however, there is enough proton density difference between gray and white matter to provide a contrast between these tissues during imaging.

The return of the net Mv to its position before the application of the RF pulse can show the composition of a particular sample. It can be characterized by two related time constants, or *processes*, called the spin-lattice relaxation process (T_1) and the spin-spin relaxation process (T_2).

The spin-lattice relaxation process (T_1) follows the time constant required for the net Mv to return to the original state, parallel to the external magnetic field. The time required depends on the nuclei giving off the extra energy quantum to their surroundings, which is usually called the lattice.

Spin-spin relaxation (T_2) occurs while the individual nuclei are oriented in the *xy* plane. These nuclei are precessing in phase with each other throughout the duration of the RF pulse. When the RF pulse is terminated, the surrounding magnetic nuclei exert an influence on the precessing nuclei and cause them to be out of phase, or to "dephase." After a period of time, this influence tends to cancel out the net Mv in the transverse (*xy*) plane. The time required for this to occur is the spin-spin relaxation time (T_2).

The two time constants T_1 and T_2 derived from the MRI signal can provide qualitative information concerning tissue conditions; this can help to determine whether the tissue or anatomic area of interest is healthy or diseased. The RF pulses that are applied to shift the magnetic nuclei can be varied to increase the contrast between different tissue areas. The variations (sequences) are saturation-recovery, inversion-recovery, spin-echo, gradient-echo, and steady-state free precession.

The saturation-recovery sequence is accomplished by sending the RF pulses with a constant time spacing between each pulse. This time constant must be longer than the spin-spin relaxation time (T_2) and approximately the same length as the spin-lattice relaxation time (T_1). In this sequence, the received signal decays to zero between each successive pulse. By making several images with different constant time spacings, T_1 values can be obtained for each image pixel. In effect, a map of T_1 values is generated. This type of sequence can demonstrate differences between adjacent areas of soft tissues.

The inversion-recovery sequence is accomplished by applying a 180° pulse that inverts the net Mv. The 180° RF pulse is followed by a short delay, which again approximates the spin-lattice relaxation time (T_1). A 90° RF pulse is then applied to provide a decay signal. This 90° RF pulse can be referred to as a "read pulse." This sequence also generates a T_1 map when the delay period is varied across the tissue sample. Inversion-recovery sequences can produce a better contrast in the tissue sample, but the imaging time is longer than in the saturation-recovery sequence.

The spin-echo sequence involves the application of a 90° RF pulse, which produces a signal in the detector coil. After a certain period, which approximates the spin-spin relaxation time (T_2), a 180° RF pulse is applied. This in effect brings the individual precessions through the 90° plane, creating what appears to be a double-sided FID signal. It can be seen that the time delay after the 180° RF pulse should be twice that of the 90° time delay (Fig. 8–8 A). The "echo" signal produced will be reduced in size because any distortions produced in the 90° RF pulse decay by molecular interactions, which are nonreversible, will be eliminated. If subsequent 180° RF pulses are applied

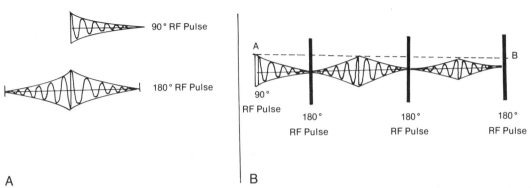

Figure 8–8. *(A)* Decay signals derived from 90° and 180° RF pulses; *(B)* schematic of a spin-echo sequence showing the subsequent reduction in the size of the echo caused by nonreversible changes from molecular interactions. The dotted line AB represents the true spin-spin relaxation time (T_2).

at twice the 90° RF pulse delay ($2T_2$), the echo signals are progressively reduced in size. A true spin-spin relaxation time can be derived by following the signal peaks in the sequence. The spin-echo sequence is usually used to measure the spin-spin relaxation times (T_2) free from imperfections.

Gradient-echo sequences are similar to spin-echo sequences except that the 180° pulse that induces the formation of the spin-echo is absent and the repetition time is kept short, which has the effect of increasing the MR signal strength. These sequences try to maintain the transverse magnetization in a steady state. The gradient-echo sequence features RF pulses that provide tip angles of less than 90°. It has been demonstrated that reduced RF tip angles can affect the image intensity and contrast. In general, the intensity of liquids (structures with larger T_2-to-T_1 ratios) is enhanced with this type of sequence.

There are several advantages to using the gradient-echo sequence—there is less heat build-up in the patient, which results in a more comfortable study, and the imaging times are faster. Two-dimensional slices can be produced in seconds rather than minutes, whereas three-dimensional imaging can be accomplished in minutes rather than hours. This decreased imaging time reduces the need for the patient to hold his or her breath for exceptionally long intervals during imaging. The shorter times result in the elimination of motion artifacts usually caused by breathing. A technique called "gradient moment nulling" makes it possible to reduce or eliminate the artifacts produced by both vascular and cerebrospinal fluid effects.

There are many proprietary varieties of the gradient-echo sequence (rapid imaging technique), and they are known by various acronyms (e.g., GRASS, FISP, FLASH, and CE-FAST). The acronyms stem from the names that the manufacturers give the technique.

Steady-state free precession provides a signal that does not decay before the next RF pulse is applied. This type of sequence can improve the signal-to-noise (SNR) ratio of the signal. Steady-state free precession sequences can produce signals of greater intensity because contributions are made from both spin-spin (T_2) and spin-lattice (T_1) relaxation times. When using this sequence, high-quality images can be produced, but the individual contributions of spin-spin (T_2) and spin-lattice (T_1) relaxations cannot be determined.

GRADIENT SYSTEM

Spatial Encoding

This is the process by which the MR signals are assigned to distinct volume elements (voxels) in the image. Gradient coils are used to produce a linear increase in the magnetic field along one spatial axis. There is a gradient coil for each of the three spatial axes. During the procedure, one of the gradient coils is activated so that the RF pulse flips the Mv from the structures in a particular slice. This gradient coil is sometimes referred to as the "slice select" gradient. The strength of the gradient system determines the minimum field of view, slice thickness, and echo time. The z gradient is used for spatial encoding along this axis and is responsible for the linear gradation of the main magnetic field.

Two processes are used to encode (identify) the MR signals of the shapes and positions of structures located within the selected slice—frequency encoding and phase encoding. Each of these processes involves the application of gradients while the MR signals are measured.

Frequency Encoding

The frequency encoding gradient, also called the read or read-out gradient, makes the Larmor frequency vary along one direction in a plane. This gradient is usually applied along the x axis and is responsible for the left-to-right gradation and spatial encoding in this plane. Structures at different locations in the plane contribute signals that oscillate at different rates. The variations in the frequency denote the position of the structures along the read axis. The frequency encoding gradient is applied while the MR signal is received.

Phase Encoding

The phase encoding gradient (y gradient) measures the anterior-to-posterior direction in the plane. It uses a third gradient coil that provides a phase change in the signals collected. The phase encoding gradient is applied for a short period of time and then terminated before collection of the data. The phase encoding sequence is repeated many times and is increased in amplitude after each successive MR signal. The number of different pulse sequences required is dependent on the spatial resolution desired and can vary from 128 to 256 phase encoding sequences.

The signals collected from these processes are subjected to computer processing to produce the completed image.

Three-Dimensional Imaging

Three-dimensional imaging is facilitated through manipulation of the gradient system during imaging. When this technique is used, data are collected from the entire imaging volume. The use of one of the varieties of the "fast imaging," gradient-echo sequences listed above is within practical limits. Three-dimensional imaging provides a greater SNR than two-dimensional techniques. Three-dimensional imaging also provides images in all three planes—axial, coronal, and sagittal—from a single set of data. The data can be reformatted by the computer to rearrange the digital information to provide multiplanar imaging.

ROOM DESIGN

MRI systems depend on the use of magnetic fields, which necessitates specific requirements for room designs. The major constraints are that the magnetic field created by the static magnetic source can be affected by the wide variety of ferromagnetic materials present in the surrounding areas and there is the possibility of interference with other mechanical and electrical devices in the facility. The type of magnet used determines the necessary architectural modifications required.

There are basically three types of magnets used in the manufacture of MRI equipment—the permanent magnet, the electromagnet, and the iron core electromagnet (hybrid). Permanent magnets are constructed from permanent magnetic materials enclosed in a massive steel frame. Electromagnets are either resistive or superconductive. These create a magnetic field by circulating electric currents through wire coils. The hybrid magnet is actually a combination of the permanent magnet and the electromagnet. It has a solenoid around a ferromagnetic substance. Each type of magnet has its own specific requirements and limitations.

Permanent magnets do not require the use of an electrical current to create the magnetic field. These can be compared with the small toy magnets used to hold items onto a metallic surface. Once magnetized, they require no special care. When these are used in MRI, they are usually encased in a special steel frame, which guides the lines of magnetic force and contains the magnetic field. This type of system is advantageous because the magnetic field is contained, so there is essentially no "fringe" magnetic field that requires extensive shielding to protect either the static magnetic field uniformity or the mechanical or electrical equipment located in the surrounding environment. The major disadvantage to the use of permanent magnets is their weight. A typical permanent magnet installation with steel frame can weigh more than 100 tons. This would not be a problem in a new installation in which the design could be adjusted to accommodate the weight. In an existing situation, however, construction expenses could be greater than those for a resistive or superconductive type magnet. Permanent magnets also have the disadvantage of having a limited field strength.

Resistive magnets use aluminum or copper wire coils to provide the static magnetic field. These types of units operate at ambient temperature. During the operation of the resistive magnet system, a great deal of heat is generated, which must be removed. In most cases, this is accomplished by circulating cold water through the coils. This type of magnet is no longer used for MRI units and is considered obsolete.

Superconductive magnets use specialized wire coils made from materials that lose their electrical resistivity when they are exposed to very low temperatures. The type II superconductors are usually alloys, such as niobium-titanium. Because this type of system requires operating temperatures of almost absolute zero, an elaborate cooling and insulating system must be provided; this system is called a *cryostat*. It cools the magnet and maintains it at the proper temperature for extended periods. The system uses both liquid nitrogen and liquid helium to provide the cold operating temperatures required. The superconductive system is considerably more complex than either of the other types of magnets discussed. It requires a high capital and operating investment to control and monitor the devices for the use of liquid helium and nitrogen.

One major disadvantage to the use of the superconductive system is the large area of "fringe" magnetic field. This fringe field can cause mechanical and electrical disturbances within a diameter range of 20 to 60 ft. Any ferromagnetic material or object within 20 ft of the units could become magnetized and disturb the homogeneity of the static magnetic field. The system has to be placed in an environment shielded from such materials. The manufacturers of superconductive equipment have architectural specifications designed to eliminate this hazard (Fig. 8–9). Care should be taken when working around this type of magnet system to remove any ferromagnetic object from the patient or staff; these objects could act as projectiles and create a dangerous "missile effect." Another disadvantage to the use of superconductive magnet systems is the possibility of the helium boiling off, causing the magnet to lose its superconductive capability. This problem is called *quenching*, and it can cause the unit to become inoperative for the length of time it takes to recool and readjust the system.

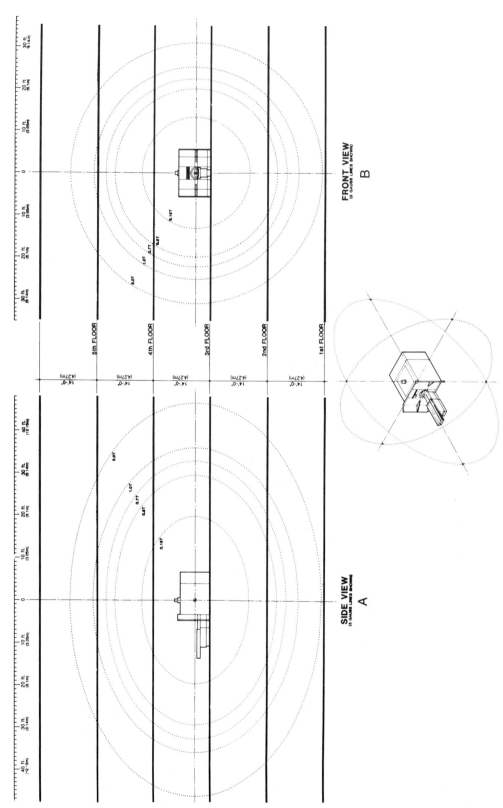

Figure 8–9. MRI system magnetic "fringe" field shown from above *(A)* and as an elevation drawing *(B)*. The fringe field extends in a three-dimensional fashion around the magnet system and is found with the resistive and superconducting types of magnet systems. (From Picker International.)

Room size varies according to the type of magnet system used and the manufacturer's specifications. The scanning-control room can be from 650 to 900 ft² in area. The computer room should be separate from the scanning area, and its location is determined by the type of magnet system used. The rooms should be climate controlled to provide optimal operating conditions for the equipment as well as a comfortable atmosphere for the patient and staff. There should be an adequate amount of room for a patient dressing room as well as a waiting room. If resistive or superconductive magnets are used, these areas must be away from the fringe magnetic field. When using these types of magnets, a metal detecting device should be installed to prevent anyone with a ferromagnetic object from entering the fringe field.

The MRI scanning room must also be shielded from RF interference. This is accomplished by using nonferrous modular panels that are constructed by laminating aluminum or copper sheets onto a suitable base, such as particle board. These panels are then applied to the interior surfaces of the room and joined together with clamping devices that effectively shield the joint spaces between the panels. Special shielded door designs are also available that provide total RF shielding. RF interference testing should be carried out after the rough shielding is in place and the interior of the room has been surfaced and finished.

Specific recommendations for room design and site planning are made by the equipment manufacturer. The type of magnet used determines the amount and variety of architectural modifications that are necessary.

EQUIPMENT

There are several equipment groups common to all types of manufactured MRI systems—the magnet, RF synthesizer, gradient coil system, shimming coil system, and computer and control-display group.

The magnet system group has already been discussed. Use of the different types of magnets necessitates a variety of design specifications for the gantry and patient couch elements (Fig. 8–10). The differences in the patient opening are a result of the magnet system used. When using permanent magnets, the magnetic field lines will pass vertically through the patient's body.

To perform MRI, a RF synthesizer must be included in the design. This system provides the RF pulses necessary to change the direction of the net Mv. The coil that produces the RF signal can also be used to detect the echo from the magnetic nuclei. The RF pulse is produced by a RF generator located some distance away from the imaging system. There are two basic designs for the RF coil—the solenoidal type and the saddle type. The solenoidal coil (Fig. 8–11) is essentially a circular loop of wire placed inside the gantry system, through which the patient passes. It is used primarily with the permanent magnet system. The saddle type of coil (Fig. 8–12) can have a single transmitter-receiver coil design or use two individual saddle coils—one separate transmitter coil and one receiver coil. These are also designed into the gantry system.

Surface coils are smaller RF coils that transmit and/or receive signals from smaller body parts. These coils must be manufactured so that they have a high degree of homogeneity in their magnetic fields. The magnetic field produced by the coil must be oriented at right angles to the main magnetic field. In the case of permanent magnets, the main magnetic field is directed vertically. This necessitates a surface coil of the solenoid coil variety that would produce a longitudinal magnetic field (Fig. 8–11). When superconducting magnets are used, the main magnetic field is longitudinal. The surface coil must generate a horizontal field (Fig. 8–12).

There are two basic types of surface coils—those that transmit and receive signals and those that only receive signals. The receive-only surface coil is used more often because greater homogeneity can be achieved with the RF body coil for the transmission of the signal.

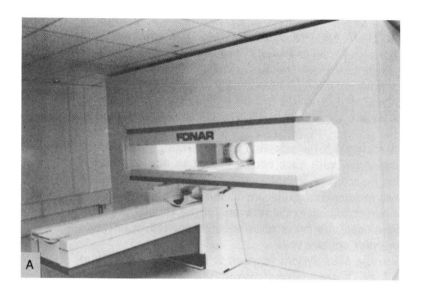

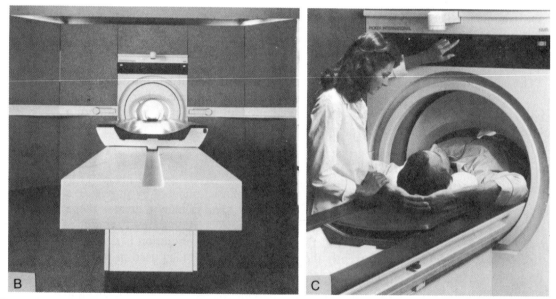

Figure 8–10. (a) Beta 3000 MRI gantry and patient couch. This unit has a 3000-gauss permanent magnet system. (b) and (c) Picker superconductive MRI system gantry and patient couch. (a from Fonar Corporation; b and c from Picker International.)

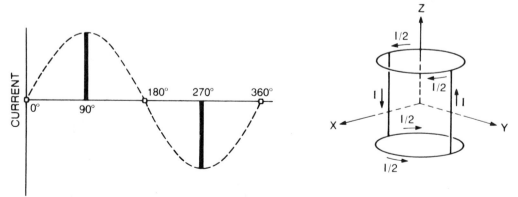

Figure 8–11. Schematic of the solenoid type RF coil and the surface current distribution for this type of coil. (From Partain, C., et al.: Magnetic Resonance Imaging, Vol II. Philadelphia, W. B. Saunders, 1988, p. 1191.)

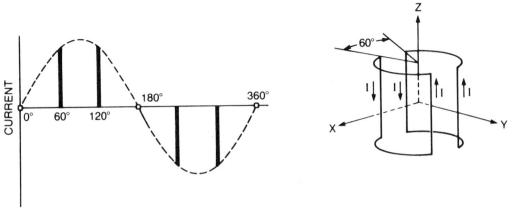

Figure 8–12. Schematic of the saddle-type RF coil and its surface current distribution. (From Partain, C., et al.: Magnetic Resonance Imaging, Vol II. Philadelphia, W. B. Saunders, 1988, p. 1191.)

Because of their smaller size, surface coils detect less noise. It can be said that the smaller the coil, the greater the SNR, which in turn can either decrease scan time or increase the resolution. These coils are usually tuned for specific anatomic locations and are currently used in studies of the spine, orbits, and musculoskeletal system.

Because the surface coils are positioned close to the patient, there is a possibility of RF burns. Stringent safety measures are necessary when these accessories are used. These coils are manufactured by a variety of companies and designed to work with specific magnet configurations. Operating and safety instructions should be carefully followed.

Gradient coil systems are necessary for the selection of the imaging plane. There are usually three sets of gradient coils, each corresponding to one of the axis lines—x, y, and z. The plane can be selected by applying a preselected field gradient over the patient. In this method, only some of the nuclei are stimulated—those perpendicular to the direction of the applied gradient. (The effects of using the gradient coil system have been discussed.)

The shimming system is necessary to provide homogeneity of the magnetic field. Two types of shimming are used—passive and active. Passive shimming is done at the time of the magnet's installation. The technique involves the placement of ferromagnetic materials around the magnet site. Active shimming is accomplished by manipulating an induced current in coils that surround the magnet. In some units, the active shimming is accomplished automatically through the computer system.

The computer units linked to the MRI system function in much the same way as those used in computer technology. These systems convert the analog information provided from the MRI scan to digital information that can be analyzed and manipulated by the computer. The computer system used is based on the type supplied by the manufacturer of the MRI equipment. The computer system will have short-term memory systems, but long-term storage should also be provided, such as the magnetic tape or floppy disc method.

The control-display system varies depending on the types of software packages that are purchased with the imaging system (Fig. 8–13). Some other peripheral equipment that could be added to the imaging system includes a printer and a multiformat imaging camera for hard copy reproduction of the MRI.

TECHNICAL CONSIDERATIONS

The MRI technique has proved its value as a diagnostic modality by providing greater contrast sensitivity than x-ray CT techniques, yielding a greater range of tissue

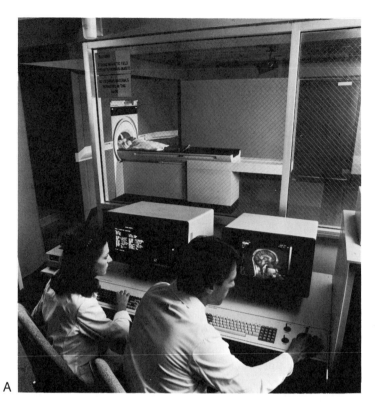

A

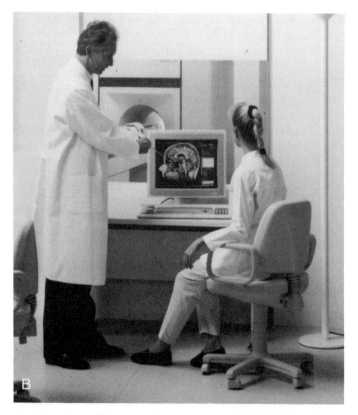

B

Figure 8–13. *(A)* Control-display console of the Picker MRI system. (From Picker International.) *(B)* The control panel and operator display at the Siemens Magnetom SP System. (From Siemens Corporation.)

discrimination. The information gained from the relaxation times T_1 and T_2 is representative of the local interactions of the nuclei. Its tissue resolution is similar to that of x-ray CT (Fig. 8–14). Currently, MRI is being used in the area of proton imaging because hydrogen nuclei are the easiest to image as they are relatively abundant in tissue and they give a measurable MRI signal.

One significant advantage to the use of MRI is that bone can be virtually eliminated from the image. When bone is imaged, it is actually the bone marrow that is being detected. This can be important when imaging areas of the spinal cord and brain, which are surrounded by bone. It has also been demonstrated that there is a difference in the relaxation times of the protons of cancerous and noncancerous tissue. Current research studies are attempting to incorporate MRI into the investigation of the chemistry and function of various tissues. Phillips Medical Systems has coupled MR spectroscopic analysis with imaging. This permits biomedical and physiological analyses as well as diagnostic imaging in a single noninvasive procedure. The technique is used in vivo ^{31}P and ^1H analysis. The results can be displayed on the operator console or printed on an optional hard copy plotter (Fig. 8–15). By the use of this method, many pathological processes can be accurately identified and monitored without using invasive procedures.

MAGNETIC RESONANCE ANGIOGRAPHY

A new technique is being applied to the imaging of intracranial and extracranial vasculature—magnetic resonance angiography (MRA). It is made possible by a software option available from Siemens Corporation. This technique provides high-resolution, three-dimensional studies of blood vessels without the invasive introduction of a contrast agent. MRA is a screening procedure for the diagnosis of intracranial aneurysms and atherosclerosis of the carotid arteries. The technique has also been used for femoral and popliteal studies. When the images are viewed in the cine mode display, the illusion of a three-dimensional image is presented, which allows for a more accurate diagnosis of the vessels in question. Figure 8–16 A and B illustrates some images acquired with this technique.

SUMMARY

MRI is a noninvasive modality that can be used to image the anatomy of the body without the use of x-radiation. The basic principle behind MRI is the use of a magnetic field and radiowaves coupled with a sophisticated computer system to produce the images. State-of-the-art MRI systems also provide the means for biomedical and physiological spectroscopic analyses during the imaging session.

Three different magnet configurations can be used to produce the main magnetic field—permanent, superconductive, and hybrid magnets. Each has advantages and disadvantages relating to its design. All MRI systems have certain equipment groups in addition to the magnet—the RF coil system, gradient coil system, shimming coil system, and computer system. Current magnets vary in strength depending on the manufacturer as well as the design. Magnet strengths currently available range from 0.4 to 1.5 T (1 T = 10,000 G).

MRI is still in the growth stage. New techniques and equipment are being developed at a rapid rate, and existing techniques are being improved. The ultimate potential of MRI in imaging is still unknown, as are the potentials of its use as a diagnostic tool. The theory presented here is a simplified explanation of the basic technical principles underlying MRI.

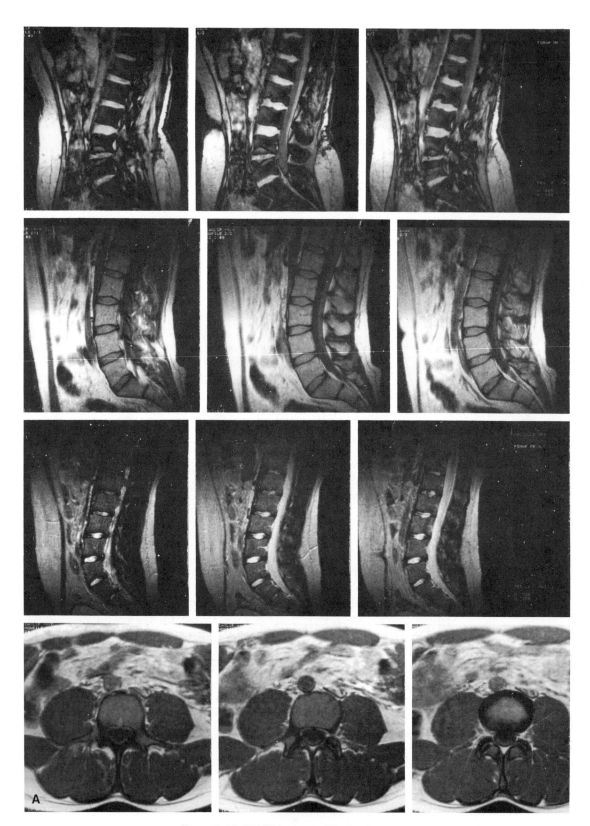

Figure 8–14. *(A)* MRI images of the lumbar spine.

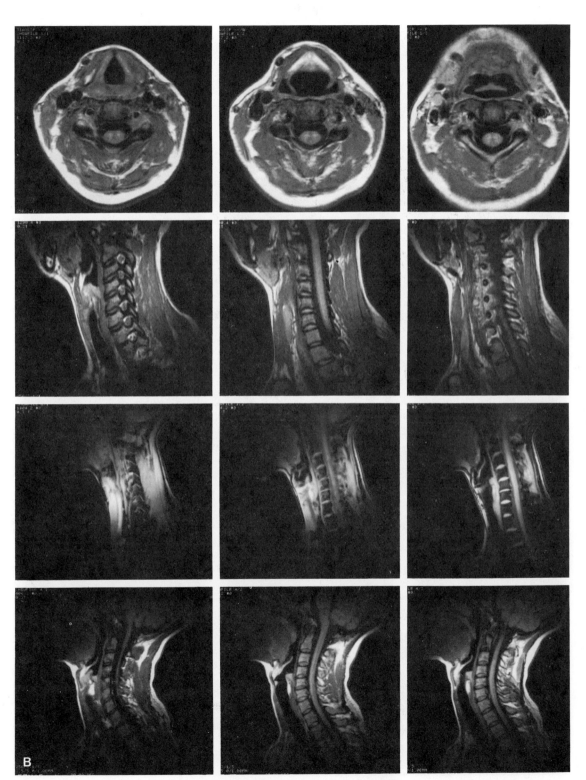

Figure 8–14 *Continued (B)* Cervical spine.

Illustration continued on following page

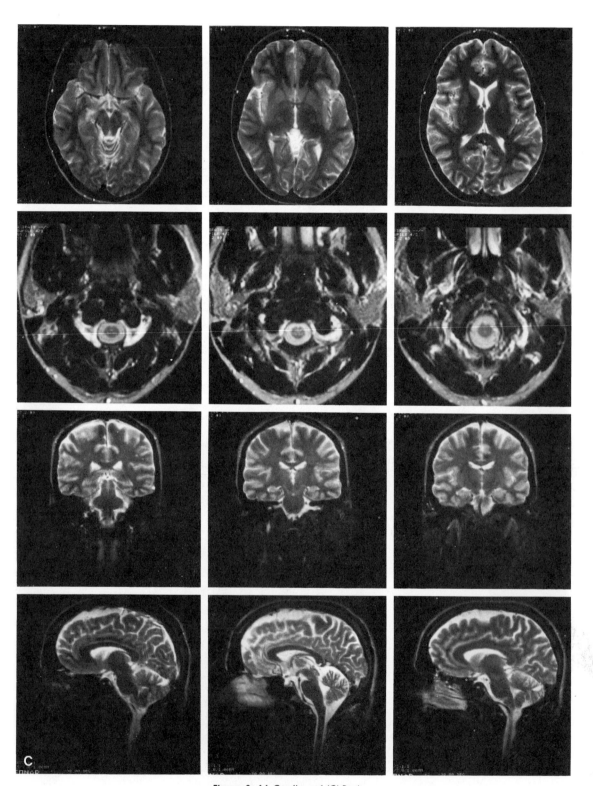

Figure 8–14 *Continued (C)* Brain.

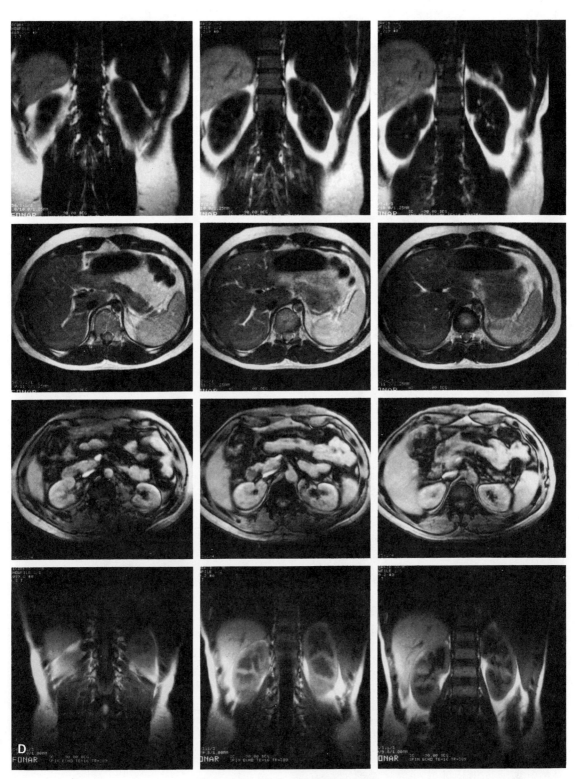

Figure 8–14 *Continued (D)* Abdomen.

Illustration continued on following page

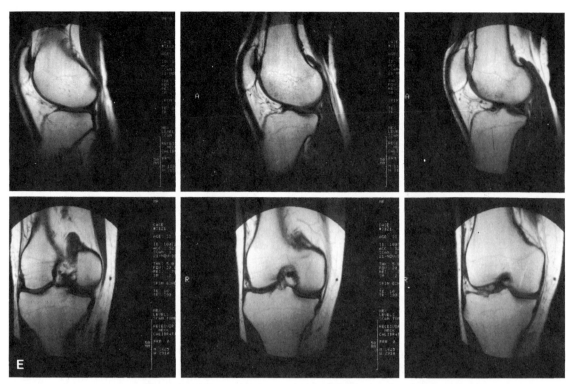

Figure 8–14 *Continued (E)* Knee. (From Fonar Corporation.)

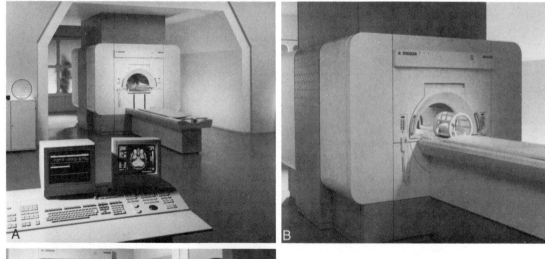

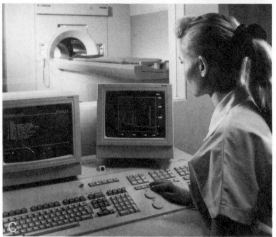

Figure 8–15. *(A)* Phillips Medical System's Gyroscan S15/ACS MRI/spectroscopy system showing operator console, gantry, and patient couch; *(B)* close-up of Gyroscan S15/ACS gantry and patient couch. Note the surface coil placed at the head of the patient couch. *(C)* Close-up of operator console showing sample spectral analysis. (From Phillips Medical Systems.)

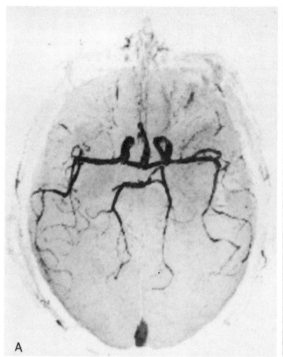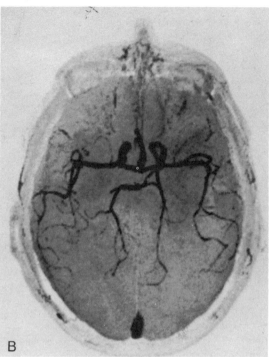

Figure 8–16. *(A)* and *(B)* Illustrations of images produced with the use of the MRA technique and software developed by Siemens Corporation. Images courtesy of Paul Ruggieri, M.D., University Hospitals of Cleveland: one of 64 partitions, 13 min, three-dimensional MRA technique. (From Siemens Corporation.)

REFERENCES

1. Hinshaw, W. S., Bottomley, P. A., and Holland, G. N.: Radiographic thin section image of the human wrist by nuclear magnetic resonance, Nature, *270*:722–723, 1977.

2. Damadian, R., Goldsmith, M., and Minkoff, L.: NMR and cancer FONAR image of the live human body, Physiol. Chem. Phys., *9*:97–100, 1977.

SUGGESTED READINGS

Abraham, A.: The Principles of Nuclear Magnetism. London, Oxford University Press, 1961.

Bangert, V., Mansfield, P., and Coupland, R. E.: Whole body tomographic imaging by NMR, Br. J. Radiol., *54*:152, 1981.

Brownell, G. L., Budinger, T. F., Lauterbur, P. C., et al.: Positron tomography and nuclear magnetic resonance imaging, Science, *215*:619, 1982.

Cooke, P., and Morris, P. G.: The effects of NMR exposure on living organisms: II. A genetic study of human lymphocytes, Br. J. Radiol., *54*:622, 1981.

Crooks, L., Arakawa, M., Hoenninger, J., et al.: Nuclear magnetic resonance whole body imager operating at 3.5K-Gauss, Radiology, *143*:169, 1982.

Crooks, L., Hoenninger, J., Arakawa, M., et al.: Tomography of hydrogen with nuclear magnetic resonance, Radiology, *136*:701, 1980.

Czervionke, L. F., Daniels, D. L., Wehrli, F. W., et al.: Magnetic susceptibility artifacts in gradient recalled echo MR imaging, Am. J. Roentgenol., *9*:1149, 1988.

Edelstein, W. A., Hutchinson, J. M. S., Johnson, G., et al.: Spin warp NMR imaging and applications to whole body imaging, Phys. Med. Biol., *25*:751, 1980.

Farrar, T. C., and Becker, E. D.: Introduction to Pulse and Fourier Transform NMR. London, Academic Press, 1971.

Fung, B. M., and Puon, P. S.: Nuclear magnetic resonance transverse relaxation in muscle water, J. Biophys., *33*:27, 1981.

Haase, A., Frahm, J., Matthaei, D., Hanicke, W., and Merbolt, K. D.: FLASH imaging: Rapid NMR imaging using low flip angle pulses, J. Magn. Reson., *67*:258, 1986.

Jack, C., Berquist, T., Miller, G. M., Forbes, G. S., Gray, J., Morin, R., and Ilstrup, D. M.: Field strength in neuro MR imaging: A comparison of 0.5 T and 1.5 T, J. Comput. Assist. Tomogr., *14*:505–513, 1990.

Kaufman, L., Crooks, L. E., and Margulis, A. R., eds.: NMR Imaging in Medicine. New York, Igaku Shoin, 1981.

Oppelt, A., Graumann, R., Barfuss, H., Fischer,

H., Hartl, W., and Schajor, W.: FISP—a new fast MRI sequence, Electromedica, *54*:15, 1986.

Pykett, I. L.: NMR imaging in medicine, Sci. Am., *256*:78, 1982.

Pykett, I. L., Newhouse, J. H., Buonanno, F. S., et al.: Principles of NMR imaging, Radiology, *143*:157, 1982.

Pykett, I. L., and Rzedzian, R. R.: Instant images of the body by magnetic resonance, Magn. Reson. Med., *5*:563, 1987.

Schmalbrock, P., Yuan, C., Chakeres, D. W.,

Kohli, J., and Pelc, N. J.: Volume MR angiography: Methods to achieve very short echo times, Radiology, *175*:861–865, 1990.

Teitelbaum, G., Yee, C., Van Horn, D., Kim, H., and Colletti, P.: Metallic ballistic fragments: MR imaging safety and artifacts, Radiology, *175*:855–859, 1990.

Wehrli, F. W.: An NMR primer: Part II. Principles of magnetic resonance imaging, NMR Images, *13*:10, 1983.

3

Angiography

nine

Principles of Angiography

HISTORICAL PERSPECTIVE
GENERAL PRINCIPLES
PREEXAMINATION HISTORY, CONSULTATION, AND INFORMED CONSENT
PREANGIOGRAPHIC PHARMACOLOGICAL AGENTS
Sedatives
    Phenobarbital (Nembutal)
    Hydroxyzine Hydrochloride (Vistaril)
    Promethazine Hydrochloride (Phenergan)
    Diphenhydramine (Benadryl)
Analgesics
    Morphine Sulfate
    Meperidine (Demerol)
    Fentanyl (Sublimaze)

Other Pharmacological Agents
    Diazepam (Valium)
    Naloxone (Narcan)
    Atropine
EQUIPMENT PREPARATION
PATIENT INSTRUCTION AND PREPROCEDURAL CARE
ESTABLISHMENT OF VESSEL ACCESS
Arterial Puncture Techniques
Venous Puncture Techniques
Direct Exposure of Artery or Vein
CONTRAST INJECTION AND FILMING
POSTPROCEDURAL CARE AND INSTRUCTIONS
Patient Discharge
Risks of Catheterization

Angiography is defined as "the x-ray visualization of the internal anatomy of the heart and blood vessels after the intravascular introduction of radiopaque contrast medium."[1] The contrast medium is introduced by an intravenous or intra-arterial injection or through a catheter that is inserted into a peripheral vessel and guided to the desired target area.

Before the discovery of x-rays, the injection of materials into the vessels of the body was performed primarily on cadavers. The procedure was limited to the injection of various vital dyes that stained the tissues of the body and facilitated the study of human anatomy after dissection. This practice was continued after Roentgen's famous discovery and extended to the introduction of radiopaque materials that permitted physicians and anatomists to record the anatomy with x-rays. The use of this technique was not successfully applied to live subjects until about 1920, when a contrast agent was developed that could be safely introduced into the vascular system.

Improvements in radiographic and ancillary equipment and the development of safer contrast agents fostered research in angiographic procedures. Angiography became a safe, reliable diagnostic technique. The angiographic catheterization procedure provided a springboard for the use of angiography for therapeutic purposes.

HISTORICAL PERSPECTIVE

"Angiography" is a general term for the radiographic examination of the blood vessels. These studies are used to image pathological and physiological changes in visceral, cerebral, peripheral, and cardiac anatomy by injecting a contrast agent into specific portions of the vascular system.

In 1844, Claude Bernard performed catheterization of both the right and left ventricles of the heart of a horse. This first step enabled investigators to develop innovative techniques that were ultimately used in human subjects. Angiography had its beginnings in the late 1800s when investigators injected radiopaque materials into the vessels of corpses to outline the anatomy. These early contrast agents were highly toxic and could not be used in living subjects.

During 1918 through 1919, Walter Dandy, a neurosurgeon at The Johns Hopkins University, developed a procedure that used air to image the ventricular system of the brain of living humans. The technique was called "pneumoencephalography." This development created an interest in the exploration of other substances that could be used to image anatomic structures not easily visualized with conventional radiography.

In early 1920, sodium iodide, a radiopaque substance, was found to be safe for use in living subjects. Egas Moniz and J. P. Caldas began performing cerebral angiography. They used sodium iodide as the contrast agent and the "radiocarousel" to image the vascular system of the brain. The radiocarousel, which was invented by Caldas, could image at the rate of one image per second for a maximum of 6 s.[1] Simultaneously, B. Brooks was investigating the use of sodium iodide in imaging the femoral arteries. This marked the beginning of the era of angiography.

Werner Forssmann searched for a method of delivering medication directly to the location of need and is credited with performing the first human cardiac catheterization. In 1929, at the age of 25, he passed a 65-cm catheter through his left antecubital vein into his right atrium. He documented this achievement with a chest x-ray demonstrating the placement of the catheter. His research was used as a foundation by many investigators for the study of cardiovascular physiology.

Various changes were made in contrast agents, equipment, and methods between these first attempts at angiography and the early 1970s. During the 1940s, rapid sequence cassette changers were further developed, and image intensifiers, generators, and x-ray tubes were beginning to be developed. In the 1950s and 1960s, automatic injection devices were used to deliver the bolus of contrast agent to the desired location. Rapid sequence imaging devices were improved, and the Schonander cut film changer was introduced.

Catheters were being investigated for the introduction of the contrast agents directly to a desired location. H. A. Zimmerman reported a successful cardiac catheterization in a human.[2] The method of choice in the early years of angiography for the introduction of the catheter was by direct approach. This involved making an incision, exposing the vessel of interest, and placing the catheter directly in its lumen.

In 1953, S. I. Seldinger described a method for the introduction of the catheter through the percutaneous replacement of the needle.[3] This technique improved the safety of angiographic studies and simplified the procedure. In 1959, J. Ross Jr. and C. Cope described the transseptal catheterization procedure.[4, 5] Cope was also perfecting a method for selective coronary arteriography, and he experimented with a variety of catheter shapes to achieve this goal.

Serial magnification techniques and subtraction were introduced during this period, and the use of computer systems in connection with radiographic equipment was beginning to be investigated.

Through the 1980s, refinements in digital techniques advanced the basic subtraction principles and launched digital subtraction angiography as the modality most often used for cardiac catheterization. The development of computed tomography and magnetic resonance as imaging tools further reduced the use of angiography as the primary tool for diagnosis. Interventional procedures were perfected during this period, and angiography shifted from a purely diagnostic tool to an adjunct to the nonsurgical intervention in many disease processes.

GENERAL PRINCIPLES

All angiographic studies are performed following the same general procedure:

1. Preexamination history, consultation, and informed consent
2. Equipment preparation
3. Patient instruction and preprocedural care
4. Establishment of vessel access
5. Contrast injection and filming and interventional treatment, if scheduled
6. Postprocedural care and instructions
7. Patient discharge

In this chapter, we consider the basic principles common to all angiographic procedures. There may be some variations during the clinical performance of the examinations owing to differing hospital and departmental protocols; however, every angiographic examination should include all of the elements listed above.

PREEXAMINATION HISTORY, CONSULTATION, AND INFORMED CONSENT

During the consultation with the physician, the indications, aims, nature, and risks of the study are discussed with the patient. This information is essential to obtaining a binding informed consent document from the patient. The patient must be aware of the intent of the consent document. The consent form is usually cosigned by witnesses to indicate that the proper procedures were followed in obtaining the patient's assent to the procedure. The consent form may be negotiated on the day of the procedure, although this depends on individual hospital protocol. At this time, the physician will obtain a history, and pertinent information will be noted on the patient's chart, such as the status of the patient's renal function, bleeding tendency, and whether there have been previous reactions to contrast agents.

The physician also indicates preprocedural instructions for the patient. These vary somewhat depending on institution and procedure protocol; however, they usually include fasting a minimum of 6 to 8 h before the procedure or restriction to clear liquids only. If the patient is taking medication, the physician determines if the patient should continue on the day of the procedure. Angiography is performed on an inpatient basis or on an outpatient basis through ambulatory surgery. If the patient has been admitted to the hospital, there will probably be orders for intravenous hydration, and the patient will arrive in the department with the intravenous line in place. Premedication is usually administered in the angiography suite after the patient's peripheral pulses and vital signs are taken.

It is important to record accurate notes concerning the patient's condition and treatment before, during, and after the study. Any reactions or difficulties must also be charted. The hospital's risk management protocol should be followed for every special procedure performed. Each member of the angiographic team should know his or her responsibilities concerning the care of the patient as well as the type and amount of records charting required for the study.

PREANGIOGRAPHIC PHARMACOLOGICAL AGENTS

Two classes of pharmacological agents are used to medicate patients before angiography—sedatives and analgesics. Some of the agents span both classes and produce effects that are considered both sedative and analgesic. In addition, certain agents have a concomitant effect when used in conjunction with other pharmacological agents.

Sedatives

Sedatives are administered to decrease the activity of the central nervous system (CNS). Excessive stimulation of the CNS can cause an individual to become more alert, anxious, and irritable. In the extreme, excessive stimulation can even cause convulsions. Sedatives reduce the desire for physical activity and have a calming or tranquilizing effect on the patient. The net effect is that the patient experiences a reduction in anxiety level relating to the procedure. Some frequently used sedatives are diphenhydramine, promethazine hydrochloride, hydroxyzine hydrochloride, and phenobarbital.

PHENOBARBITAL (NEMBUTAL)

This agent is classified as a barbiturate and a nonspecific CNS depressant. Barbiturates produce what is considered to be dose-dependent depression of the CNS. The action of this agent is short in duration (4 to 6 h). An intramuscular dose of 150 to 200 mg can produce a "hypnotic" effect. The average intramuscular dose for angiography premedication ranges from 75 to 100 mg. Phenobarbital is contraindicated in patients with hepatic disease, emphysema, other breathing disorders, or porphyria.

HYDROXYZINE HYDROCHLORIDE (VISTARIL)

Hydroxyzine is indicated for the relief of the anxiety, tension, and psychomotor agitation experienced by the patient before a diagnostic or interventional angiographic procedure. It also controls the nausea and vomiting that can be attendant with the administration of the contrast agent. The only contraindication is previous sensitivity to the agent. It should be noted that hydroxyzine has a concomitant effect when used in conjunction with other CNS depressants. The usual dose is 25 to 100 mg administered intramuscularly.

PROMETHAZINE HYDROCHLORIDE (PHENERGAN)

This drug belongs to the family of drugs generically called the phenothiazines and functions primarily as an antihistaminic agent. It also has an antiemetic, anticholinergic (drying) effect. One of the major side effects of this drug is its ability to produce sedation. The duration of its action is short (4 to 6 h). It is usually contraindicated when large amounts of other types of CNS depressants have been administered; it can be given in combination with other CNS depressants, but concomitant effects usually occur. Promethazine can intensify the action of the other drugs, and dosages should be adjusted to counter its influence. The usual dose ranges from 25 to 50 mg administered orally or intramuscularly.

DIPHENHYDRAMINE (BENADRYL)

This drug is also primarily an antihistaminic agent. Diphenhydramine's sedative side effect makes it useful as premedication for angiographic procedures. It exhibits a marked anticholinergic effect that may be undesirable. Its usual dose ranges from 25 to 50 mg administered intramuscularly or orally.

Analgesics

Analgesics are agents administered to reduce pain and are classified as narcotics (strong) and nonnarcotics (mild).

Narcotic analgesics are either derived from opium or synthetically produced to create the same pharmacological effect. These agents can relieve pain without producing a loss of consciousness and can cause a physical dependence. Morphine, codeine, and hydromorphone (Dilaudid) are some naturally occurring opioids. Meperidine (Demerol), fentanyl (Sublimaze), and propoxyphene (Darvon) are representative of synthetic narcotic analgesic agents.

The narcotic analgesics primarily affect the CNS and the gastrointestinal system. They can alter the patient's mental alertness, are usually antitussive, and have the potential to cause physical dependence if used for chronic treatment. The narcotic analgesics usually produce nausea and vomiting as well as a depression of the respiratory system. The effects of the narcotic analgesics can be reversed with naloxone (Narcan). Among the contraindications to the use of this class of analgesics are a hypersensitivity to morphine, severe CNS depression, bronchial asthma, head injury, acute alcoholism, cardiac arrhythmias, biliary obstruction, convulsive disorders, and increased intracranial pressure.

The agents most often used as premedication analgesics are morphine, meperidine, and fentanyl.

MORPHINE SULFATE

This analgesic is a naturally occurring opioid. The amount of agent used in the normal adult ranges from 2 to 20 mg administered intramuscularly. The onset of the analgesic effect usually occurs within 15 to 20 min, and its duration is from 3 to 6 h. The effect on the patient's respiratory and gastrointestinal systems is moderate.

MEPERIDINE (DEMEROL)

This agent is also administered intramuscularly and has a dose range of from 75 to 150 mg. It acts within 10 to 15 min and lasts for 2 to 4 h. Meperidine has a moderate probability of causing respiratory depression and gastrointestinal distress. This agent is usually administered with diazepam (Valium) to offset its negative effects.

FENTANYL (SUBLIMAZE)

Fentanyl is a reasonably fast-acting analgesic, with effects occurring within 5 to 15 min. It is also administered intramuscularly in the dose range of from 0.05 to 0.1 mg. This drug has a high risk of causing respiratory depression, and the patient should be carefully monitored throughout the procedure.

Other Pharmacological Agents

Each institution has its own armamentarium of drugs that are used before, during, and after the procedure. The list may differ from the group of agents discussed in this text; however, the radiographer or cardiovascular and interventional technologist should become familiar with each of the agents and their action, dose, and adverse reactions. If the biliary tree is undergoing study, the patient may also be given antibiotic treatment before the procedure begins. The initial dose is administered as a preventative measure, and treatment is usually continued for 24 h after an uncomplicated procedure.

Several other pharmacological agents can have significant use in the special procedure suite—diazepam (Valium), naloxone (Narcan), and atropine.

DIAZEPAM (VALIUM)

This drug is used to relieve the anxiety the patient experiences before the procedure. Diazepam can reduce the requirement for opioid analgesics and is an adjunct for the relief of painful acute musculoskeletal conditions. It can be administered in conjunction with some of the narcotic analgesics, such as meperidine.

NALOXONE (NARCAN)

Narcan is a narcotic antagonist that prevents or reverses the effects of the opioid narcotic analgesic agents. Its action can be demonstrated within 2 min. Its usual dose range for an adult is from 0.4 to 2 mg administered intravenously.

ATROPINE

This drug can reduce the effect of laryngospasm. Although it has not found a place as a premedication for special procedures, it is a bronchodilator and is sometimes given as a preoperative agent to reduce salivation and excessive secretions in the respiratory tract. Atropine can prevent the cholinergic effects of some of the pharmacological agents, such as cardiac arrhythmias, hypotension, and bradycardia.

EQUIPMENT PREPARATION

The specific equipment, contrast agents, and accessories needed for angiography have been discussed. It is essential for the radiographer to prepare the angiographic suite before the patient arrives for the procedure. The equipment should be checked to ensure that it is functional, and the accessory items necessary to the procedure should be set out. There should be an adequate supply of these items in the angiographic suite to be used as replacements as needed. The radiographer should discuss the procedure with the physician to determine if there is a possibility of intervention. If so, the radiographer should ensure that the items required for the interventional procedure are also available.

PATIENT INSTRUCTION AND PREPROCEDURAL CARE

When the patient arrives in the department, he or she should be properly identified. The radiographer should consult the chart for information pertinent to the procedure. At this time, the order for the study should be confirmed. The procedure should be explained to the patient to establish a rapport and ensure the patient's cooperation during the procedure. The various members of the special procedure team should also be introduced.

If the study is being done through ambulatory surgery, the patient should be instructed to change into a hospital gown and transported to the angiographic suite.

The special procedure nurse will check the patient's peripheral pulses and secure a set of baseline vital signs. If any premedication has been ordered, the nurse will administer it at this time.

ESTABLISHMENT OF VESSEL ACCESS

Angiography is usually accomplished by accessing a vessel, introducing a catheter into its lumen, and manipulating it so that it arrives at the desired location. The arterial approach is used most often.

In the early days of angiography, the vessel had to be surgically exposed to accomplish this task. In 1953, Seldinger developed a technique that has become the basis for modern angiographic catheterization (Fig. 9–1). The technique is applied to both arterial and venous catheterization techniques. The technique is accomplished through the Seldinger procedure as follows:

1. The arterial pulse is identified, and the puncture site is chosen.
2. The site is shaved, surgically prepared, and draped.
3. Local anesthetic is applied to the area, and a nick is made in the skin to facilitate needle access.
4. An 18-gauge Seldinger needle or its variant is inserted into the vessel, the stylet is removed, and pulsatile blood flow is sought.
5. A guide wire is inserted through the lumen of the needle.
6. The needle is withdrawn.
7. The catheter is then threaded over the guide wire and advanced into the lumen of the vessel.
8. The guide wire is removed, and the catheter is advanced in the vessel to the desired location.

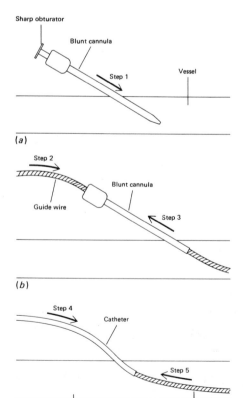

Figure 9–1. Schematics illustrating the Seldinger method of percutaneous puncture. *(a)* The puncture needle has been inserted into the vessel (Step 1); *(b)* the guide wire has been inserted into the vessel through the needle (Step 2); the needle is withdrawn, with the guide wire remaining in the vessel (Step 3); *(c)* a catheter is threaded into the vessel over the guide wire (Step 4); the guide wire is then removed and the catheter is advanced in the vessel (Step 5).

9. During the procedure, the catheter is flushed with heparinized saline, if not contraindicated, to prevent thrombosis.

10. At the conclusion of the study, the catheter is removed, and pressure is maintained at the site until hemostasis is achieved.

In actual practice, the procedure may undergo some minor variation depending on the type of needle used, whether an obstruction is encountered, whether the insertion is being done at the site of a previous graft, or whether vascular dilators or sheaths are needed.

Arterial Puncture Techniques

Several approaches are used for the arterial catheterization procedure—through the common femoral, brachial, or axillary artery. The most frequent approach is through the femoral artery.

The femoral artery can be approached both antegrade and retrograde. The antegrade approach is less desirable in obese patients owing to the difficulty in maneuvering the needle around large abdominal folds. The retrograde puncture method is accomplished approximately 1 cm below the inguinal ligament; the exact location can be determined by manually palpating for the best femoral arterial pulse. The needle is inserted between the index and middle fingers at an angle of 25 to 30° toward the midline (Fig. 9–2). This angle should correspond to the longitudinal axis of the vessel. Once the vessel is cannulated, a catheter can be introduced.

The axillary and brachial approaches are used when both femoral arteries are compromised or in cases of aortic occlusion. These approaches are also reserved for procedures in which access from above is desirable. Brachial and axillary catheterization techniques pose the risks of cerebral embolization, neural injury, spasm, and arterial thrombosis. The risks of complications using these methods are twice that of the femoral approach.[6]

Axillary puncture is accomplished in the lateral axillary fold (Fig. 9–3). The arm can be fully abducted with the hand placed under the head. The needle is inserted into the artery at the point of maximal pulse. As in the other puncture techniques, the needle

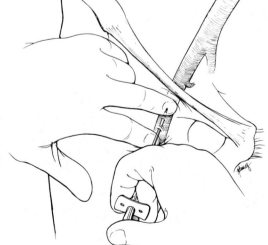

Figure 9–2. Method used for retrograde femoral artery puncture. (From Kadir, S.: Diagnostic Angiography. Philadelphia, W. B. Saunders, 1986, p. 39.)

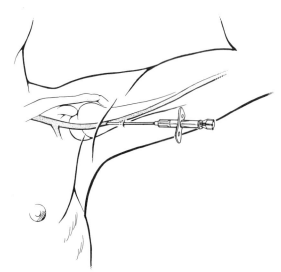

Figure 9–3. Technique used for an axillary arterial puncture. (From Kadir, S.: Diagnostic Angiography. Philadelphia, W. B. Saunders, 1986, p. 40.)

is inserted between the index and the middle fingers. Once cannulation is effected, a guide wire can be introduced. The catheter can then be introduced into the vessel over the guide wire to complete the procedure.

The brachial approach involves the introduction of the needle into the midportion of the humerus (bicipital groove) (Fig. 9–4). The arm is abducted 90°, and the brachial artery is located by palpation. The needle is inserted in the same manner as for the previous approaches. The angle the needle forms with the plane of the arm should be approximately 45°. The brachial artery is a superficial vessel, and the needle does not have to be inserted very deep for cannulation.

Another approach used to place the catheter in cases where there is suspected aneurysm or occlusion of the aorta is the translumbar approach (Fig. 9–5). This procedure can be done at either of two levels—the high approach (lower border of T12) or the low approach (lower border of L2). (A complete discussion of this technique is given in Chapter 10.) This approach is not as desirable owing to its attendant risks. Patient selection is limited to individuals who can maintain a prone position for approximately 2 h.

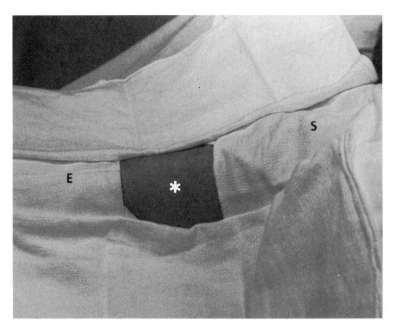

Figure 9–4. Photograph showing the patient prepared with the arm positioned for a brachial artery puncture. E, elbow; S, shoulder; * puncture site. (From Kadir, S.: Diagnostic Angiography. Philadelphia, W. B. Saunders, 1986, p. 40.)

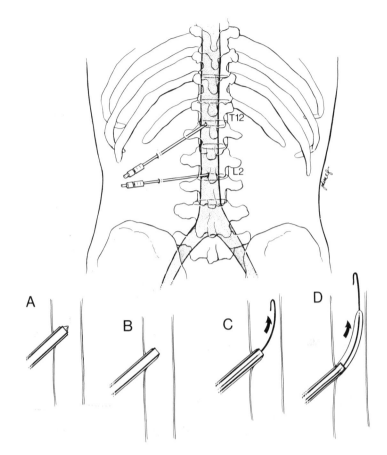

Figure 9–5. Schematic of a translumbar puncture. The patient is placed in the prone position, and the needle is inserted in the left flank. *(A)* The needle and obturator are inserted into the aorta. *(B)* After successful insertion, the obturator is removed. *(C)* A guide wire is then inserted through the needle into the aorta. *(D)* Next, a catheter is threaded over the guide wire into the aorta. (From Kadir, S.: Diagnostic Angiography. Philadelphia, W. B. Saunders, 1986, p. 42.)

If angiography of the venous system is required, the catheter is inserted into the lumen of the vena cava. This catheterization approach is usually through the femoral vein, but the study can be accomplished by using the right jugular vein or the cubital vein of the upper extremity. The Seldinger method is also used to introduce the catheter into the lumen of the vessel.

Venous Puncture Techniques

These techniques are usually used during venous angiographic procedures. Any of the arterial puncture needles can be used for venous access. The usual approach is through the femoral vein; however, the cubital and internal jugular veins can also be used. The basic technique is the same as that for arterial puncture. After the vessel has been transfixed, the needle stylet is removed, and a flexible connector with a syringe is attached to the needle hub. As the needle is withdrawn, suction is applied using the syringe. When blood is seen in the tubing, the sheath is advanced into the vessel. A guide wire can then be inserted into the vessel, and a catheter is threaded into the lumen of the vein in a manner similar to that used in arterial catheterization.

The femoral vein can be found 1 to 2 cm below the inguinal ligament and 0.5 cm medial to the femoral artery. A small skin incision is made over the area. The femoral artery is secured and moved away from the puncture site with the fingers before the needle is inserted.

The cubital vein can be accessed via the antecubital fossa. The cannulation is usually accomplished with an angiocatheter sheath needle; specially designed needles are available for this procedure.

Puncture of the internal jugular vein is usually made on the right side; this provides the best access to the superior vena cava. A small skin incision is made in the area of the sternocleidomastoid muscle. A syringe is attached to an Amplatz needle, and suction is applied throughout the insertion procedure. This allows the physician to know when he or she has achieved successful cannulation of the vessel. A Valsalva maneuver can be used to distend the internal jugular vein for better visibility. When the vessel is cannulated, a catheter introducer sheath is inserted, and catheterization can proceed.

Direct Exposure of Artery or Vein

Sometimes it is desirable to directly expose the artery or vein to introduce the catheter. The technique is basically the same for any vessel. It begins with the isolation of the vessel of interest by palpation. Local anesthetic is introduced initially through a short 25 to 27-gauge needle to raise a superficial intradermal wheal. This is followed by deep introduction into the subcutaneous, deep fascial, and periosteal tissues using a 1 1/2-in 22-gauge needle. When the proposed catheter insertion site is anesthetized, a transverse incision is made in the area of interest. The tissues are separated using a blunt instrument to expose the desired vessel, which is then brought to the surface. The vessel is secured both proximally and distally with silk suture material, umbilical tape, or silicone elastomer tape.

If an artery has been exposed, the incision into it is made with a scalpel blade (cutting edge up); the catheter is then inserted and moved to the desired location. A vein can be incised using small scissors. The catheter is inserted and moved to the location of choice.

At the end of the procedure, the vessels are repaired, and the incision is closed and dressed.

CONTRAST INJECTION AND FILMING

This part of the study is procedure specific and varies by institution and physician. Almost all of the angiographic procedures require the use of an automatic injection device to deliver the contrast agent at the desired flow rate. The image recording or filming will depend on the type of equipment available in the angiographic suite. General angiographic procedures such as renal arteriography, cerebral angiography, and peripheral arteriography are imaged on conventional film using a rapid serial changer. During cardiac catheterization, the procedure is usually imaged digitally and by cinefluorography.

If interventional radiology is to be performed, it is usually accomplished with conventional angiography as a mapping and planning procedure. Interventional techniques may require that the patient return to the department at a later time for a follow-up angiogram. In these cases, the documentation provided at the time of the original study is valuable in ensuring the safety of the patient during subsequent examinations.

POSTPROCEDURAL CARE AND INSTRUCTIONS

When the study has been completed, the catheter is removed. When the catheter has a shaped tip, the guide wire must be reinserted to remove the catheter. Manual pressure is applied to the puncture site until bleeding has stopped. Any abnormal condition of the patient requires that notation be made on the chart and the physician be notified.

The patient is then moved to a designated location and remains on bedrest for a minimum of 4 h. Continuous monitoring of the patient should be carried out during this period of time; this includes recording the pulse on the side of entry four times during the first hour at 15-min regular intervals and twice an hour for the remaining 3 h. Vital signs should be checked at these intervals and recorded on the patient's chart. The puncture site should be observed as part of the monitoring process for possible internal or external bleeding.

The patient should be urged to take fluids by mouth even if intravenous hydration is being applied. If the patient appears to be stable after the prescribed period of bedrest and has someone who can care for him or her for a 24-h period, the patient can be discharged.

Patient Discharge

If the examination was done on an outpatient basis, the patient can be released if stability has been achieved after the 4-h mandatory bedrest period. The patient should be advised to increase and maintain fluid intake, restrict movement for the following 24-h period, and immediately report any difficulties such as fever, pain or bleeding at the site of entry, coldness, numbness, or tingling of the extremities.

Angiography is a relatively safe procedure. The risks attendant with these procedures fall into two major categories—catheterization and contrast-related risks.

Risks of Catheterization

Complications that can occur as a result of the catheterization procedure include bleeding (internal and external), thrombus formation, cholesterol embolization, arterial dissection, and rupture of an aneurysm. The cardiac, renal, or neurological blood flow can be compromised during the procedure, resulting in ischemia, permanent organ damage, or death. Continuous monitoring of the patient's vital signs and pulse can result in an early warning of complications, and any abnormality should be immediately brought to the attention of the physician.

Complications related to the administration of the contrast agents are discussed in Chapter 4.

SUMMARY

Angiography requires the placement of a catheter into a vessel to inject a contrast agent to obtain the necessary information. The most common method of introducing the catheter is the Seldinger method. This is a percutaneous technique that can be accomplished easily and relatively safely.

The importance of obtaining a signed consent form cannot be overstressed. Patient cooperation can be secured by thoroughly educating the patient as to the study process and the procedures to follow both before and after the study. Complications can occur as a result of the catheterization process, catheter manipulation, or contrast agent administration.

REFERENCES

1. Seldinger, S. I.: Catheter replacement of the needle in percutaneous arteriography, Acta Radiol. [Diagn], *39*:368–376, 1953.
2. Zimmerman, H. A., Scott, R. W., and Becker, N. D.: Catheterization of the left side of the heart in man, Circulation *1*:357, 1950.
3. Seldinger, S. I.: Catheter replacement of the needle in percutaneous arteriography: A new technique, Acta Radiol., *39*:368, 1953.
4. Ross, J. Jr.: Transseptal left heart catheterization: A new method of left atrial puncture, Ann. Surg. *149*:395, 1959.
5. Cope, C.: Technique for transseptal catheterization of the left atrium: Preliminary report, J. Thorac. Surg., *37*:482, 1959.
6. Hessel, S. J., and Adams, D. F.: Complications of angiography, Radiology, *138*:273–281, 1981.

SUGGESTED READINGS

Barnhart, E. R.: Physicians Desk Reference, 44th ed. Oradell, NJ, Medical Economics Company, 1990.

Hitner, H., and Nagle, B.: Basic Pharmacology for Health Occupations, 2nd ed. Mission Hills, California, Glencoe/McGraw-Hill, 1980.

McEvoy, G. K., and Pharm. D., eds.: AHFS Drug Information. American Society of Hospital Pharmacists, 1991.

ten

Aortography

ANATOMIC CONSIDERATIONS
INDICATIONS AND
   CONTRAINDICATIONS
CONTRAST MEDIA
PROCEDURE

Translumbar Aortography
Percutaneous Catheter Aortography
EQUIPMENT
PATIENT POSITIONING

Aortography is the radiographic examination used to diagnose vascular pathology of the aorta and lower extremities. There are several methods of aortography, with each differing primarily in the technique of injection. This often necessitates differences in patient positioning. "Aortography," then, is a general term describing radiography of the aorta. However, to be more accurate, it is frequently referred to by the method of injection; the methods of aortography are translumbar aortography, which involves injection of the contrast agent via direct needle puncture of the abdominal aorta, and catheter aortography, which involves catheterization via the femoral (retrograde aortography) or brachial artery (antegrade aortography).

ANATOMIC CONSIDERATIONS

The aorta can be subdivided into three parts—the ascending aorta, aortic arch, and descending aorta.

The ascending aorta originates at the base of the heart with the root of the aorta. The aortic sinuses are found in the wall of the root of the aorta. These are related to the cusps of the aortic valve and are named for them—right, left, and posterior. Two of these sinuses—the right and the left—contain the orifices of the coronary arteries. The ascending aorta extends anterosuperior from the base of the heart and slightly to the right for approximately 5 cm and terminates by becoming the arch of the aorta, which is usually at the level of the sternal angle (Fig. 10–1).

The aortic arch courses from right to left as well as from anterior to posterior. It lies in almost a true sagittal plane (Fig. 10–2).[1] From the sternal angle, the aortic arch ascends toward the left. As it ascends, it is directed posterior. The upper portion of the arch courses posterior to the left of the trachea and esophagus. At about the level of the fourth thoracic vertebra, it turns inferior and runs a short distance before becoming the descending aorta.

There are three major branches given off by the aortic arch—the brachiocephalic trunk, the left common carotid artery, and the left subclavian artery (Fig. 10–1). These branches supply the head and upper extremities with blood.

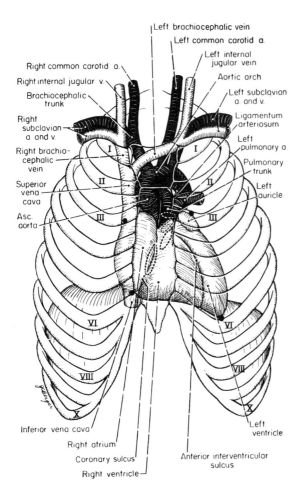

Left brachiocephalic vein
Left common carotid a.
Left internal jugular vein
Aortic arch
Right common carotid a.
Right internal jugular v.
Brachiocephalic trunk
Left subclavian a. and v.
Right subclavian a. and v.
Ligamentum arteriosum
Right brachiocephalic vein
Left pulmonary a.
Superior vena cava
Pulmonary trunk
Left auricle
Asc. aorta
Inferior vena cava
Right atrium
Coronary sulcus
Right ventricle
Left ventricle
Anterior interventricular sulcus

Figure 10–1. Schematic of the heart and great vessels within the bony thorax. Note that the ascending aorta changes to the aortic arch at the level of the sternal angle. (From Woodburne, R. T.: Essentials of Human Anatomy, 4th ed. New York, Oxford University Press, 1969.)

Figure 10–2. Schematic of the aortic arch in the anterior view. From this aspect the aortic arch is almost in a direct sagittal plane. (From Gardner, E., Gray, D. J., and O'Rahilly, R.: Basic Human Anatomy. 4th ed., Philadelphia, W. B. Saunders, 1975.)

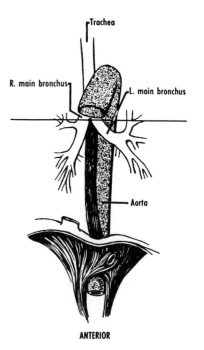

Trachea
R. main bronchus
L. main bronchus
Aorta

ANTERIOR

The descending aorta extends from its origin at the level of the intervertebral disk between the fourth and fifth thoracic vertebrae to about the fourth lumbar vertebra. It can be subdivided into a thoracic portion and an abdominal portion.

The branches of the descending aorta can be classified as either parietal or visceral and may be summarized as follows:

Thoracic aorta
  Parietal branches
    Posterior intercostal arteries
    Subcostal arteries
    Superior phrenic arteries
    Vas aberrans artery
  Visceral branches
    Bronchial arteries
    Esophageal arteries
    Pericardial artery
    Mediastinal artery
Abdominal aorta
  Parietal branches
    Inferior phrenic arteries
    Lumbar arteries
    Common iliac arteries
    Median sacral artery
  Visceral branches
    Middle suprarenal arteries
    Renal arteries
    Gonadal arteries
    Celiac trunk
    Superior mesenteric artery
    Inferior mesenteric artery

The parietal branches supply the body wall of the thoracic cavity, whereas the visceral branches supply the organs contained within the thoracic cavity. The thoracic portion of the aorta runs from the origin of the descending aorta to the aortic hiatus in the diaphragm (Fig. 10–3), which is about the level of the 12th thoracic vertebra. As the thoracic aorta passes through the opening in the diaphragm, it becomes the abdominal portion of the descending aorta.

The abdominal aorta courses toward the midline anterior to the vertebral column. At the level of the fourth lumbar vertebra, the abdominal aorta bifurcates into the right and left common iliac arteries (Fig. 10–4). The bifurcation can be topographically located slightly inferior and to the left of the navel. This point is considered the termination of the aorta. The common iliac arteries are the major arteries of the pelvis. Each common iliac artery divides into an internal and an external iliac artery. The external iliac arteries then form the femoral arteries of the lower extremities.

During aortography, it is not uncommon for some of the branches to visualize. Frequently, the circulatory supply of the kidneys will be well demonstrated.

INDICATIONS AND CONTRAINDICATIONS

Aortography is indicated when information concerning the aorta and its major branches becomes necessary for diagnostic or therapeutic purposes. It offers the surgeon a means by which an accurate preoperative evaluation concerning the nature, number, and course of the great vessels of the chest and abdomen can be made.

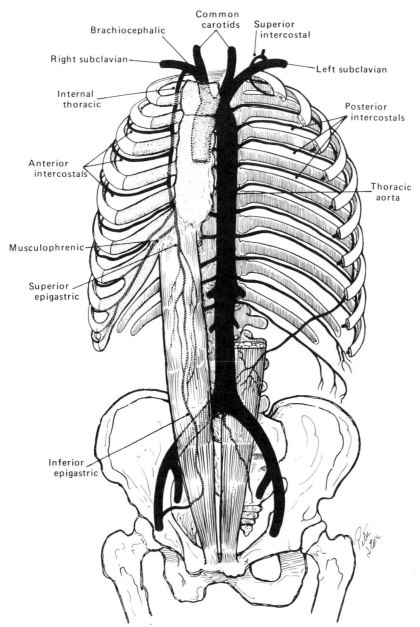

Figure 10–3. Schematic of the route of the descending aorta in the body. (From Langley, L. L., Telford, I. R., and Christensen, J. B.: Dynamic Anatomy and Physiology, 4th ed. New York, McGraw-Hill, 1974. © Copyright Mosby-Year Book, Inc.)

Some specific indications for the procedure include suspected aneurysms, congenital anomalies, and many acquired diseases affecting the thoracic or abdominal aorta. The following is a summary of the specific indications for aortography:

Congenital anomalies
    Abnormal position of specific vessels
    Abnormal number of specific vessels
    Patent ductus arteriosus
    Coarctation and pseudocoarctation of the aorta
    Aortic pulmonary window
    Aortic arch anomalies

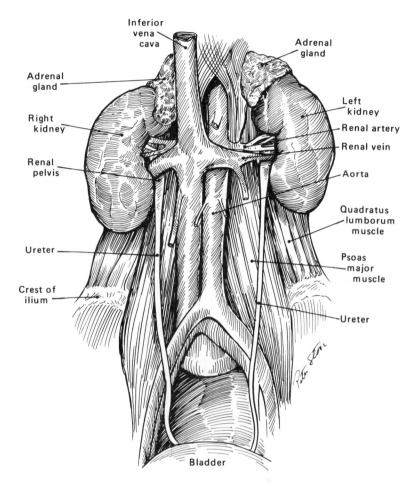

Figure 10–4. Schematic showing the location of the abdominal portion of the descending aorta and its bifurcation and their relationships with the inferior vena cava and abdominal viscera. (From Langley, L. L., Telford, I. R., and Christensen, J. B.: Dynamic Anatomy and Physiology, 4th ed. New York, McGraw-Hill, 1974. © Copyright Mosby-Year Book, Inc.)

Pulmonary sequestration
Truncus arteriosus
Aortic diverticula
Ruptured aortic sinus aneurysm
Aortic stenosis
Acquired diseases
Preoperative mapping of aneurysms of the aorta and brachiocephalic vessels
Aortic stenosis
Obstructive disease of the aorta
Aortic insufficiency
Buckling of the aorta and brachiocephalic vessels

The contraindications to aortography can be divided into those that are physiological in nature and those that are related to the toxic effects of the contrast agents. Physiological contraindications, which are also related to the specific procedural techniques used, include femoral arteriosclerosis, which contraindicates the retrograde transfemoral approach to avoid intimal damage, and aneurysms at the injection site, which contraindicate the use of the direct puncture technique.

Sensitivity to iodine is an example of a toxic effect of a contrast agent that contraindicates the procedure. Patients with severe hepatorenal disease should be carefully evaluated to determine the advisability of performing the study. This, however, is not an absolute contraindication to aortography.

CONTRAST MEDIA

Aortography requires a large amount of a highly concentrated contrast agent to produce accurate diagnostic information. In choosing a contrast agent for use in the presence of severe hepatorenal disease, the relative toxicities of the various media available should be evaluated to avoid unnecessary complications. However, the ultimate choice of contrast agent rests, as usual, with the physician performing the procedure.

The amount of contrast agent delivered to the patient during catheter aortography varies with the type of study being done. Translumbar aortography requires from 10 to 35 ml of contrast agent in a single injection. If more than one injection is carried out, the total should not exceed 60 to 80 ml. Thoracic aortography usually requires from 45 to 70 ml over a 2-s interval. Abdominal aortography requires a total of 40 to 70 ml. See Chapter 3 for specific volume and flow rate recommendations.

PROCEDURE

Aortography can be performed to visualize the thoracic or abdominal aorta. In both cases, the contrast medium is injected into the lumen of the aorta through either translumbar aortography or percutaneous catheter aortography. With the percutaneous catheter approach, both flush and selective studies of the visceral vasculature can be accomplished via aortography depending on the level of catheter placement within the lumen of the aorta. The abdominal aorta is the major route for studies of the vasculature of the lower extremity and renal vessels; these studies are considered separately in Chapters 12 and 13.

Translumbar Aortography

The direct puncture approach is also a nonselective procedure, and visualization of the branches of the aorta depends on the concentration of contrast material within the aorta.

The specific technique of direct puncture of the aorta differs according to the physician performing the procedure. There are two basic variations—high and low— and the approach chosen depends on the anatomic information desired. The procedure is accomplished with a specially designed 18-gauge catheter with a 6F sheath. The patient is placed into the prone position. The insertion point can be at the level of the 12th thoracic vertebra (high approach) or at the third lumbar vertebra (low approach), and it is always made from the left flank approximately one hand's width from the spinous process.

In the low approach, the needle is directed in the axial plane at an angle of approximately 40°. This approach provides opacification of the vessels of the lower extremity without superimposition of the vessels of the abdominal viscera.

The high approach is used when there is a suspected aortic aneurysm or occlusion. The needle is directed cranially to avoid accidental injury to the renal artery. The angle is similar to that of the low approach, but there is the added risk of inducing a pneumothorax through accidental puncture of the lung. This approach is less desirable than the low approach because of the opacification of the vessels of the abdominal viscera.

Once aortic puncture has been accomplished, a length of polyethylene tubing is connected to the needle. The tubing and needle are then flushed with heparinized saline solution. A test injection is made with 5 ml of contrast material to determine the placement and location of the needle tip within the aortic lumen. If the test injection indicates proper placement of the needle, the injection can be made. The amount of contrast material used will vary with the information desired; however, injection of 10 to 20 ml over 2 to 3 s is usually enough to opacify the proximal aorta and visceral branches, whereas 20 to 25 ml is required for good visualization of the distal aorta and its parietal branches.[2] The injection can be made manually or with an automatic injection device; the method chosen depends on preference and/or availability of the necessary equipment.

Percutaneous Catheter Aortography

This method of aortography can be done either retrograde via the femoral artery or antegrade via the brachial or carotid arteries. It is a nonselective catheterization that allows placement of a catheter at any level within the lumen of the aorta. Selective catheterization of one of the major branches of the aorta may be performed immediately after a nonselective catheter aortogram if more detailed information regarding a specific area is desired.

The most common technique of catheter insertion is the Seldinger method of percutaneous arterial puncture.[3] The advantage of the Seldinger technique is that smaller needles are used to effect the puncture, and a catheter approximately the same size as the needle is then inserted over a previously placed guide wire. This proves to be less traumatic to the vessel than the technique previously described by Pierce in 1951, whereby the catheter is inserted through a large-bore needle.[4] The following is a summary of the basic steps of the Seldinger approach:

1. Under local anesthetic, puncture the femoral artery directly.
2. Insert a guide wire through the needle into the artery.
3. Remove the needle. Apply pressure proximal to the puncture site to control bleeding.
4. Thread a catheter over the guide wire into the artery.
5. Remove the guide wire.
6. Advance the catheter to the desired level within the lumen of the aorta.

Once catheter placement has been successfully accomplished, the catheter is flushed with heparinized saline solution, and a test injection of a small amount of contrast agent may be made to check catheter placement. When the procedure is complete and the catheter has been removed, pressure should be applied to the puncture site for a minimum of 5 min.

A comparison of the various methods described is given in Table 10–1.

Table 10–1. COMPARISON OF VARIOUS METHODS OF AORTOGRAPHY

Method	Advantages	Disadvantages
Translumbar aortography	Method of choice for wide variety of pathologic conditions of abdominal aorta Relatively simple puncture technique	Lack of flexibility in control of contrast agent Patient must remain motionless during procedure
Percutaneous catheter aortography	Flexible in regard to contrast agent placement Patient may be moved without risk during procedure Extravascular injection minimized Method of choice for both thoracic and abdominal aortography	Cannot be performed in cases of intraluminal pathology

EQUIPMENT

The equipment required for aortography varies with the method chosen. A properly equipped special procedure room should be available for aortography to yield the maximum amount of information from the procedure.

A rapid sequence film changer should be used to record the flow of contrast material through the aorta, and it should have the capabilities of from one to six exposures per second, with a minimum of 10 to 20 films.

An automatic injector is useful during most methods of aortography. Typical parameters are given in Chapter 3. If a manual injection is to be made, a protective device should be available for the person making the injection.

Each procedure requires various syringes and needles. The specialized needles required for the intravenous and translumbar methods should be sterilized in advance and kept in the department. For the percutaneous catheter technique, a sterile catheterization tray should be available that contains all necessary materials.

An emergency cart should be available as part of the special procedure suite.

PATIENT POSITIONING

The radiographic positioning for aortography depends on the injection procedure chosen and the information desired. Preliminary films should be taken so that proper positioning, technique, and coverage of area of interest can be determined before the injection is made, thereby minimizing the possibility of subjecting the patient to another injection.

Because of the means of injection, translumbar aortography requires that the patient

Table 10–2. SUMMARY OF POSITIONS FOR AORTOGRAPHY

Procedure	Projection	Patient Position	Central Ray	Anatomy
Translumbar aortography	Posteroanterior	Patient prone, centered to table, arms next to body, lower legs supported	Vertical beam to center of rapid sequence changer, area of interest over film changer	Aorta and major branches
Percutaneous catheter midstream aortography	Anteroposterior	Patient supine, arms next to body (single plane), arms above head (biplane)	Vertical beam to center of rapid film changer, area of interest centered to changer	Aorta and major branches in area of interest demonstrated in frontal view
	Lateral	Patient in true lateral position, arms above head (single plane)	Vertical beam to center of rapid film changer	Aorta and major branches in area of interest demonstrated in lateral view
		Patient supine, centered to table (biplane)	Horizontal beam to center of upright film changer	
	Posterior obliques	Patient in supine oblique position	Vertical beam to center of rapid sequence changer	Anatomy best demonstrated by posterior oblique projections (same as intravenous aortography, above)

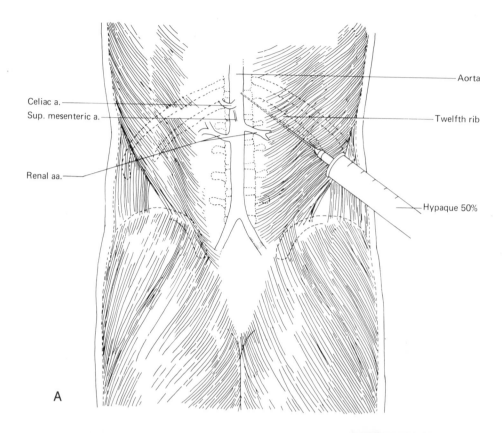

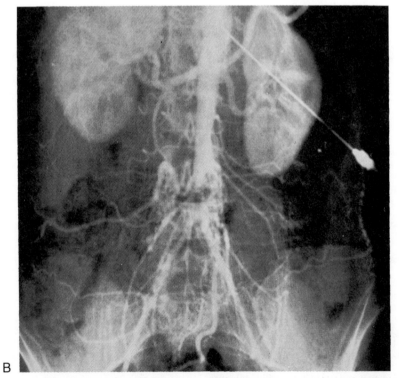

Figure 10–5. *(A)* Schematic showing the location of the translumbar puncture for aortography; *(B)* radiograph showing needle placement during translumbar aortography. *(A* from Winthrop Laboratories; *B* from Radiol. Clin. North Am., *2:426, 1963–1964.)*

remain in the prone position (Fig. 10–5). The area of the aorta and its branches to be radiographed depend on the nature of the specific underlying disease.

Intravenous aortography is the most flexible of the various procedural methods in regard to positioning of the patient. The position used should yield the maximum amount of information from the study. The positions that may be used during intravenous aortography are anteroposterior, lateral, and posterior oblique. The area of interest is another factor that depends on the nature of the pathology.

Catheter aortography begins with the patient in the supine position for the introduction of the catheter. After successful placement, the patient may be rotated into the right posterior oblique position for demonstration of the brachiocephalic vessels during thoracic aortography. This is usually the position of choice for the delineation of any type of aneurysm. If a biplane study is done, the patient is maintained in the supine position, and anteroposterior and lateral projections can be taken with one injection. With catheter aortography, the selective injection of any of the major branches may be done easily, if necessary.

Table 10–2 summarizes the positioning for the various aortographic methods.

REFERENCES

1. Gardner, E., Gray, D. J., and O'Rahilly, R.: Anatomy: A Regional Study of Human Structure, 4th ed. Philadelphia, W. B. Saunders, 1975.
2. Cooley, R. N., and Schreiber, M. H.: Radiology of the Heart and Great Vessels, 3rd ed. Baltimore, Williams & Wilkins, 1978.
3. Seldinger, S. I.: Catheter replacement of the needle in percutaneous arteriography, Acta Radiol., *39*:368, 1953.
4. Pierce, E. C.: Percutaneous femoral artery catheterization in man with special reference to aortography, Surg. Gynecol. Obstet., *93*:56, 1951.

SUGGESTED READINGS

PERCUTANEOUS CATHETER AORTOGRAPHY

Amplatz, K.: Percutaneous arterial catheterization and its application, Am. J. Roentgenol. Radium Ther. Nucl. Med., *87*:265, 1962.
Barcia, T. C., et al.: Indications for angiography in blunt thoracic trauma, Radiology, *147*:15, 1983.
Bell, D. D., et al.: Routine aortography before abdominal aortic aneurysmectomy: A prospective study, Am. J. Surg., *144*:191, 1982.
Grollman, J. H. Jr., and Marcus, R.: Transbrachial arteriography: Techniques and complications, Cardiovasc. Intervent. Radiol., *11*:32–35, 1988.
Kozak, B. E., and Rosch, J.: Curved guide wire for percutaneous pulmonary angiography, Radiology, *167*:864–865, 1988.
McLellan, G. L., and Scalapino, M. C.: Pulmonary artery catheterization: A modified technique, Radiology, *169*:264–265, 1988.
Newton, T. H.: The axillary artery approach to arteriography of the aorta and its branches, Am. J. Roentgenol. Radium Ther. Nucl. Med., *89*:275, 1963.
Shaw, P. J., et al.: Percutaneous transfemoral lumbar aortography as an outpatient procedure, Br. Med. J. [Clin. Res.], *286*:604, 1983.
Sprayregen, S., Veith, F. J., and Bakal, C. W.: Catheterization and angioplasty of the non-opacified peripheral autogenous vein bypass graft, Arch. Surg., *123*:1009–1012, 1988.

Rose, S. C., and Moore, E. E.: Angiography in patients with arterial trauma: Correlation between angiographic abnormalities, operative findings and clinical outcome, Am. J. Roentgenol., *149*:613–619, 1987.

TRANSLUMBAR AORTOGRAPHY

Beall, A. C. Jr., et al.: Translumbar aortography: A simple safe technique, Ann. Surg., *157*:882, 1963.
Beranbaum, S. L., and Meyers, P. H.: Special Procedures in Roentgen Diagnosis. Springfield, IL, Charles C Thomas, 1964.
Cooley, R. N., and Agnew, C. H.: Technique of translumbar aortography, Tex. State J. Med., *55*:945, 1959.
Frick, P. C.: Translumbar aortography, Radiol. Technol., *39*:261, 1968.

ACCESSORIES

Akisada, M., et al.: A new type of cross-hatched wedged grid for biplanar serial angiography of the abdomen, Invest. Radiol., *16*:305, 1981.
Odman, P.: The radiopaque polyethylene catheter, Acta Radiol., *52*:52, 1959.

eleven

Venous Angiography

ANATOMIC CONSIDERATIONS

INDICATIONS AND
CONTRAINDICATIONS

CONTRAST MEDIA

PROCEDURE

Upper Extremity and Superior Vena
Cava

Azygos and Hemiazygos System

Inferior Vena Cava and Pelvis

Lower Extremity

EQUIPMENT

PATIENT POSITIONING

Venous angiography is the radiographic demonstration of the veins of the body. This procedure is also known as venography or phlebography and can be performed in all areas of the body. The most common site and purpose for venography is in the lower extremity for the diagnosis of deep vein thrombosis of the leg. Venography is also used to study the veins of the upper extremity, azygos and hemiazygos system, renal venous system, inferior and superior venae cavae, and iliac and pelvic veins. The procedure can be accomplished through direct injection or catheterization.

ANATOMIC CONSIDERATIONS

The veins of the body collect the blood from the systemic circulation and return it to the heart and lungs for reoxygenation. The venous system of the body is extensive, and consideration is given here only to major veins with significance in venous angiography. The venous system of the body ultimately empties into two major veins—the inferior and superior venae cavae—which direct the venous blood into the right atrium of the heart (Fig. 11–1). All of the major veins are tributaries of these vessels and compose the venous circulation. The superior vena cava receives blood from the upper portion of the body, and the inferior venae cavae serves the lower portion.

The venous system of the upper extremity consists of both superficial and deep veins. The deep veins are usually small and paired; they accompany the arteries and ultimately drain into the axillary vein. The veins of the upper extremity contain valves that prevent backflow of the blood and aid in movement of the blood to the heart.

There are three major superficial veins of the upper extremity—the cephalic vein, the basilic vein, and the median antebrachial vein of the forearm (Fig. 11–2). These vessels are the primary means of drainage in the upper extremity. The cephalic vein starts in the distal forearm, receives the drainage from the dorsal aspect of the hand, runs along the lateral aspect of the arm, and ends just below the clavicle. At this point, the vein courses medially and joins the axillary vein. The median cubital vein forms a

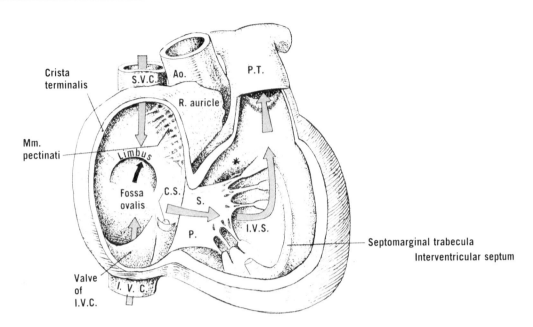

Figure 11–1. The external and internal anatomy of the heart. A, Right atrium and right ventricle, showing the tricuspid orifice. The arrows indicate the circulation of the blood. An arrow in the fossa ovalis represents "probe patency" of the foramen ovale. The membranous part of the interventricular septum lies mostly under cover of the septal cusp. The asterisk indicates the supraventricular crest. The septomarginal trabecula is frequently called the moderator band. S.V.C., superior vena cava; Ao., aorta; R., right; P.T., pulmonary trunk; I.V.S., interventricular septum; S., septal cusp of tricuspid valve; P., posterior cusp of tricuspid valve; C.S., opening of the coronary sinus. (From O'Rahilly, R.: Anatomy. Philadelphia, W. B. Saunders, 1983.)

connection between the cephalic and the basilic veins of the upper extremity and is located on the anterior aspect of the arm at the level of the elbow. This vein is the usual location for blood sampling, intravenous injection, blood transfusion, and introducing catheters for contrast radiography. The basilic vein runs up from the distal forearm toward the medial side of the arm, where it ultimately becomes the axillary vein. The median vein collects the venous return from the palmar aspect of the hand. It then courses over the anterior of the arm until it joins the basilic vein. In another variant of the normal anatomy, the median vein can also join the median cubital vein. The axillary vein continues a short distance and becomes the subclavian vein at approximately the level of the first rib. The subclavian vein is then joined by the internal jugular vein to form the brachiocephalic vein. The brachiocephalic vein also collects blood from the vertebral, internal mammary, intercostal, and thyroid veins.

The left and right brachiocephalic veins, which are formed by the union of the internal jugular and subclavian veins, join to form the superior vena cava. The superior vena cava then courses down on the right side of the ascending aorta, where it receives the azygos vein before entering the right atrium of the heart.

The azygos and hemiazygos system comprises unpaired vessels that lie on each side of the spine (Fig. 11–3). There are several normal variants of the anatomic presentation of this system of veins.

The azygos vein arises at about the level of the right renal vein and courses up to the right of midline. It collects venous blood from a variety of vessels, including the intercostal, subcostal, mediastinal, esophageal, right ascending lumbar, pericardial, bronchial, accessory hemiazygos, and hemiazygos veins. The hemiazygos and accessory hemiazygos veins are located to the left of midline and are considered to correspond

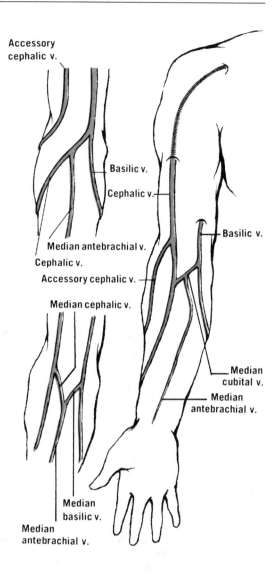

Figure 11–2. Diagram of some common patterns of the superficial veins of the upper limb. Only the larger channels at the elbow are shown: these are the ones most likely to be visible through the skin. (From O'Rahilly, R.: Anatomy. Philadelphia, W. B. Saunders, 1983.)

to the azygos vein. These vessels collect blood from a variety of vessels on the left side of the body and ultimately empty into the azygos vein for transport to the heart.

The venous system of the lower extremity comprises both deep and superficial veins. Unlike in the upper extremity, here the deep veins provide the primary drainage. There is some communication throughout the venous system of the lower extremity; however, this is limited to one-way flow from the superficial system to the deep veins.

The superficial veins are represented primarily by the great and small saphenous veins. The accessory saphenous vein also contributes to the return of blood from the lower extremity, when it is present. It is usually located over the posteromedial aspect of the thigh and communicates with both the great and small saphenous veins. The great saphenous vein originates at the medial side of the foot at the level of the median marginal vein. It continues in front of the medial malleolus, ascends along the anteromedial aspect of the lower leg and thigh, and ends in the common femoral vein. The location of this vessel at the medial malleolus provides an excellent avenue for intravenous administration of medications, if necessary. The small saphenous vein, also called the lesser saphenous vein, originates on the lateral side of the foot at the level of the lateral marginal vein. It then courses toward the posterior of the lower leg and

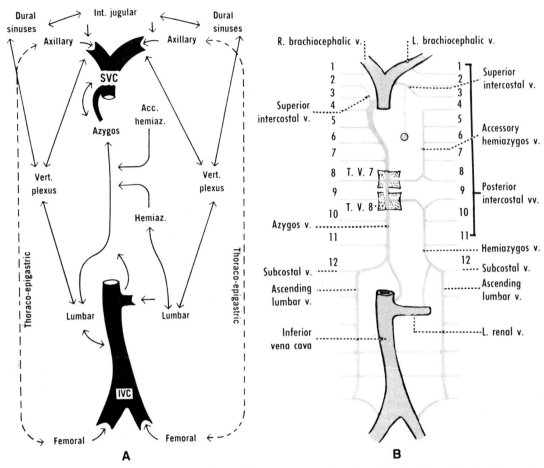

Figure 11–3. *(A)* Scheme of the main connections of the azygos, caval, and vertebral systems of veins. Connections of the azygos and hemiazygos veins with the posterior intercostal veins also occur. *(B)* The main veins of the thorax. An interrupted blue line indicates the course of a left superior vena cava (a rare anomaly) on its way to the coronary sinus. (From O'Rahilly, R.: Anatomy. Philadelphia, W. B. Saunders, 1983.)

ascends to above the knee joint. Several normal variants may be present at this level, and the small saphenous vein joins the popliteal, greater saphenous, or deep muscular calf veins (Fig. 11–4).

The deep veins of the lower extremity consist primarily of the femoral and popliteal. These are usually paired and accompany the arteries. These normally originate with the vessels in the plantar surface of the foot and follow the course of the anterior tibial, posterior tibial, and peroneal arteries. The anterior and posterior tibial veins ascend to just below the level of the knee, where they anastomose to form the popliteal vein (Fig. 11–5). At approximately the level of midthigh, the popliteal veins become the superficial femoral vein. This vein ascends until it is joined by the deep femoral vein. This occurs about 5 to 10 cm below the inguinal ligament; the resultant vessel is called the common femoral vein. The common femoral vein becomes the external iliac vein above the inguinal ligament. It connects with the internal iliac vein to become the common iliac vein. At about the level of the fifth lumbar vertebra, the left and right iliac veins join to become the inferior vena cava.

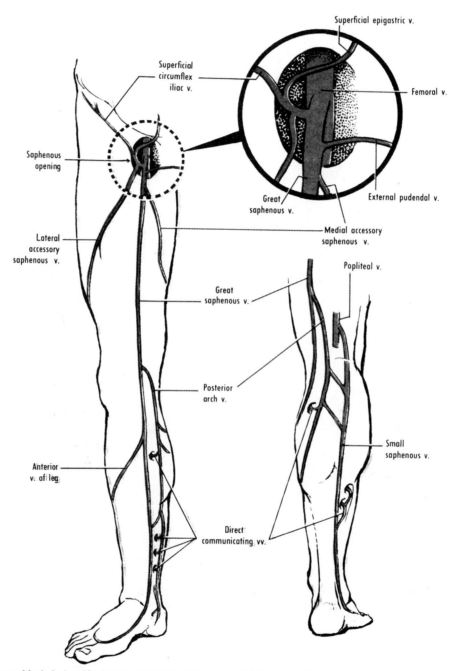

Figure 11–4. A simplified representation of the superficial veins of the lower limb. The major tributaries and also the major communicating veins above the ankle are shown according to Dodd and Cockett. Details of the veins of the foot have been omitted. (From O'Rahilly, R.: Anatomy. Philadelphia, W. B. Saunders, 1983.)

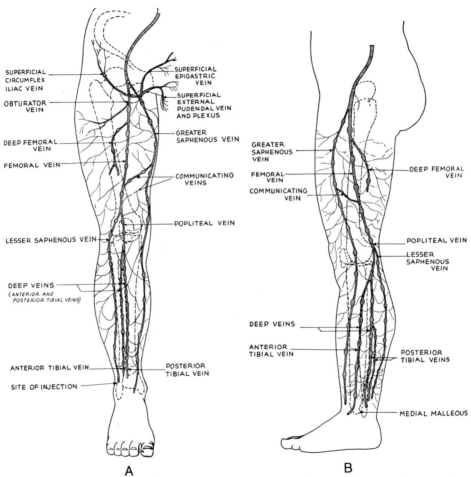

Figure 11–5. Schematic drawing of the major veins of the lower leg as they would appear in a normal venogram. *(A)* Anteroposterior projection. *(B)* Lateral projection. (From Meschan, I.: Normal Radiographic Anatomy, 2nd ed. Philadelphia, W. B. Saunders, 1959.)

INDICATIONS AND CONTRAINDICATIONS

Venous angiography is used primarily to diagnose thrombosis and occlusion of the vessels. Central selective catheter visceral venography is also done to enable the physician to perform blood sampling and pressure measurements within the vessel. Extremity venography has been useful in trauma cases to determine the extent of vessel damage. In the lower extremity, the examination is used primarily to determine the presence or absence of deep vein thrombosis. The study is relatively safe but not without risk. The possibility of a reaction to the contrast agent cannot be ignored. The examination is unpleasant for the patient and can produce complications such as thrombosis secondary to the examination, nausea, vomiting, dizziness, superficial phlebitis, skin reactions, edema, and localized pain.[1]

The only contraindications for this examination are a known sensitivity to the contrast media or the patient's being an "at-risk" case, that is, a patient for whom the risk of the procedure outweighs the risk of the associated pathology.

CONTRAST MEDIA

The water-soluble contrast agents can be used for this procedure; the choice of ionic versus nonionic is the physician's. It is recommended that a 60% concentration be used for upper extremity and superior vena cavography and a 76% concentration be used for all other types of studies. If digital subtraction angiography is being performed, the concentration of the contrast agent can be reduced to 20%. The amount of material used varies with physician's preference, the area being examined, and hospital protocol.

PROCEDURE

Venous angiography can be performed with the catheter technique or by direct injection. The choice of method is dictated by area of interest, physician preference, and type of pathology present. Preprocedural patient care is the same as for all angiographic procedures.

Upper Extremity and Superior Vena Cava

In the upper extremity, the site of puncture is dependent on the area of investigation. If the entire arm is to be imaged, a distal forearm vein is punctured. The physician may use either a 19-gauge butterfly needle or a small angiocath. The median cubital vein is usually the site of choice for evaluation of the axillary vein or central structures. This route is the same as that for the evaluation of the superior vena cava and can be done by direct injection or catheterization. The patient is prepared with the palm facing up and the arm abducted 90° from the body. A tourniquet is applied proximal to the puncture site for manual injection methods. The contrast agent is then injected. During the last 5 ml of the injection, the tourniquet is released, and filming can proceed.

If the study is for diagnosis in the superior vena cava, the injection can be performed using a simultaneous bilateral direct injection of contrast agent into the median cubital vein. Catheter angiography in this area can be accomplished through catheterization of the median cubital vein, the jugular vein, or the femoral vein; the usual routes are the cubital and femoral approaches. An automatic injection device is used, and visualization of the contrast can be accomplished with fluoroscopy; filming can be accomplished in a single plane or biplane mode.

Azygos and Hemiazygos System

To visualize the vessels in the azygos and hemiazygos system, selective catheter venography is used. A catheter is maneuvered from the median cubital or femoral vein and selectively positioned in the azygos vein. An automatic injector is used to deliver the contrast agent at a rate of 15 ml/s for a total volume of 30 ml. Filming is usually accomplished in the biplane mode.

Inferior Vena Cava and Pelvis

The inferior vena cava is imaged with the median cubital or femoral approach. The technique involves the introduction of a catheter into the inferior vena cava. The type and size of the catheter depend on the approach and physician's preference. The cubital vein approach is contraindicated if thrombosis is suspected. Contrast agent is delivered by automatic injection at a rate of 20 ml/s for a total volume of 40 ml.

The veins of the pelvis, including the iliac veins, are usually imaged using a catheter sheath technique from a femoral vein approach. The external iliac vein can also be studied by catheter insertion at the median cubital vein. The rate and total volume of contrast agent vary with the site to be examined. A summary of these rates is given in Table 11–1.

Table 11–1. SUMMARY OF VENOGRAPHIC PROCEDURES

Anatomic Area	Puncture Site	Injection Manual	Injection Automatic	Rate (ml/s) Volume (ml)	Film Sequence Rate (s^{-1})	Film Sequence Total	Plane Single	Plane Biplane
Upper extremity	Site dependent on area to be investigated	×		NA/30 ml	1	8	×	
Superior vena cava	Bilateral Cubital vein injection	×		NA/25 ml each arm	1	8		×
	Catheter angiography Cubital		×	15/30 ml	2	6		×
	Femoral		×	15/30 ml	1	2		×
Azygos and hemi-azygos system	Catheter angiography Cubital		×	5/12 ml	1	6		×
	Femoral		×	5/12 ml	1	6		×
Inferior vena cava	Catheter angiography Cubital		×	20/40 ml	1	4		×
	Femoral		×	20/40 ml	4	8		×
Pelvis	Catheter sheath angiography Bilateral femoral		×	20/40 ml	2	8		×
Lower extremity	Superficial dorsal pedis vein	×		NA/75–150 ml	*	*	×	
Iliac veins, External	Femoral vein Ipsilateral		×	10/20 ml	2	8	×	
	Contralateral		×	10/20 ml	2	8	×	
	Cubital vein		×	10/20 ml	2	8	×	
Internal	Femoral		×	8/15 ml	2	8	×	

*Observation by fluoroscopy; filming done with 100- to 105-mm cine camera and/or large-format film such as 14- × 17- or 14- × 36-in films.

Lower Extremity

A number of techniques are used for contrast venography of the lower extremity. In general, the patient is positioned supine on a tilting radiographic table. The opposite leg is placed on a support that allows the leg of interest to be suspended or non–weight bearing. Tourniquets can be used to slow the progress of venous return; they can also help compress the superficial veins, allowing the contrast easier access to the deep veins. When this method is used, one tourniquet is placed above the ankle and the other is affixed slightly above the knee. A dorsal pedis vein is chosen for the puncture site, and a 23-gauge butterfly needle is used for the cannulation. The contrast agent is injected into the vein by manual injection or using an automatic injector with a slow rate. It is imperative that the injection site be monitored for extravasation into the surrounding tissues; the study should be aborted and recannulation attempted if extravasation occurs.

Descending venography can be performed with the catheter approach from a femoral vein puncture.[2] In the case of a unilateral study, the catheter is placed in the ipsilateral vein. When bilateral studies are done, a single femoral puncture will produce satisfactory images while reducing patient discomfort. The patient is placed in a 60° semierect position with the contralateral leg supported to provide non–weight-bearing status for the leg under study. From 30 to 100 ml of contrast agent is slowly injected into the catheter at a rate of 50 to 75 ml/min. Contrast flow can be followed by fluoroscopy, and filming is accomplished by spot film or cine camera.

If the equipment does not permit placement of the patient in the angled position, supine venography can be performed. The puncture site is the same, and tourniquets are used to slow the venous blood flow. The contrast agent is injected manually. After 50% of the contrast agent has been injected, the lower tourniquet is removed, and

Table 11–2. SUMMARY OF POSITIONING FOR VENOUS ANGIOGRAPHY

Procedure	Patient Position
Upper extremity	Anteroposterior projection
Superior vena cava	Single plane Anteroposterior projection

	Biplane
	  Anteroposterior projection
	  Lateral projection

Inferior vena cava	Single plane Anteroposterior projection

	Biplane
	  Anteroposterior projection
	  Lateral projection

Azygos and hemiazygos system	Single plane Anteroposterior projection

	Biplane
	  Anteroposterior projection
	  Lateral projection

Pelvis	Anteroposterior projection
Lower extremity Lower leg	Anteroposterior projection Internal oblique projection External oblique projection
Knee and distal femur	Anteroposterior projection
Femur and pelvis	Anteroposterior projection

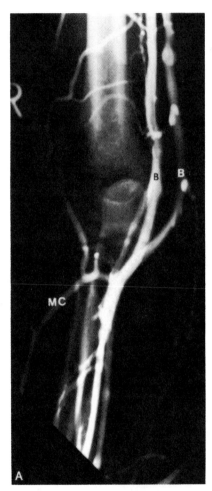

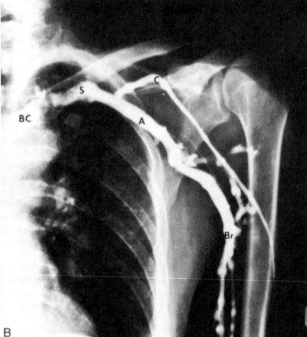

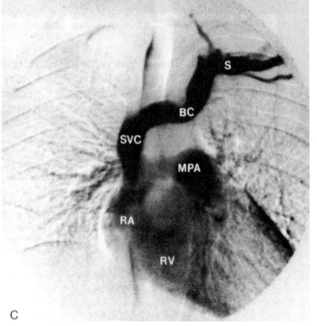

Figure 11–6. *A* to *C,* Normal upper extremity venograms. The basilic vein is duplicated. A, axillary; B, basilic; BC, brachiocephalic; Br, brachial; C, cephalic; MC, median cubital; MPA, main pulmonary artery; RA, right atrium; RV, right ventricle; S, subclavian vein; SVC, superior vena cava.

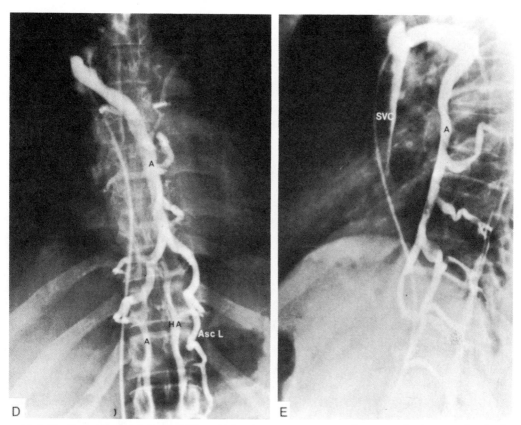

Figure 11–6 *Continued D* and *E,* Normal AP and lateral azygos venogram. A, azygos; Asc L, ascending lumbar; HA, hemiazygos veins; SVC, superior vena cava.

Illustration continued on following page

filming can proceed. As the contrast agent moves up the leg, the upper tourniquet is removed, and overhead films can be made of the upper leg and pelvis. The study should include imaging of the iliac vein and the inferior vena cava.

In both descending and ascending venography, filming can be accomplished with a cine camera or large-format film radiography. The use of a "stepping" table is an advantage for this type of study.

EQUIPMENT

Venography can be performed in any radiographic fluorographic room that is equipped for fluoroscopy and has some type of imaging system. It is advantageous for specialized equipment such as a stepping table or large-format cassette changer to be available. Biplane film changers are recommended when central venography is performed; this will alleviate some patient discomfort and reduce the risks attendant with a second injection of contrast agent. Automatic injection should be used when the study requires that a rapid injection of contrast agent be accomplished, such as in venacavography. The use of digital subtraction can enhance the study while providing a reduction in patient discomfort because of the decrease in the concentration of the contrast agent used.

If catheter studies are performed, a variety of different catheters should be available, including a 5F or 6F pigtail catheter for superior and inferior vena cavography, a cobra

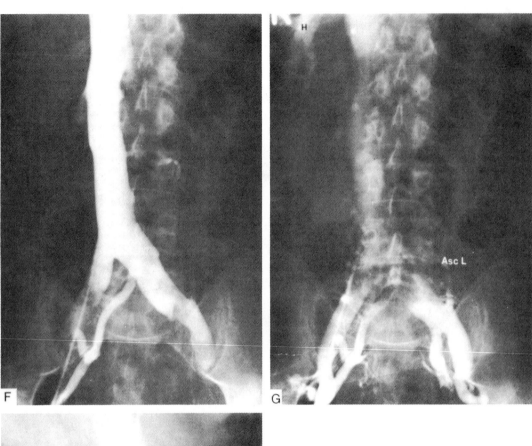

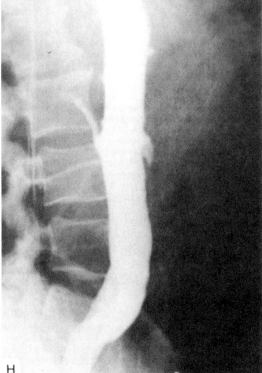

Figure 11-6 *Continued* Normal inferior vena cavagram. *F*, Early phase. *G*, Later film shows reflux of contrast medium into pelvic and hepatic (H) veins. *H*, Lateral film shows the normal relation of the inferior vena cava to the spine. Asc L, ascending lumbar vein.

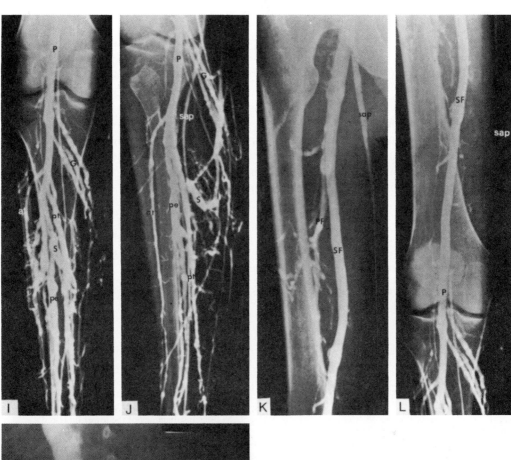

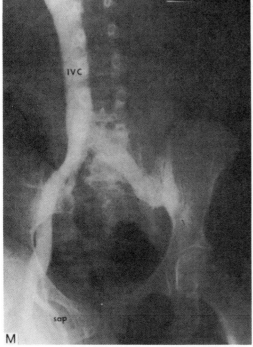

Figure 11–6 *Continued* Normal leg venogram. *I*, Anteroposterior and *J*, lateral distal leg. *K* and *L*, Proximal and distal thigh. *M*, Iliac vein and inferior vena cava. at, anterior tibial; G, gastrocnemius; IVC, inferior vena cava; P, popliteal; pe, peroneal; PF, profunda femoris; pt, posterior tibial; S, soleal; sap, saphenous; SF, superficial femoral veins. (From Kadir, S.: Diagnostic Angiography. Philadelphia, W. B. Saunders, 1986.)

catheter with end and side holes for the veins of the pelvis and azygos system, and the multipurpose 100-cm catheter for the cubital vein approach when imaging the iliac veins. A variety of angiocath systems and various gauge butterfly needles should be maintained as a part of the general equipment.

PATIENT POSITIONING

The patient's position varies with the type of study being done. Table 11–2 summarizes the positions necessary for the various types of venous angiography. These positions may vary with the institution and the physician performing the study. In general, the patient is supine, and the part is imaged in the anteroposterior projection in single-plane studies and in both anteroposterior and lateral projections in biplane studies. Figure 11–6 provides some examples of venous angiography.

REFERENCES

1. Lensing, A., Prandoni, P., Buller, H. R., Casara, D., Cogo, A., and Wouter ten Cate, J.: Lower extremity venography with iohexol: Results and complications, Radiology, 177:503–505, 1990.

2. Morano, J. U., and Raju, S.: Chronic venous insufficiency: Assessment with descending venography, Radiology, 174:441–444, 1990.

SUGGESTED READINGS

Albrechtsson, U., and Olsson, C. G.: Thrombotic side effects of lower limb phlebography, Lancet, 1:723–724, 1976.

Clarke, J. C., and McIlrath, E. M.: The role of emergency venography in the diagnosis and management of deep venous thrombosis, Ulster Med. J., 59:46–50, 1990.

Grassi, J., and Polak, J. F.: Axillary and subclavian venous thrombosis: Follow up evaluation with color Doppler flow US and venography, Radiology, 175:651–654, 1990.

Martin, E. D., Koser, M., and Gordon, D. H.: Venography in axillary-subclavian vein thrombosis, Cardiovasc. Radiol., 2:261–266, 1979.

Raju, S.: Venous insufficiency of the lower limb and stasis ulceration, Ann. Surg., 197:688–697, 1983.

Ramsay, L. E.: Impact of venography on the diagnosis and management of deep vein thrombosis, Br. Med. J., 286:698–699, 1983.

Salzman, E. W.: Venous thrombosis made easy, N. Engl. J. Med., 314:847–848, 1986.

twelve

Femoral Arteriography

ANATOMIC CONSIDERATIONS
Arterial Supply
Veins
INDICATIONS AND
    CONTRAINDICATIONS

CONTRAST MEDIA
PROCEDURE
EQUIPMENT
PATIENT POSITIONING

Femoral arteriography involves demonstration of the circulation of the lower extremity. This procedure has gained importance in the identification of many vascular abnormalities, including embolism, aneurysm, and arterial injury, and many bone and soft tissue lesions.

The procedure involves the entire lower extremity and can be accomplished with a single-film technique, digital subtraction angiography (DSA), single-plane serial radiography, or biplane serial radiography. The single-film technique usually does not supply an adequate amount of diagnostic information and therefore is not considered here as a major method.

ANATOMIC CONSIDERATIONS

Arterial Supply

At about the level of the fourth lumbar vertebra, the abdominal aorta terminates in a bifurcation. At this point, the aorta becomes the common iliac arteries. These arteries travel for a short distance (about 5 cm), and at about the upper level of the sacrum, they divide into the external and internal iliac arteries.

The internal iliac arteries supply blood to the pelvic region, whereas the external iliac arteries are the origin of the blood supply to the lower extremities (Fig. 12–1). The external iliac artery courses for about 10 cm before becoming the femoral artery at a point midway between the anterior superior iliac spine and the symphasis pubis. This is also the level at which the femoral artery enters the lower extremity. The branches of the femoral artery are divided into superficial and deep branches, as summarized in Table 12–1.

As the femoral artery passes into the popliteal space, it becomes the popliteal artery. It courses in a lateral oblique direction to its termination, where it divides into the anterior and posterior tibial arteries. The popliteal artery usually has six major branches—lateral superior genicular, medial superior genicular, middle genicular, lateral inferior genicular, medial inferior genicular, and sural arteries.

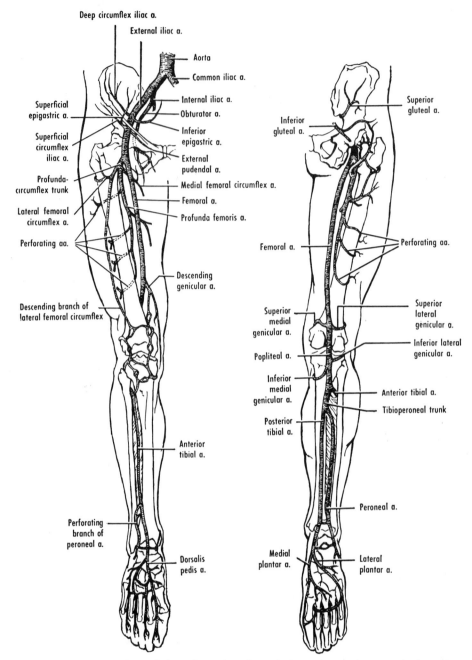

Figure 12–1. Arteries on the lower limb as shown from the anterior and posterior aspects. (From Gardner, E., Gray, D. J., and O'Rahilly, R.: Anatomy, 3rd ed. Philadelphia, W. B. Saunders, 1969.)

Table 12–1. MAJOR BRANCHES OF THE FEMORAL ARTERY

Superficial	Deep
Epigastric	Muscular branches
Circumflex iliac	Deep external pudendal
External pudendal	Deep femoral
	Lateral circumflex
	Medial circumflex
	Descending genicular

The anterior tibial artery courses forward from its origin to descend into the interosseous membrane of the lower leg to the level of the anterior aspect of the ankle joint, where it becomes the dorsalis pedis artery. The major branches of the anterior tibial artery are located around the knee and ankle joints, and many smaller muscular branches are given off along its descending route. The anterior tibial artery is the smaller of the two branches of the popliteal artery.

The posterior tibial artery is a direct continuation of the popliteal artery. Coursing downward toward the ankle, it passes between the medial malleolus of the tibia and the calcaneus and terminates in the foot. As in the anatomy of the anterior tibial artery, the major branches of the posterior tibial artery—the peroneal, nutrient, communicating, posterior medial malleolar, and medial calcaneal arteries—are concentrated around the knee and ankle joints.

A summary of the circulation from the level of the anterior and posterior tibial arteries is given in Figure 12–2.

Veins

As in all veins, those of the lower extremity have thinner walls than the arteries and are equipped with valves to prevent the backflow of blood. The veins of the lower extremity begin as small channels; they are both superficial and deep-set in the foot. There are more valves in the deep-set veins; the veins become progressively larger along their ascending courses. These veins run with the arteries and are named similarly. The veins of the superficial group collect in the great and small saphenous veins.

The veins of the deep-set group and those of the small saphenous vein empty into the popliteal vein, whereas the great saphenous vein drains into the femoral vein. From

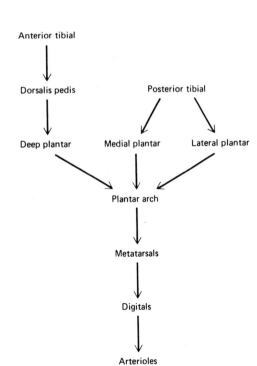

Figure 12–2. Flow chart summarizing the arterial circulation of the lower leg.

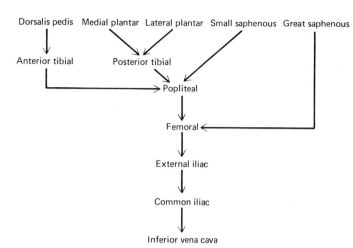

Figure 12-3. Flow chart summarizing the venous circulation of the lower extremity.

this point, the blood flows up through the external and common iliac veins and ultimately into the inferior vena cava to the heart.

A summary of the venous circulation of the lower extremity is given in Figure 12-3.

INDICATIONS AND CONTRAINDICATIONS

The indications for femoral arteriography include many vascular disorders of the lower extremities. The most common condition diagnosed by this procedure is arteriosclerosis obliterans, a disease that results in vascular occlusion. Trauma to the lower extremity with clinical evidence of vascular involvement requires femoral arteriography for injury assessment. The procedure is also useful in the diagnosis of bone and soft tissue tumors. The following is a summary of the indications for femoral arteriography:

Vascular lesions
   Arteriosclerosis obliterans
   Thromboangiitis obliterans
   Embolism
   Aneurysms
   Arteriovenous fistula
   Arteriovenous malformation
   Arterial trauma
   Grafts
   Arterial spasm
Bone tumors
   Chondroma
   Osteoma
   Angioma
   Giant cell tumor
   Osteosarcoma
   Chondrosarcoma
   Intraosseous sarcoma
   Ewing's tumor
   Reticulum cell sarcoma
   Osteoid osteoma

Soft tissue tumors
  Fibroma
  Lipoma
  Myxoma
  Neurofibroma
  Fibrosarcoma
  Differentiated (blastic) sarcoma
  Undifferentiated (ablastic) sarcoma

The procedure is relatively safe and not specifically contraindicated. Contraindications that usually apply for the intravascular injection of a contrast agent also apply to this procedure.

CONTRAST MEDIA

The contrast media used for femoral arteriography are the water-soluble organic iodine compounds. If the ionic contrast agents are used, either sodium or meglumine may be used; however, the N-methylglucamine salts are better tolerated for intravascular injection. Highly concentrated compounds, in the range of 50 to 76 per cent, are recommended. Low osmolality or nonionic iodine compounds can also be used.

The amount of contrast agent injected depends on the method chosen. If the injection is made into the distal aorta through percutaneous catheter insertion or translumbar aortography, a total of 40 to 60 ml is introduced at a rate of 10 to 15 ml/s over 3 to 4 s. Direct puncture of the femoral artery requires 20 to 30 ml injected at a rate of 8 to 10 ml/s for 2 to 3 s. If a specialized large-field cassette changer or cineradiography is used, the amount injected can be reduced because the entire system can then be recorded with a single injection. When DSA is performed, the total amount of contrast agent required for adequate arterial opacification is 20 to 25 ml.

PROCEDURE

The contrast agent can be introduced by translumbar aortography or percutaneous arterial puncture with or without catheterization to demonstrate the vascular system of the lower extremity. Percutaneous arterial puncture via the femoral artery is the method of choice. If this approach is not possible, catheterization via the axillary artery or translumbar aortography may be used.

The techniques of translumbar aortography and percutaneous catheter insertion by the Seldinger method have been discussed previously. The percutaneous transfemoral approach involves certain important variations in methodology. Opacification of the lower extremity may be accomplished by direct puncture of the femoral artery, with the needle directed either caudally or cephalad. The only advantage of the former method is that the entire amount of contrast agent is delivered into the arterial system of the lower extremity. Catheterization with the Seldinger technique is another variation, with the catheter placed in the femoral artery or distal aorta. Catheterization techniques should always be performed with strict aseptic technique. The ultimate choice of injection technique is left to the preference of the radiographer.

EQUIPMENT

Femoral arteriography requires filming of the entire lower extremity to provide an adequate diagnostic study. Filming can be accomplished through a single-film or serial film technique. Each method requires some specialized equipment.

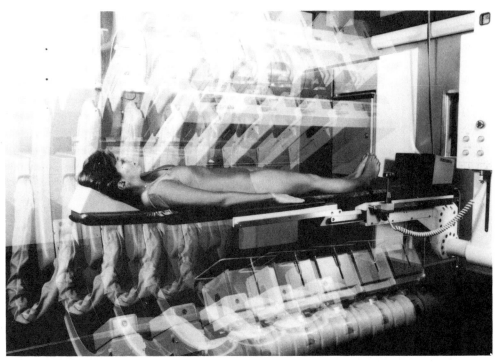

Figure 12–4. Siemens Angioskop D33 X-ray unit with optional stepping device that allows the patient to remain immobile during the study. It can be seen that the x-ray unit moves to position the desired anatomy for imaging. (From Siemens Corporation.)

The single-film technique requires a 14- × 36-in (35- × 90-cm) cassette to expose the lower extremity. Because there is variation in density between the lower leg and the femur, some compensation in technique is required to produce adequate films. Filters may be used at the tube for compensation. Another method of compensation is to load the cassette with two sheets of 14- × 17-in (35- × 42.5-cm) film of different speeds. The disadvantage of the single-film technique is that a second injection is usually required to record details that were missed with the first injection.

The serial filming method has become commonplace in most institutions that are equipped with a special procedure suite. All varieties of rapid sequence changers, including cut film and specialized large cassette changers, are available. The cut film changer usually uses a standard 14- × 14-in (35- × 35-cm) field size with a movable tabletop that automatically shifts the patient to obtain successive views of the lower extremity. Figure 12–4 shows the operation of the Siemens Angioskop D33 x-ray system equipped with the optional stepping device.

The main advantage of the serial radiographic technique of femoral arteriography is that the study can usually be accomplished with one injection. The method of injection is governed to some extent by the method of filming chosen. More contrast is necessary for the single-film technique than for serial filming.

DSA has some advantages over the previously discussed techniques. The contrast agent can be observed in real time, that is, as it is actually flowing through the vessels. In this way, both the adequacy of filling and any pathology can be observed almost immediately. DSA also requires the use of a smaller amount of contrast agent to opacify the vessels, reducing the severity of any subjective and objective symptoms that may occur.

The disadvantage with use of DSA is that only a single field may be observed at a time, with additional injections required to complete the entire procedure. Given these

Table 12–2. CONTENTS OF TYPICAL CATHETER ARTERIOGRAPHY TRAY

Item	Amount and/or Size
Luer-Lok syringe	1 (10 ml)
Luer-Lok syringes	4 (20 ml)
Surgical drape	1
Gauze squares	15–20 (4 × 4 in)
Small scissors	1
Towel clips	2
Towels	4
Forceps (sponge)	2
Scalpel handle and blade	1
Metal container	1
Glass container	1
Small hemostat (straight)	1

factors, the total amount of contrast agent injected and the time involved to perform the study are about the same as for the other techniques.

The necessary injection device depends on the particular method of introducing the contrast agent. Translumbar aortographic techniques usually require manual injection. Automatic injection devices are required for most injection techniques in current use.

Sterile trays are required for all methods of contrast introduction. Needles specialized for the specific procedure should be included in the tray (i.e., translumbar or Seldinger approach). Table 12–2 lists the equipment in a typical catheter arteriogram sterile tray.

PATIENT POSITIONING

The only basic position used in femoral arteriography is anteroposterior. The patient is placed on the radiographic table in the supine position with the legs together and the toes pointed up.

A variation of this position is used to provide a better visualization of the popliteal vessel and its branches. The patient is positioned as described above, but the toes are rotated approximately 30° internally. The heels can be spread apart to facilitate the internal rotation. The feet should be immobilized to prevent the possibility of motion during filming.

If the study is performed with 14- × 17-in (35- × 42.5-cm) cassettes in a conventional radiographic table, two or more injections are necessary. Careful positioning of each segment is necessary to avoid retakes. In these cases, the abdomen, pelvis, thigh, and lower leg must be filmed in the anteroposterior position.

Table 12–3. SUMMARY OF POSITIONS FOR FEMORAL ARTERIOGRAPHY

Projection	Patient Position	Central Ray	Anatomy
Anteroposterior	Patient in supine position, legs together with toes pointed up, feet immobilized to prevent motion	Directed at right angles to film	Arterial circulation of lower extremity
	Patient in supine position, legs together with toes internally rotated approximately 30°, feet immobilized to prevent motion	Directed at right angles to film	Arterial circulation of lower extremity with better visualization of popliteal artery and its branches

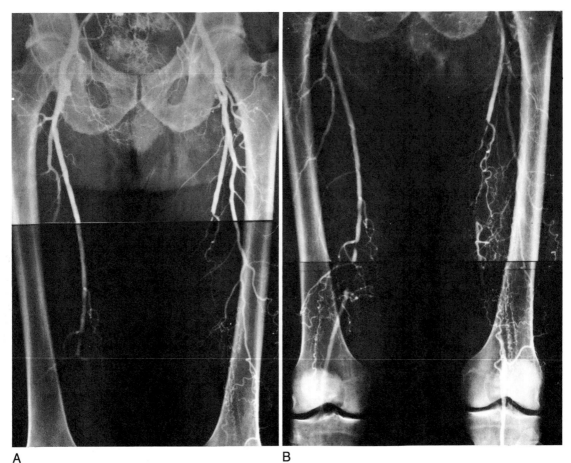

A   B

Figure 12–5. Selected radiographs from a femoral arteriogram depicting the travel of the contrast medium in the lower extremity. *(A)* Severe atherosclerotic disease with bilateral occlusions of superficial femoral arteries; *(B)* collaterals fill popliteal vessels distally. (From Juergens, J. L., Spittell, J. A., Jr., Fairbairn, J. F., II: Allen-Barker-Hines Peripheral Vascular Disease, 5th ed. Philadelphia, W. B. Saunders, 1980. Copyright Mayo Clinic, Rochester, MN.)

Figure 12–5 radiographically depicts the travel of the contrast medium through the lower extremity during femoral arteriography. Table 12–3 is a summary of positioning for femoral arteriography.

When DSA is used, the C-arm can be rotated to provide additional projections, if necessary. The additional projections are usually patient specific and may vary from procedure to procedure.

SUGGESTED READINGS

Almen, T.: Peripheral angiography with metrizamide, Diagn. Imag., *48*:206, 1979.

Baum, S., and Abrams, H. L.: A J-shaped catheter for retrograde catheterization of tortuous vessels, Radiology, *83*:436, 1964.

Berk, M. E.: Arteriography in peripheral trauma, Clin. Radiol., *14*:235, 1963.

Chermet, J.: Arteriography of lower limbs with blocked circulation ("dry-limb" arteriography), Radiology, *140*:826, 1981.

Chesney, D. N., and Chesney, M. D.: Care of the Patient in Diagnostic Radiography, 4th ed. Oxford, Blackwell Scientific Publications, 1973.

Cohen, M. I., and Vogelzang, R. L.: A comparison of techniques for improved visualization of the arteries of the distal lower extremity, Am. J. Roentgenol., *147*:1021–1024, 1986.

Fu, W. R.: Angiography of Trauma. Springfield, IL, Charles C Thomas, 1972.

Frykberg, E. R., Vines, F. S., and Alexander, R. H.: The natural history of clinically occult arterial injuries: A prospective evaluation, J. Trauma, *29*:577–583, 1989.

Gavant, M. L.: Digital subtraction angiography of the foot in atherosclerotic occlusive disease, South Med. J., *82*:328–334, 1989.

Kozak, B. E., Bedell, J. E., and Rosch, J.: Small vessel leg angiography for distal vessel bypass grafts, J. Vasc. Surg., *8*:711–715, 1988.

Lang, E. K.: A survey of the complication of percutaneous retrograde arteriography: Seldinger technique, Radiology, *81*: 257, 1963.

Love, L., and Braun, T.: Arteriography of peripheral vascular trauma, Am. J. Roentgenol., *102*:431, 1968.

McLean, G., et al.: Angiography of skeletal disease. Orthop. Clin. North Am., *14*:257, 1983.

Passiariello, R., et al.: Digital video subtraction angiography for routine peripheral arteriography, Ann. Radiol. (Paris), *25*:455, 1983.

Sethi, G. K., Scott, S. M., and Takaro, T.: Multiple plane angiography for more precise evaluation of aortoiliac disease, Surgery, *78*:154–159, 1975.

Speck, U., et al.: Contrast media and pain in peripheral arteriography, Invest. Radiol., *15*(Suppl. 6):335, 1980.

Turnipseed, W. D., et al.: Intra-arterial digital angiography: A new diagnostic method for determining limb salvage by-pass candidates, Surgery, *92*:322, 1982.

Weigen, J. F., and Thomas, S. F.: Complications of Diagnostic Radiology. Springfield, IL, Charles C Thomas, 1973.

Whitley, J. E., and Whitley, N. O.: Angiography: Techniques and procedures. St. Louis, Warren H. Green, 1971.

thirteen

Renal Angiography

ANATOMIC CONSIDERATIONS
Arterial Supply
Venous Drainage
INDICATIONS AND
    CONTRAINDICATIONS

CONTRAST MEDIA
PROCEDURE
Renal Venography
EQUIPMENT
PATIENT POSITIONING

Although radiographic visualization of the renal arteries usually occurs during aortography, it usually is not suitable for a detailed study of the renal arterial circulation (Fig. 13–1). Selective renal arteriography, however, gives an accurate radiographic demonstration of the renal artery anatomy. This is usually accomplished by one of two methods (Fig. 13–2A and B). With a catheter positioned within the aorta at the level of the renal arteries, the supply to both kidneys can be visualized, as can the status of the aorta and any pathological condition that may be obscured by the catheter tip. If this method fails to yield the necessary information, selective catheterization of a single renal artery can be performed. Intravenous digital subtraction angiography through catheter placement in the inferior vena cava has also been used successfully to evaluate certain renal masses.

The newer modalities such as computed tomography, magnetic resonance imaging and ultrasonographic techniques have almost completely replaced renal angiography as a diagnostic technique for renal pathology. Renal angiography, however, remains a viable tool in the study of certain renal abnormalities.

ANATOMIC CONSIDERATIONS

The kidneys are bean-shaped organs that lie in the abdomen next to the vertebral column at the level of the 12th thoracic vertebra to the second or third lumbar vertebra. The renal hilum, an indented area on the medial border of the kidneys, can usually be found at the level of the interspace of the first and second lumbar vertebrae. This level can vary by as much as one vertebral body in either direction. It is here that the major vessels and ureters enter and leave the kidney.

The internal structure of the kidney is divided into two areas—the cortex, or outer area, and the medulla, or inner portion. The cortex contains the glomeruli, which are capsules that enclose a convoluted group of capillaries. The glomeruli are portions of the nephrons, the functional units of the kidney (Fig. 13–3). The cortex also comprises other portions of the nephron, the convoluted tubules, and portions of the origins of the collecting ducts.

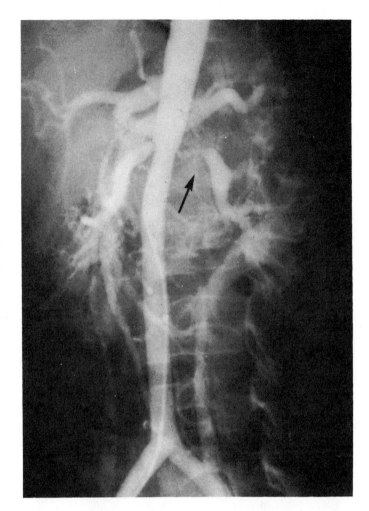

Figure 13–1. Radiograph of an aortogram showing the filling of the renal vessels. (From Witten, M. U.: Emmett's Clinical Urography: An Atlas and Textbook of Roentgenologic Diagnosis, 4th ed. Philadelphia, W. B. Saunders, 1977.)

The medulla comprises straight tubules, continuations of the convoluted tubules called Henle's loop, and collecting ducts.[1] The medulla has the appearance of many pyramids, the apex of which terminates in the cuplike indentation of the minor renal calyx (Fig. 13–4).

The nephrons filter blood plasma and permit selective reabsorption of water and dissolved materials necessary for maintaining the ionic balance of the blood back into the circulation. There are 1 million or more of these nephrons in each kidney. During renal arteriography, the interlobular arteries are not outlined as separate channels but instead appear as a diffuse accumulation over the entire kidney. This is usually called the nephrogram phase of the arteriogram.

Arterial Supply

The renal arteries originate as branches of the abdominal aorta at about the level of the interspace of the first and second lumbar vertebrae. They course transversely toward each kidney, with the right renal artery passing posterior to the inferior vena cava. The superior mesenteric artery is just above the origin of the renal arteries.

The renal artery gives off an extrarenal branch called the inferior suprarenal artery, which supplies the largest portion of the adrenal gland. Other portions are supplied by

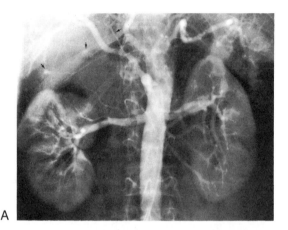

A

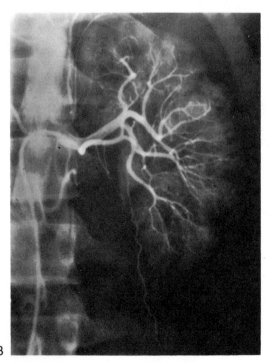

B

Figure 13–2. *(A)* Radiograph of a renal arteriogram made by the flush method. Note that the catheter is placed at the level of the renal vessels. Both kidneys are visualized in this manner. *(B)* Selective angiogram (arterial phase) showing wrapping of normal vessels around upper pole mass. Note the location of the catheter in the orifice in the renal artery. (From Witten, M. U.: Emmett's Clinical Urography: An Atlas and Textbook of Roentgenologic Diagnosis, 4th ed. Philadelphia, W. B. Saunders, 1977.)

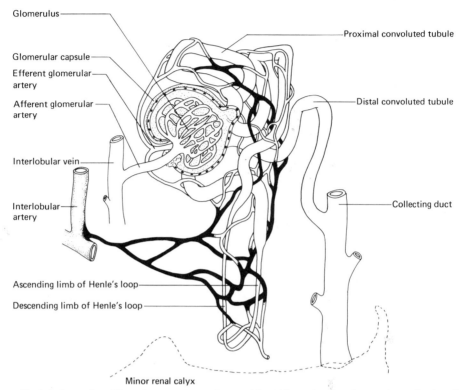

Glomerulus

Glomerular capsule

Efferent glomerular artery

Afferent glomerular artery

Interlobular vein

Interlobular artery

Ascending limb of Henle's loop

Descending limb of Henle's loop

Proximal convoluted tubule

Distal convoluted tubule

Collecting duct

Minor renal calyx

Figure 13–3. Schematic of the microscopic anatomy of the kidney showing the nephron, the functional unit of the organ.

the superior and middle suprarenal arteries, which are branches originating directly from the aorta. The adrenal glands are usually demonstrated during renal angiography.

Before the renal arteries enter the hilum of the kidney, each divides into five branches corresponding to the five renal segments. These enter the renal sinus and course both anteriorly and posteriorly to the renal pelvis (Fig. 13–5). The renal sinus is a recess containing the renal vessels and the renal pelvis, the upper expanded portion of the ureter.

In the renal sinus, the larger branches of the renal artery subdivide to form smaller interlobar branches. These vessels course between the lobes, in the renal columns, toward the periphery of the kidney. At the level of the renal cortex, the interlobar branches become the arcuate arteries. These arteries course along the line between the cortex and medulla and give off branches called the interlobular arteries.

Figure 13–4. Schematics of the gross internal structure of the kidney showing the renal pyramids and their termination in the renal calyx. (From Gardner, E., Gray, D. J., and O'Rahilly, R.: Anatomy, 3rd ed. Philadelphia, W. B. Saunders, 1969.)

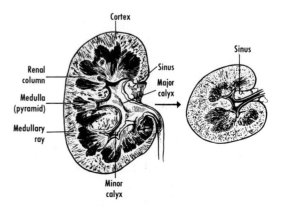

Cortex

Renal column

Medulla (pyramid)

Medullary ray

Minor calyx

Sinus

Major calyx

Sinus

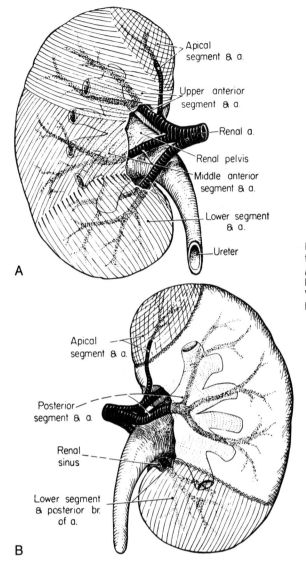

A

B

Figure 13–5. Schematics of the segmental branches of the renal arteries shown in the anterior *(A)* and posterior *(B)* aspects. Note that the renal artery gives branches both anteriorly and posteriorly to the renal pelvis. (From Woodburne, R. T.: Essentials of Human Anatomy, 4th ed. New York, Oxford University Press, 1969.)

The interlobular arteries subdivide into the afferent arterioles that course into the glomerulus (see Fig. 13–3). In the glomerulus, the afferent arteriole becomes an efferent arteriole and then forms a capillary plexus surrounding the straight and convoluted tubules.

Venous Drainage

The efferent arteriole plexus is continuous with small venules that unite to form interlobular and medullary veins. These drain into the arcuate veins, which course along the boundary of the cortex and medulla. Interlobar veins are formed by the arcuate veins and converge to form the renal vein, which ultimately drains into the inferior vena cava.

Table 13–1 summarizes, in order of filling, the vessels seen during the various phases of renal arteriography. It should be noted that when renal masses are evaluated with intravenous digital subtraction angiography, the catheter is placed in the inferior vena cava via the femoral approach. This technique demonstrates the patency of the inferior

Table 13–1. SUMMARY OF RENAL CIRCULATORY PATTERN

Phase	Vessels Observed
Arterial	Abdominal aorta (nonselective studies only), renal artery with extrarenal branches, segmental branches, interlobular arteries
Nephrogram	Arcuate arteries, interlobular arteries, afferent arterioles, efferent arterioles, venules, interlobular and medullary veins, arcuate veins, interlobular veins
Venous	Main renal veins

vena cava during the initial phase of the study. The later phases appear as stated in Table 13–1.

INDICATIONS AND CONTRAINDICATIONS

Renal angiography is indicated for the diagnosis of various vascular lesions[2] and as an adjunct to surgery or interventional therapy. Renovascular hypertension is the greatest indication for the use of this procedure. The following is a list of some of the renovascular problems that cause renal hypertension and that can be diagnosed with this procedure:

Atherosclerosis
   Stenosis
Fibromuscular disease
   Medial fibroplasia with mural aneurysm
   Perimedial fibroplasia
   Intimal fibroplasia
   Periarterial fibroplasia
Selective venous sampling for renin

In addition, this procedure is indicated for the presurgical mapping of renal neoplasms and for renal transplantation.

Renal angiography is also indicated in certain aspects of renal trauma. Although computed tomography and excretory urography are used extensively to diagnose renal contusions, tears, and infarctions, these studies are not as sensitive as renal angiography in determining renal arterial involvement. Angiography is usually indicated when arterial involvement such as laceration or occlusion is suspected.

Although the renal veins can usually be seen during the venous phase of the angiogram, renal venography via selective catheterization is the procedure of choice when the diagnosis of renal vein thrombosis is warranted.

The contraindications for renal angiography are few. Because the excretory pathway of most angiographic contrast agents is through glomerular filtration, severe renal diseases should be major contraindications.[3] However, severe renal disease is not a definite contraindication for renal angiography because complications are rare. Renal angiography has been performed on patients with severe renal disease without resulting in any major reactions. Catheter techniques may be contraindicated in the presence of certain vascular disease states. In these cases, other routes or methods of demonstrating the renal vascular anatomy may be used.

CONTRAST MEDIA

To opacify the renovascular system, water-soluble organic iodine contrast agents are usually used. Fully substituted tri-iodinated benzoic compounds can be used; however, the possibility of renal injury as the result of the contrast agent increases with its concentration within the organ. The use of low osmolality or nonionic contrast agents greatly reduces the incidence of reaction. These should be the media of choice for high-risk patients.

Renal injury can also occur if certain drugs are administered before injection of the contrast agent. If the vessel has been completely occluded by the catheter, as can occur during selective renal angiography, the possibility of a toxic reaction increases. Occlusion of the renal vessels by the catheter prevents the rapid flushing of the contrast agent through the renal circulation, causing an increase in the concentration over a larger period of time.

The amount of contrast agent injected depends on the technique used. Nonselective procedures require 25 to 30 ml of a 60, 75, or 76 per cent contrast agent, whereas selective techniques require 6 to 8 ml of a suitable radiopaque agent to opacify the renal vasculature.

PROCEDURE

The procedure methods of renal angiography can be classified as nonselective or selective. The nonselective techniques include translumbar injection and percutaneous nonselective catheterization (Fig. 13–6). The selective method also involves percutaneous catheterization. It differs from the nonselective catheterization method in that the catheter is placed within the lumen of a renal artery rather than in the aorta. Catheterization techniques have gained popularity because of their simplicity and safety, and they have become the common method by which the renal vascular system is opacified.

The translumbar approach is not usually used for renal angiography for several reasons, including the problems associated with the puncture technique itself and the fact that the patient must remain in the prone position during the procedure. The latter reason is important because the orifices of the renal vessels are located dorsally, and their opacification is made more difficult because of the position of the patient and the specific gravity of the contrast agent.

When the percutaneous catheterization method is used, it is possible to visualize the renal vasculature nonselectively or selectively. Nonselective renal studies require that the catheter be placed in the aorta at a level slightly above the orifices of the renal

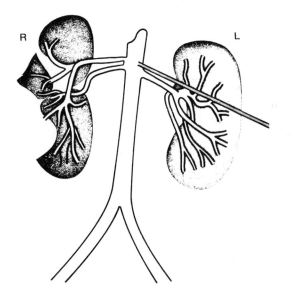

Figure 13–6. Schematic showing the location for the translumbar puncture in relation to the renal vessels. (From X-Ray Focus 12(2), 1973. Copyright Ilford, Inc.)

arteries. An injection made at this level will usually yield good filling of the renal arteries because it opacifies the vessels of both kidneys simultaneously. This type of study is indicated when comparison of the main renal arteries is desired; it can also be used to complement a selective study.

The selective renal angiogram involves placing the tip of the catheter within the lumen of the main renal artery. The catheter should be positioned so that it does not occlude the vessel into which it is placed. This is important to ensure that the contrast agent is flushed rapidly through the renal circulation.

Occasionally, a kidney may be supplied by more than one renal artery. In such a case, a single selective injection will not adequately demonstrate the complete renal vasculature, and a midstream aortogram is required. Usually, a midstream aortogram is done before selective opacification of the renal vasculature. This delineates the course and number of the main renal vessels and provides important information regarding the origin of these vessels.

As the contrast medium passes through the renovascular system, three phases can be

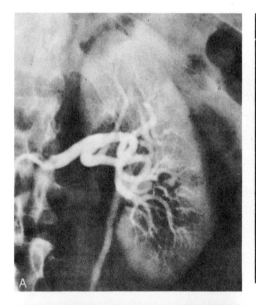

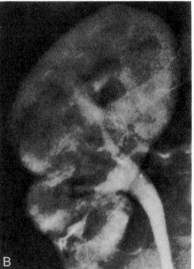

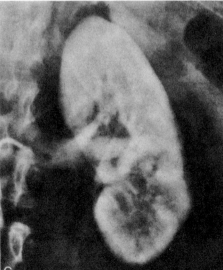

Figure 13–7. Radiographs of the phases of renal arteriography: *(A)* arterial phase; *(B)* early nephrogram phase; *(C)* venous phase. (*A* and *C* from Meschan, I.: Synopsis of Radiologic Anatomy with Computed Tomography, Philadelphia, W. B. Saunders, 1980; *B* from Witten, M. U.: Emmett's Clinical Urography: An Atlas and Textbook of Roentgenologic Diagnosis, 4th ed. Philadelphia, W. B. Saunders, 1977.)

demonstrated radiographically—the arteriogram, nephrogram, and venous phases (Fig. 13–7). During the arteriogram phase, exposures should be made at a frequency of at least two per second. An exposure frequency of one per second is satisfactory for the nephrogram and venous phases of renal angiography.

The nephrogram phase is caused by capillary opacification and the presence of the contrast agent in the excretory portion of the kidney. It best demonstrates the contour of the kidney and the renal hilum.

The venous phase begins during the nephrogram phase and can be best visualized from 5 to 9 s after injection. The exposure frequency should be programmed to include all three phases to yield a diagnostic renal angiogram.

Renal Venography

Renal venography is accomplished by passing a catheter from the femoral or cubital vein into the lumen of a main renal vein. When the catheter is positioned, the physician can perform venous sampling for renin levels, and contrast venography can be performed.

If renal venography is done, the physician may choose to partially occlude the renal artery to provide more homogeneous distribution of the contrast agent in the renal venous system. This can be accomplished chemically such as through the use of epinephrine diluted with 5 per cent glucose solution or mechanically such as through partial balloon occlusion of the renal artery. A representative filming sequence is three films per second for 2 s followed by one film per second for 4 s, with an injection rate of 15 to 18 ml/s for a total of 30 to 36 ml of contrast agent.

The venous sampling process is usually accomplished over a period of 30 min. Three separate blood samples are taken at 10-min intervals. The first two samples are drawn and placed into vials containing calcium disodium edetate. Immediately after the second sampling, the patient is given 20 mg Lasix to stimulate renin secretion from the kidney.

Postprocedural care is the same as for any angiographic procedure.

EQUIPMENT

The equipment requirements for angiographic special procedures are basically similar. In all cases, a method of recording the events of the procedure is necessary. Rapid sequence changers with minimum capabilities of from two to six exposures per second are recommended. The use of a cinerecording device is advantageous for recording the passage of the bolus of contrast agent through the system. Programming the exposure frequency of the rapid sequence changer should be done to yield the maximum amount of information about the procedure. The phases of renal angiography and the nature of the underlying disease should be considered when planning the sequence of exposures to be used. It should be remembered that maximum visualization of the venous phase generally occurs between 5 and 10 s after the start of the injection, and unless a vast amount of information is required about the venous drainage of the kidney, the filming can be completed within 9 s of the injection.

Injection equipment required for renal angiography varies with the procedural method chosen. With the translumbar approach, the contrast agent can be injected by hand or automatic injector. Catheter techniques usually require that the injection be made automatically. The optional electrocardiograph-triggering device that is available for automatic injection devices permits the injection to be made at the optimum point in the cardiac cycle (i.e., immediately before diastole). If the injection is made at diastole, the contrast medium maintains a satisfactory level of concentration, thereby requiring a smaller amount for adequate opacification. With the subsequent contraction of the heart, the contrast agent is flushed through the remaining renal vessels as a less-diluted bolus, providing optimum opacification during the later phases of the procedure.

Sterile trays and packs are required for the procedure; these should include the specialized puncture needle if the translumbar approach is to be used. For the catheterization procedures, a special catheterization pack is required. The catheter required varies with the procedure; the catheter required for a midstream aortogram is shaped differently than that used for selective renal angiography. The selective method requires a curve in the distal end of the catheter to facilitate entrance into the renal vessel orifice, whereas the catheter used for midstream techniques has no curve at its distal end. The curved distal end of the selective renal catheter must be large enough for the tip to be in the renal vessel while the curve lies on the opposite wall of the aorta. This prevents the catheter from being ejected from the vessel during injection of the contrast agent.

The catheterization procedures require use of an image intensification device to follow the placement of the catheter, either in the aorta or selectively into a renal vessel. This is also essential if cinerecording or videotaping of the procedure is to be done.

As in all angiographic procedures, complications may occur. Therefore, emergency equipment and supplies should be available in the special procedure suite before the examination to offset any crisis situation that may arise.

PATIENT POSITIONING

Patient positioning for renal angiography is somewhat dependent on the injection procedure used. If the translumbar approach is selected, the positioning is limited to the prone position. The needle location precludes any other position or excessive movement of the patient. The patient is centered on the table with the arms next to the body in a comfortable position. The shins should be supported, and the legs should be placed in internal rotation. The kidneys usually extend between the 12th thoracic and third lumbar vertebrae when the patient is recumbent. The central ray should be adjusted so that it passes through the abdomen at the level of the hilum of the kidney.

If percutaneous methods are used, the most common position is recumbent supine. The technique of catheter placement, however, allows more flexibility in patient positioning than the previous method. Occasionally, obliques may be required for

Table 13–2. SUMMARY OF POSITIONS FOR RENAL ANGIOGRAPHY

Procedure	Projection	Patient Position	Central Ray	Anatomy
Translumbar puncture	Posteroanterior	Patient prone, centered on table, arms at side of body, head in lateral position, shins supported, slight internal rotation of legs	Vertical beam to center of film changer, through midsagittal plane at level of kidney hilum	Renal arteries, aorta, and associated major branches
Percutaneous catheter	Anteroposterior	Patient supine, kidney of interest centered over changer (selective study); patient centered on table (midstream technique)	Vertical beam to center of film changer at level of kidney hilum	Renal arterial supply, accessory renal arteries
	Posterior oblique	Patient supine, rotated into right or left posterior oblique (position dependent on side to be studied)	Vertical beam to center of film changer at level of kidney hilum	Origin of renal arteries

better demonstration of the origin of the renal vessels. Again, the location of the central ray should be at the level of the hilum of the kidney. This is usually at the level of the first lumbar vertebra. Topographically, this point is approximately 2 in (5 cm) inferior to the xyphoid process.

Selective renal angiography requires that the particular kidney in question be centered over the film changer. Again, as in the previous methods, the central ray should pass through the hilum of the kidney. Table 13–2 is a summary of positioning for renal angiography.

REFERENCES

1. Woodburne, R. T.: Essentials of Human Anatomy, 7th ed. New York, Oxford University Press, 1983.
2. Bunnell, I. L.: Selective Renal Arteriography. Springfield, IL, Charles C Thomas, 1968.
3. Cattell, W. R.: Excretory pathways for contrast media, Invest. Radiol., 5:176, 1970.

SUGGESTED READINGS

RENAL ANGIOGRAPHY

Abrams, H. L. (ed.): Angiography: Vascular and Interventional Radiology, 3rd ed., Boston, Little, Brown & Co., 1983.

Bollack, C., et al.: Arteriography and cancer of the kidney, Prog. Clin. Biol. Res., 100:349, 1982.

Chait, A.: Current status of renal angiography, Urol. Clin. North Am., 12:687–698, 1985.

Cho, K. J.: Current role of angiography in the evaluation of adrenal disease causing hypertension, Urol. Radiol., 3:249, 1982.

Fu, W. R.: Angiography of Trauma, Springfield, IL, Charles C Thomas, 1972.

Gedroyc, W. M. W., Reidy, J. F., and Saxton, H. M.: Arteriography of renal transplantation, Clin. Radiol., 38:239, 1987.

Hanto, D. W., and Simmons, R. L.: Renal transplantation: Clinical considerations, Radiol. Clin. North Am., 25:239, 1987.

Harrington, D. P., et al.: Compound angulation for the angiographic evaluation of renal artery stenosis, Radiology, 146:829, 1983.

Hudson, E.: Renal arteriography, X-Ray Focus, 12:43, 1973.

Lang, E. K., Sullivan, J., and Frentz, G.: Renal trauma: Radiological studies, Radiology, 154:1–6, 1985.

Leiter, E., and Brendler, H.: Percutaneous transfemoral renal angiography, J. Mt. Sinai Hosp., 32:51, 1965.

Letourneau, J. G., Day, D. L., Ascher, N. L., et al.: Imaging of renal transplants, Am. J. Roentgenol., 150:833, 1988.

Mardis, H.: Technical considerations in renal arteriography: Some modifications of retrograde femoral catheterization technique, J. Urol., 93:627, 1965.

SPECIAL TECHNIQUES

Hillman, B. J.: Renovascular hypertension: Diagnosis of renal artery stenosis by digital video subtraction angiography, Urol. Radiol., 3:219, 1982.

Petty, W., Spigos, D. G., Abejo, R., et al.: Arterial digital angiography in the evaluation of potential renal donors. Invest. Radiol., 21:122–124, 1986.

Picus, D., Neeley, J. P., McClennan, B. L., et al.: Intraarterial digital subtraction angiography of renal transplants, Am. J. Roentgenol., 145:93, 1985.

Smith, C. W., et al.: Evaluation of digital venous angiography for the diagnosis of renovascular hypertension, Radiology, 144:564, 1982.

Winsett, M. Z., Amparo, E. G., Fawcett, H. D., et al.: Renal transplant dysfunction: MR evaluation, Am. J. Roentgenol., 150:319, 1988.

4 Cardiac Catheterization

fourteen

Selective Angiocardiography

ANATOMIC CONSIDERATIONS
Coronary Vascular System
Left Main Coronary Artery
Right Main Coronary Artery
Venous Drainage
INDICATIONS AND
    CONTRAINDICATIONS

CONTRAST MEDIA
PROCEDURE
Selective Angiocardiography
Coronary Arteriography
EQUIPMENT
PATIENT POSITIONING

Selective angiocardiography is the radiographic demonstration of the heart and its vasculature. Coronary arteriography is the specific procedure used to delineate the coronary artery system. These studies are usually performed in the cardiac catheterization suite and can be grouped under the general heading of "cardiac catheterization." Cardiac catheterization is used for the diagnosis, assessment of abnormalities, and evaluation of the effects of a pathological condition on the heart and great vessels.

The procedures are accomplished with standard angiographic catheterization techniques. They are relatively safe and may be used as diagnostic studies to determine the nature of the anatomy and any pathology and in conjunction with interventional procedures to effect a nonsurgical treatment.

ANATOMIC CONSIDERATIONS

The heart is a hollow muscular organ that lies obliquely in the left median portion of the lower thoracic cavity. It adjusts the circulation of the blood to the metabolic rate of the tissue cells; in essence, it is a pump.

The heart has an apex and a base. The apex is located approximately 8 cm from the median plane at about the level of the fifth or sixth interspace; this level is approximately 2.5 cm inferior to the left nipple. The base of the heart is the most superior portion. It faces up and to the right, and from it emerge the greater vessels (Fig. 14–1).

An obliquely placed septum divides the heart into right and left halves. Each half consists of two chambers—an atrium and a ventricle (Fig. 14–2).

The atria receive blood from the veins, and the ventricles propel blood into the arteries. Blood from the heart flows in two circuits—a short circulation called the pulmonary (or lesser) and a longer, more extensive one called the systemic (or greater).

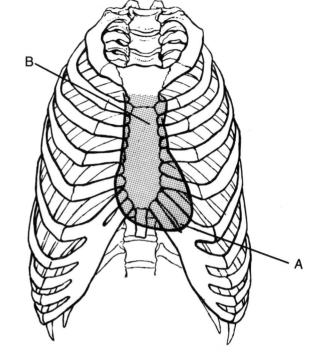

Figure 14–1. Schematic of the heart within the thoracic cavity showing *(A)* the apex, *(B)* the base, and their relationship to the bony thorax. (From Gardner, E., Gray, D. J., and O'Rahilly, R.: Anatomy, 4th ed., Philadelphia, W. B. Saunders, 1975.)

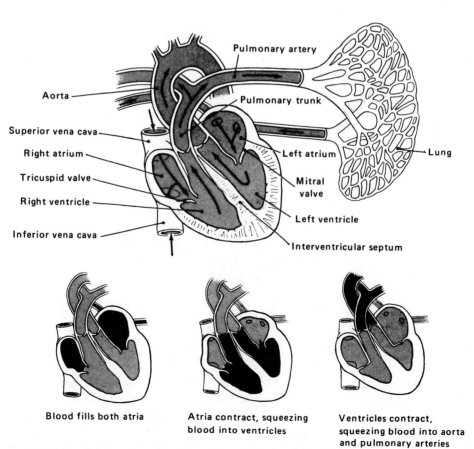

Blood fills both atria

Atria contract, squeezing blood into ventricles

Ventricles contract, squeezing blood into aorta and pulmonary arteries

Figure 14–2. Schematic of the heart showing the four chambers, the valves, the great vessels associated with it, and the flow of blood through it. (From Langley, L. L., Telford, I. R., and Christensen, J. B.: Dynamic Anatomy and Physiology, 4th ed., New York, McGraw-Hill, 1974. © Copyright Mosby-Year Book, Inc.)

The anatomy of the heart is easily understood if it is related to the flow of blood through it. Therefore, the anatomy of the heart is presented in relation to the blood flow, beginning with the drainage from the systemic circulation.

Blood returning from the systemic veins drains into the venae cavae. These great veins—the superior and inferior venae cavae—empty into the right atrium of the heart (Fig. 14–3). A small amount of venous blood drains from the myocardium directly into the right atrium; however, in general, the greatest portion of venous blood from the systemic circulation drains into the superior and inferior venae cavae.

With the contraction (systole) of the right atrium, the blood is forced into the right ventricle through the right atrioventricular aperture. This aperture is equipped with a valve, the tricuspid valve, that prevents the backflow of blood to the right atrium during systole of the ventricle. As the ventricle contracts, the blood is forced past the pulmonary semilunar valve into the pulmonary trunk and the lesser circulation. The arterial, or outflowing, portion of the right ventricle is called the conus arteriosus.[1] The pulmonary artery divides into right and left sides, which take the blood through the lungs. Here, the blood gives off carbon dioxide and becomes oxygenated. It is then transported by the four pulmonary veins to the left atrium (Fig. 14–4).

When the left atrium contracts, it forces the blood through the left atrioventricular valve into the left ventricle. This is the largest chamber of the heart, and its walls are considerably thicker than those of any of the previous chambers. The thicker walls and larger capacity are necessary to offset the arterial pressure in the aorta. The upper anterior portion of the left ventricle is called the aortic vestibule.[1] As the left ventricle contracts, the blood is pushed through the aortic semilunar valve into the aorta and through the systemic circulation (Fig. 14–5). The blood returns from the body tissues through the systemic veins, which ultimately drain into the superior and inferior venae cavae; then, the cycle begins again.

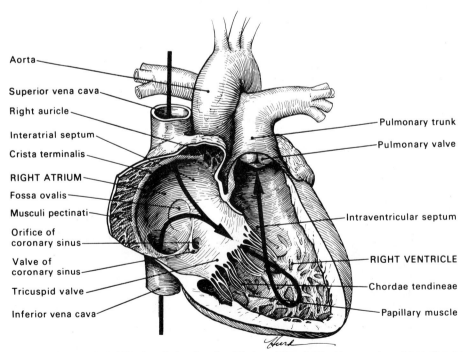

Aorta
Superior vena cava
Right auricle
Interatrial septum
Crista terminalis
RIGHT ATRIUM
Fossa ovalis
Musculi pectinati
Orifice of coronary sinus
Valve of coronary sinus
Tricuspid valve
Inferior vena cava

Pulmonary trunk
Pulmonary valve
Intraventricular septum
RIGHT VENTRICLE
Chordae tendineae
Papillary muscle

Figure 14–3. Schematic of the heart showing the interior of the right atrium and ventricle. The heavy arrows indicate the flow of blood from the venae cavae to the right atrium and from the right atrium to the right ventricle. (From Langley, L. L., Telford, I. R., and Christensen, J. B.: Dynamic Anatomy and Physiology, 4th ed., New York, McGraw-Hill, 1974. © Copyright Mosby-Year Book, Inc.)

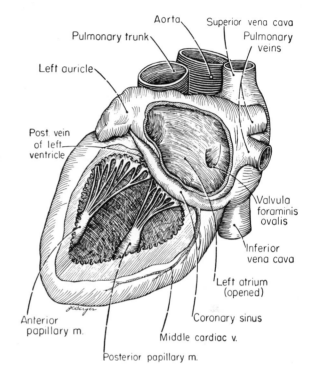

Figure 14–4. Schematic of the heart showing the left atrium and ventricle. The blood flows from the pulmonary veins to the left atrium, through the mitral valve into the left ventricle, and from there into the systemic circulation. (From Woodburne, R. T.: Essentials of Human Anatomy, 4th ed., New York, Oxford University Press, 1969.)

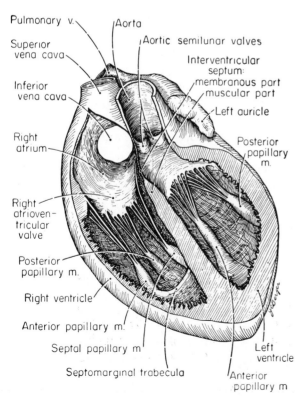

Figure 14–5. Schematic of the internal anatomy of the heart. The blood from the left ventricle passes through the aortic valve and into the general circulation. (From Woodburne, R. T.: Essentials of Human Anatomy, 4th ed., New York, Oxford University Press, 1969.)

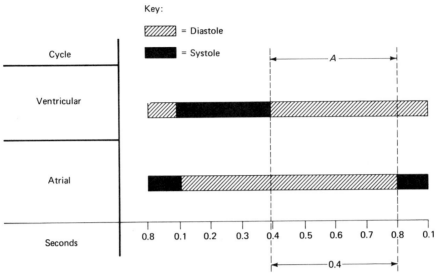

Figure 14–6. A graph of the cardiac cycle showing atrial and ventricular systole and diastole. It can be seen that the actual period of diastole is 0.7 s for the atria and 0.15 s for the ventricles. These periods overlap, giving the heart a period of 0.4 s complete quiescence *(A)*.

The cardiac cycle is repeated about 75 times per minute, and the time required for each cycle is about 0.8 s. The cycle consists of three phases—atrial contraction (systole), ventricular contraction (systole), and complete rest (diastole) (Fig. 14–6).[2]

Coronary Vascular System

The coronary arteries are the source of blood supplying the heart. We begin our discussion with the coronary anatomy at the aorta, which is the origin of the two main coronary arteries (Fig. 14–7). Three small dilations, or sinuses, are located in the root of the aorta. They lie opposite the corresponding cusps of the aortic valve. The coronary arteries arise from two of these, so they are considered coronary sinuses. The third sinus is considered a noncoronary sinus because it does not connect directly with any coronary arteries.

The left main coronary artery arises from the left posterior aortic sinus, and the right main coronary artery originates from the anterior, or right, aortic sinus. These sinuses are called the aortic sinuses, or Valsalva's sinuses.[3]

Left Main Coronary Artery

This artery originates in the left aortic sinus. It arises from a single opening in the upper portion of the sinus, and its length can vary from 2 to 3 mm to 3 to 4 cm. It divides to form the anterior interventricular branch (left anterior descending artery) and the left circumflex branch (Fig. 14–8).[4] These branches occupy the anterior interventricular sulcus and the atrioventricular sulcus, respectively. This oversimplification of the bifurcation of the left main coronary artery is provided because usually no more than two large branches of this artery can be found.[5]

The anterior interventricular branch is considered a direct continuation of the left main coronary artery. It courses toward the apex of the heart in the anterior interven-

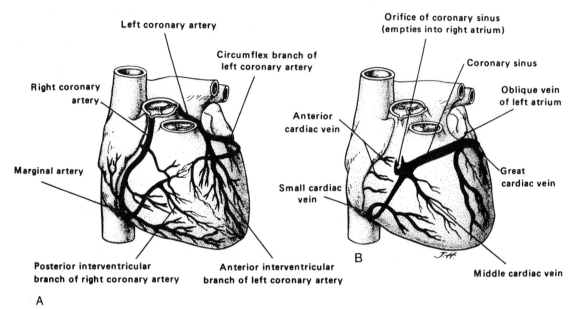

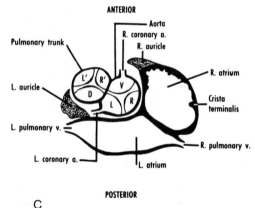

Figure 14–7. The coronary arteries. *(A)* An external view of the heart, showing the course of the left and right coronary arteries from their origin at the root of the aorta; *(B)* an external view of the heart showing the venous vasculature; *(C)* schematic of the three aortic sinuses at the root of the aorta, the origin of the coronary arteries, and their relation to the surrounding cardiac anatomy. (*A* and *B* from Langley, L. L., Telford, I. R., and Christensen, J. B.: Dynamic Anatomy and Physiology, New York, McGraw-Hill, 1974; © Copyright Mosby-Year Book, Inc. *C* from Gardner, E., Gray, D. J., and O'Rahilly, R.: Anatomy, 3rd ed., Philadelphia, W. B. Saunders, 1969.)

tricular sulcus. In the frontal view, the left anterior interventricular branch plus the left main coronary artery form a gently reversed S curve.[4] After reaching the apex of the heart, the left anterior interventricular branch continues up into the posterior interventricular sulcus and anastomoses with the terminal branches of the posterior interventricular branch of the right coronary artery.[2] Along its route, the left anterior interventricular branch gives off a variable number of arteries that course into the interventricular septum. At the level of the pulmonary valve, smaller branches are given off that supply the right ventricle. One or more of these branches form a curve around the heart and meet similar branches of the proximal right coronary artery. This circle is called Vieussens' ring, and it is an important means of collateral circulation between the right and left coronary arteries.[5] Some larger branches are given off to supply the free wall of the left ventricle. At times, one or more of these branches arise at the point of division of the left main coronary artery; these are usually called the diagonal left ventricular arteries.[5]

The left circumflex coronary artery, which is the second major branch of the left main coronary artery, courses at a sharp angle from its origin toward the left atrioventricular sulcus. It travels in this groove around to the back of the heart toward the right coronary artery, where anastomosis of these arteries frequently occurs. The circumflex artery gives off a large branch called the left marginal artery. As its name

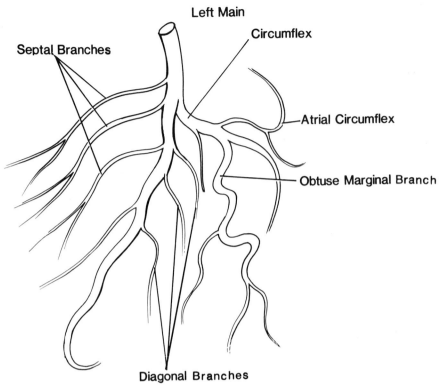

Figure 14–8. Left coronary artery in left anterior oblique projection with cephalad angulation. (From Gedgaudas, E., et al.: Cardiovascular Radiology, Philadelphia, W. B. Saunders, 1985, p. 235.)

implies, this artery courses along the left margin of the heart to supply the left ventricle. Branches of the left marginal artery course over the free wall of the left ventricle somewhat parallel to those given off by the left anterior interventricular branch (left anterior descending artery).

Right Main Coronary Artery

Frequently, the right main coronary artery has two aortic ostia, which may arise from the anterior aortic sinus and from a smaller adjacent ostium. When present, the second ostium is very small—about 1 mm in diameter. This is called the conus artery of the right coronary system (Fig. 14–9). It is this artery that frequently anastomoses with an opposing branch from the left anterior interventricular artery, forming Vieussens' ring. When the right main coronary artery arises from a single ostium in the aortic sinus, the first ventricular branch is considered the conus artery.

From its origin in the aortic sinus, the right main coronary artery courses in the right atrioventricular sulcus (coronary sulcus) to the diaphragmatic surface of the heart. At the acute margin of the heart, the right coronary artery gives off an artery called the right marginal branch, which courses almost to the apex of the heart. On the diaphragmatic surface of the heart, the right coronary artery makes a U turn and courses toward the apex of the heart in the posterior interventricular sulcus. This terminal portion of the right coronary artery is called the posterior interventricular branch (posterior descending artery).

The U turn of the right coronary artery is located at the crux of the heart. This is the point at which the right and left atrioventricular sulci cross the posterior interatrial and interventricular sulci. It is also here that the atrioventricular node artery originates from the right coronary artery.

On reaching the apex of the heart, the posterior interventricular branch frequently anastomoses with the anterior interventricular branch of the left coronary artery.

Venous Drainage

The venous drainage of the heart is considered to consist of three separate groups, rather than one.

The first group from the area of the left ventricle drains into the coronary sinus. Some prominent veins in this system are the anterior interventricular, posterior interventricular (middle cardiac), and left marginal veins. As it enters the atrioventricular sulcus, the anterior interventricular vein becomes the great cardiac vein, which in turn becomes the coronary sinus. The posterior interventricular vein usually drains directly into the right atrium; however, it often joins the coronary sinus just before entering the atrium. The left marginal vein and associated smaller vessels drain from the left ventricle into the great cardiac vein and coronary sinus.[5]

In the second group, several large veins called the anterior cardiac veins transport venous blood from the area of the right ventricle and drain directly into the right atrium. The most prominent of these veins—the right marginal vein—drains the lower margin of the heart.

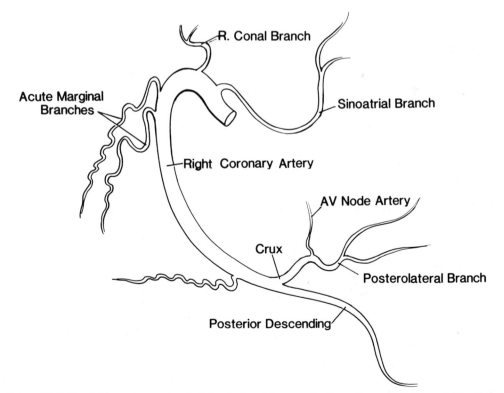

Figure 14–9. The right coronary artery in left anterior oblique projection with cephalad angulation. Note that the crux is well visualized. (From Gedgaudas, E., et al.: Cardiovascular Radiology, Philadelphia, W. B. Saunders, 1985, p. 233.)

The third group consists of many very small veins—the venae cordes minimal or thebesian veins.[1] These begin in the myocardium and mainly terminate by draining directly into the atria. They occur often on the right side of the heart but seldom on the left side.

INDICATIONS AND CONTRAINDICATIONS

Angiocardiography is useful in the diagnosis of septal defects; it provides a detailed appraisal of complex congenital diseases, such as truncus arteriosus or transposition of the great vessels.

Coronary arteriography has a wide variety of indications; however, the main purpose of the study is to provide a clear-cut definition of the coronary anatomy. Coronary arteriography provides information regarding the angiographic appearance of the coronary vascular system that can be used in conjunction with clinical findings and symptoms to obtain an accurate diagnosis of many congenital and acquired coronary diseases. The study can be used to assess the necessity and approach for interventional techniques and to present information about the condition and distribution of the coronary anatomy in patients undergoing cardiac surgery. The following is a summary of some of the indications for angiocardiography and coronary arteriography:

Coronary atherosclerosis
   Evaluation of collateral pathways
   Preoperative evaluation of disease
   Assessment of surgical results
   Evaluation of drug therapy
Chest pain of uncertain origin
Congenital coronary abnormalities
   Septal defects
   Aortic arch anomalies
   Increased cardiac size
   Anomalous left coronary artery
   Primary endocardial fibroelastosis
   Tetralogy of Fallot
   Peripheral pulmonary arterial stenosis
   Valvular pulmonary stenosis
Acquired valvular heart diseases
Acquired vascular diseases
Preoperative and postoperative evaluations of patients undergoing cardiac surgery

Among the few contraindications for these procedures are severe hepatorenal disease and active infection or bacterial endocarditis. Use of nonionic contrast agents reduces the risks associated with the administration of a contrast agent. Also, any factor that limits the catheterization procedure, such as the absence of a pulse in an extremity, is a contraindication for catheterization in that extremity.

These procedures are relatively safe, but they are not entirely without risk, and careful, continuous monitoring of the patient is needed throughout the procedure to ensure maximum safety.

CONTRAST MEDIA

Positive contrast (radiopaque) agents are usually used for angiocardiography, but carbon dioxide, a negative contrast material, can be used to diagnose tumors of the right atrium or pericardial effusion.[6, 7] However, this is not usually done, and conse-quently is not discussed here.

The positive contrast agents used must possess a low viscosity, be relatively nontoxic, and be highly radiopaque. The ideal contrast agent does not exist, but many contrast agents are satisfactory for use in this procedure. If a contrast agent with a high viscosity is used, it should be warmed to body temperature before use. The use of nonionic contrast agents reduces the risk of contrast-related reactions. The choice of the contrast agent is made by the physician performing the procedure and/or the protocol of the institution. For some typical parameters, see Tables 3–2 and 3–3.

PROCEDURE

Selective Angiocardiography

Selective angiocardiography is performed by inserting a catheter into any of the chambers of the heart or into the pulmonary artery. This procedure is more time consuming than the intravenous method, but the results are superior because of the lack of superimposition of the other opacified anatomic regions and the nominal amount of contrast media dilution. Selective cardiac catheterization is divided into right- and left-sided catheterization.

Selective right cardiac catheterization of the atrium or ventricle is accomplished by inserting a catheter into a peripheral vein of the upper or lower extremity and advancing it into the chambers of the right heart or pulmonary artery. Placement of the catheter should be monitored with an image intensifier.

Selective left cardiac catheterization of the left ventricle and atrium can be accom-plished through various methods. (A detailed description of each method of left heart catheterization is beyond the scope of this text; therefore, selected references devoted to these methods are given at the end of the chapter.)

Coronary Arteriography

Before discussing the various procedures used for coronary arteriography, an under-standing of the circulatory physiology of the coronary artery system is necessary.

Unlike other vascular filling that occurs during the systolic phase of the cardiac cycle, the coronary arteries accept blood only during diastole. This is understood easily if you recall the location of the ostia of the coronary arteries at the root of the aorta. In this location, as the systolic phase occurs, the comparatively small coronary vessels are compressed, preventing the forward flow of blood through the coronary vascular system. During the diastolic phase, however, this compression is released, and the forward flow of blood in the coronary vascular system can occur. Therefore, the optimum time for injection of contrast medium is during cardiac diastole. This phase is relatively short, and simply attempting to inject during this phase is inadequate without improving the forward flow of the contrast medium by other means. An obvious improvement is to prolong the diastolic phase, with a corresponding increase in the inflow of the coronary vascular system.

Another factor affecting the visualization of the coronary vascular system is the cardiac output during systole. If an injection of contrast medium is made at the root of the aorta, considerable dilution occurs as a result of the high velocity of blood flow from the heart. A method by which the high concentration of contrast can be maintained is the reduction of the velocity of blood flowing from the heart, which in essence reduces cardiac output.

Successful opacification of the coronary vessels also depends on the flow of contrast agent into and through the coronary vascular system itself. Therefore, it is necessary to increase forward flow through the coronary vascular system by decreasing coronary resistance and increasing aortic diastolic pressure. This can be accomplished with the use of coronary vasodilators and occlusion of the aorta, respectively. One result of the injection of the contrast medium into the vascular system is vasodilation, which promotes an increase in flow.[8]

The methods used to opacify the coronary vascular system can be divided into two broad categories—the nonselective, or aortic flush, methods and the selective catheterization methods.

All of the nonselective methods involve the injection under high pressure of a large amount of contrast agent at the root of the aorta. Variations in the efficiency of the method occur when modifications of techniques are used. The simplest nonselective method consists of a random injection of a large amount of contrast agent at the root of the aorta. This method is grossly inefficient because of the physiological factors discussed above. Various modifications of the basic nonselective injection technique have been used in an attempt to create ideal physiological conditions during the injection. Among these have been the addition of the ECG-activated automatic syringe, which can phase the injection of contrast agent with the diastolic phase of the cardiac cycle. This technique results in improved coronary visualization with the use of smaller amounts of contrast agents.

The specialized nonselective coronary "loop" catheters introduced by Bellman et al. in 1959 and elaborated on by Paulin have resulted in improved visualization of the coronary vascular system.[9, 10]

Other modifications of the random nonselective injection that improve visualization of the coronary artery system include the use of acetylcholine-induced cardiac arrest, which effectively prolongs the diastolic phase and improves filling of the coronary vessels; aortic occlusion with specialized balloon catheters; and a decrease in cardiac output by using increased intrabronchial pressure or by having the patient perform a Valsalva maneuver during the injection.[11]

All of the aortic flush methods have the limitation of superimposing the aortic root over the coronary ostia and proximal portions of the coronary arteries.

Selective coronary arteriography was first performed by Sones et al.[12] Modifications of the original technique have been used since its introduction (see "Suggested Readings" at the end of the chapter). Of these modifications, two have emerged as those most widely used today—the Amplatz and Judkins techniques. The basis of the original Sones technique involves the passage of a catheter from a peripheral artery to the root of the aorta. Through various manipulations, it is placed in the orifice or in a coronary artery. The required catheter has a specially tapered tip that is unsuitable for automatic injection devices. It is important that the catheter does not occlude the coronary artery.

Both the Amplatz and the Judkins technique involve differently shaped catheters for each coronary artery. The physician can locate the arterial orifice with a minimum of catheter manipulation.

Some complications that may occur during selective coronary arteriography are ventricular fibrillation, asystole, coronary spasm, and death. Because the procedure presents some risk, the patient should be monitored throughout the examination, and emergency care equipment should be available in the special procedure room in case any problems arise.

EQUIPMENT

The equipment required for cardiac catheterization and interventional cardiology is much more sophisticated than that for other angiographic studies. Certain measurements, such as measurement of the oxygen content of the chambers of the heart and great vessels, blood flow, and intracardiac pressure, and many other specialized tests can be made with the patient in a resting state. However, it is sometimes essential to the diagnosis to know the patient's cardiac response to physical stress. To accomplish this, the cardiac catheterization suite may have associated stress testing laboratories and/or specialized testing apparatus. These can be simple or sophisticated depending on the institution. The specifics of the cardiac catheterization suite are discussed in Chapter 1.

The system requires that the physician be able to manipulate the equipment to image the heart in a variety of complex projections (Fig. 14–10). Magnification radiography is also often performed, and the equipment should facilitate its use. In addition, biplane radiography is essential to the performance of the study. This enables the physician to keep the volume of contrast agent to a minimum. In most cases, cardiac catheterization suites are equipped with digital radiography units capable of performing subtraction.

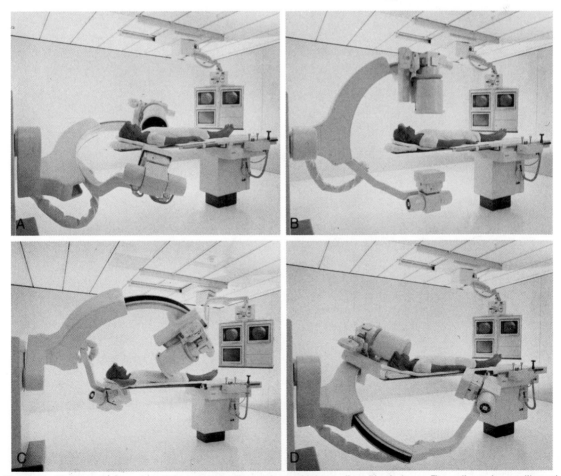

Figure 14–10. Siemens Coroskop C for angiocardiography and interventional techniques. The unit can be positioned with high speed to provide a wide variety of different positions without moving the patient. (A) Right and circumflex coronary arteries and mitral and tricuspid valves; (B) left coronary artery; (C) left coronary artery and atrial septum; (D) four-chamber view. (From Siemens Corporation.)

Table 14–1. STERILE PACK FOR CARDIAC CATHETERIZATION

Equipment	Amount, Type, and/or Size
Mosquito forceps	Straight
Mosquito forceps	Curved
Retractors	
Tissue forceps	
Probe	
Gowns	
Scalpel blades and handle	
Scissors	Dressing
Scissors	Operating
Variety of needles	
Syringe	1 (10 ml)
Syringe	1 (5 ml)
Syringes	3 (30 ml)
Three-way stopcock and rubber tubing connections	
Small glass containers	
Sponges	4 × 4 in
Sterile draping material and towels	
Suturing material	

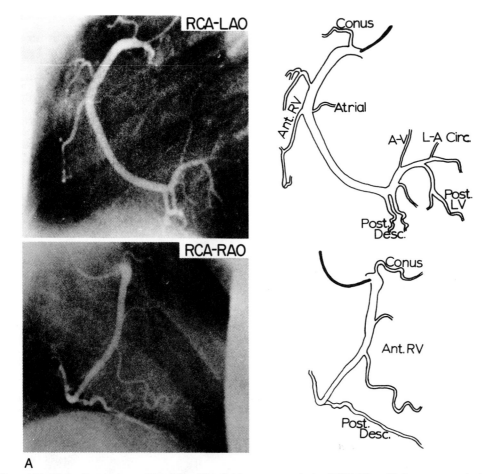

A

Figure 14–11. Radiographs and tracings of the right coronary arteries (RCA) *(A)* and left coronary arteries (LCA) *(B)* in the left anterior oblique (LAO) and right anterior oblique (RAO) projections. (From Cooley, R. N., and Schreiber, M. H.: Radiology of the Heart and Great Vessels, 2nd ed. © 1967, the Williams & Wilkins Co., Baltimore.)

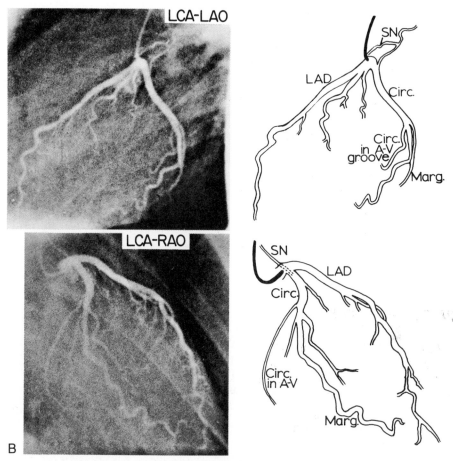

B

Figure 14–11 *Continued (B) See legend on opposite page*

The study is usually recorded using cineradiography and can be archived on digital media or magnetic tape.

Sterile catheterization trays should contain the surgical equipment necessary for the procedure. Table 14–1 is a list of supplies found in a sample sterile tray for catheterization. A sufficient number and variety of vascular catheters should be available for the procedure. Additional equipment necessary for cardiac catheterization includes the following:

Skin cleanser
Normal saline solution
Heparinized saline solution
Contrast media
Anesthetic agent
Emergency drug cart
Cardiopulmonary resuscitation equipment

An automatic injection device is also an essential piece of equipment for the suite. The unit should be equipped with an electrocardiogram trigger and the capabilities for phased injections.

Table 14–2. SUMMARY OF TYPICAL POSITIONS USED DURING SELECTIVE CORONARY ARTERIOGRAPHY

Left Coronary Artery	Right Coronary Artery
Anteroposterior	Anteroposterior
Perpendicular	Cephalic angulation
Cephalic angulation	Right anterior oblique 45°
Caudal angulation	Cephalic angulation
Right anterior oblique 45°	Caudal angulation
Perpendicular	Left anterior oblique 30°
Cephalic angulation	Perpendicular
Caudal angulation	
Left anterior oblique 45°	
Cephalic angulation	
Caudal angulation	
Left anterior oblique 60°	
Perpendicular	
Left lateral	
Perpendicular	

PATIENT POSITIONING

In general, single-projection studies are inadequate for the proper demonstration of the cardiac and coronary vascular anatomy. The exact positioning is determined by the pathology and the physician performing the study. Most studies require a combination of projections, which can be achieved with the radiographic equipment in a cardiac catheterization suite (Fig. 14–11). A biplane C-arm system can facilitate obtaining the projections. Table 14–2 is a summary of some typical positions used during selective coronary arteriography.

REFERENCES

1. Gardner, E., Gray, D. J., and O'Rahilly, R.: Anatomy: A Regional Study of Human Structure, 4th ed., Philadelphia, W. B. Saunders, 1975.
2. Woodburne, R. T.: Essentials of Human Anatomy: 7th ed. New York, Oxford University Press, 1983.
3. Kimber, D. C., et al.: Anatomy and Physiology, 15th ed. New York, Macmillan, 1966.
4. Schobinger, R. A., and Ruzicka, F. F., Jr.: Vascular Roentgenography. New York, Macmillan, 1964.
5. James, T. N.: Anatomy of the Coronary Arteries. New York, Harper & Row, 1961.
6. Paul, R. E., et al.: Intravenous carbon dioxide for intracardiac gas contrast in the roentgen diagnosis of pericardial effusion and thickening, Am. J. Roentgenol., 78:224, 1957.
7. Viamonte, M., Jr.: CO_2 angiocardiography: Im-
proved technique and results, Am. J. Roentgenol., 88:31, 1962.
8. Friesinger, G. C., et al.: Hemodynamic consequences of the injection of radiopaque material, Circulation, 31:730, 1965.
9. Bellman, S., et al.: Coronary arteriography: Differential opacification of the aortic stream by catheters of special design—experimental development, N. Engl. J. Med., 262:325, 1960.
10. Paulin, S.: Coronary angiography—a technical, anatomic and clinical study, Acta Radiol. [Suppl.] (Stockh.), 233:1, 1964.
11. Dotter, C. T., and Frische, L. H.: Visualization of the coronary circulation by occlusion aortography: A practical method, Radiology, 71:502, 1958.
12. Sones, F. M., et al.: Cine-coronary arteriography, Circulation, 20:773, 1959.

SUGGESTED READINGS

SELECTIVE ANGIOCARDIOGRAPHY

Biermann, M. D.: Selective Arterial Catherization. Springfield, IL, Charles C Thomas, 1969.

Block, P. C., et al.: A prospective randomized trial of outpatient versus inpatient cardiac catheterization, N. Engl. J. Med., 319:1251, 1988.
Bonzel, T., et al.: Isocentric biplane angiocardiog-

raphy for hemiaxial left ventricular volume estimation: First results, Cardiology, *1*(Suppl.):127, 1981.

Buonocore, E., et al.: Anatomic and functional imaging of congenital heart disease with digital subtraction angiography, Radiology, *147*:647, 1983.

Cooley, R. N., and Schreiber, M. H.: Radiology of the Heart and Great Vessels, 3rd ed. Baltimore, Williams & Wilkins, 1978.

Erikson, U.: Safety in angiography: II. Catheters, Ann. Radiol., *22*:351, 1979.

Gertz, E. W., et al.: Improved radiation protection for physicians performing cardiac catheterization, Am. J. Cardiol., *50*:1283, 1982.

Lowe, C. A.: Trends in angiocardiography in congenital heart disease, Radiology, *47*:97, 1981.

Mahrer, P. R., Young, C., and Magnusson, P. T.: Efficacy and safety of outpatient catheterization, Cathet. Cardiovasc. Diagn., *13*:304, 1987.

Meschan, I.: Radiographic Positioning and Related Anatomy, 2nd ed. Philadelphia, W. B. Saunders, 1978.

Rahimtoola, S. H.: The need for cardiac catheterization and angiography in valvular heart disease is not disproven, Ann. Intern. Med., *97*:433, 1982.

Stockton, D. L.: Cardiac catheterization and angiocardiography at the National Institutes of Health: Development, progress and techniques, Radiol. Technol., *40*:25, 1968.

Watson, J. C.: Patient Care and Special Procedures in Radiologic Technology, 3rd ed. St. Louis, C. V. Mosby, 1969.

Verel, M. D., and Grainger, M. D.: Cardiac Catheterization and Angiocardiography: An Introductory Manual, 3rd ed. New York, Churchill Livingstone, 1978.

SELECTIVE CORONARY ARTERIOGRAPHIC TECHNIQUE

Amplatz, K., and Harner, R.: New subclavian artery catheterization technic: Preliminary report, Radiology, *78*:963, 1962.

Cumberland, D. C.: Amipaque in coronary angiography and left ventriculography, Br. J. Radiol., *54*:203, 1981.

Grollman, J. H., Jr., Hanafel, W., and MacAlpin R.: Guided coronary arteriography and left ventriculography, Radiology, *91*:315, 1968.

Johnson, L. W., et al.: Coronary arteriography 1984—1987: A report of the Registry of the Society for Cardiac Angiography and Interventions. I. Results and complications, Cathet. Cardiovasc. Diagn., *17*:5, 1989.

Judkins, M. P.: Percutaneous transfemoral selective coronary arteriography, Radiol. Clin. North Am., *6*:467, 1968.

Koppes, G. M.: Complication rate of power coronary angiography injection, Angiology, *31*:130, 1980.

Lee, G. B., and Amplatz, K.: Coronary arteriography: Selective vs. non-selective methods, Minn. Med., *51*:343, 1968.

Lee, G. B., and Amplatz, K.: Selective coronary arteriography, J.A.M.A., *204*:444, 1968.

Lehman, J. S., et al.: Selective coronary arteriography, Radiology, *83*:846, 1964.

Meyerowitz, P. D., et al.: Digital subtraction angiography as a method of screening for coronary artery disease during peripheral vascular angiography, Surgery, *92*:1042, 1982.

Ricketts, H. J., and Abrams, H. L.: Percutaneous selective coronary cine arteriography, J.A.M.A., *181*:620, 1962.

Schroeder, S. A.: The complications of coronary arteriography: A problem that won't go away, Am. Heart J., *99*:139, 1980.

Sewell, W. H.: Coronary arteriography by the Sones technique—technical considerations, Am. J. Roentgenol., *95*:673, 1965.

Sheldon, W. C.: Technics for coronary arteriography, Cathet. Cardiovasc. Diagn., *5*:191, 1979.

Takaro, T., et al.: Coronary arteriography: Indications, techniques, complications, Thorac. Surg., *5*:213, 1968.

Viamonte, M., Gosselin, A. J., and Sommer, L. S.: Coronary arteriography, Am. J. Roentgenol., *92*:872, 1964.

5

Neuroradiography

Innovations in radiographic equipment and techniques have resulted in changes in the way nervous system disorders are diagnosed and treated. Computed tomography and magnetic resonance imaging are used more frequently to image pathology of the nervous system and will continue to increase in importance as improvements are made in the specificity of contrast media (organ versus disease), equipment, and procedures. Techniques such as myelography and angiography still have a place in a physician's diagnostic armamentarium; however, these studies will make increasing use of digital radiographic techniques. Interventional neuroradiology will grow in importance as newer advances develop.

This textbook focuses on myelography and cerebral angiography in its discussion of the special procedures used for neuroradiologic diagnosis because use of these techniques is relatively stable. The newer techniques, as applied to magnetic resonance imaging and computed tomography, have been discussed as they apply to special procedure radiography in general. The dramatic changes occurring in these areas preclude any in-depth presentations of techniques that in all probability will be obsolete as this book goes to print.

fifteen

Cerebral Angiography

ANATOMIC CONSIDERATIONS
Arterial Supply
   Internal Carotid Artery
   Vertebrobasilar System
   Circle of Willis
Venous Drainage
INDICATIONS AND
  CONTRAINDICATIONS

CONTRAST MEDIA
PROCEDURE
Direct Puncture Technique
EQUIPMENT
PATIENT POSITIONING

The demonstration of the cerebrovascular system through the use of contrast material is called "cerebral angiography." It had its official beginnings in 1927 when it was presented to the Neurologic Society of Paris by Egas Moniz, a Portuguese neurologist.[1] Since its presentation, there have been many improvements in technique, contrast media, and equipment. Recent advances have centered around catheter technique, contrast media, computed tomography, magnetic resonance imaging, the use of digital subtraction, and interventional neuroradiology techniques. The interest in cerebral angiography throughout the years has been responsible for the development of the specialized field of neuroradiology.

ANATOMIC CONSIDERATIONS

Cerebral angiography provides the physician with a wealth of information regarding the anatomy of the cerebral vascular system as well as indirect information regarding the superficial and deep-lying structures of the brain. A great deal of knowledge has been compiled concerning the anatomy of the cerebrovascular system, most of which is not discussed in this text. However, a general summary of the major vessels of the cerebrovascular system is presented. The variations in arteries and veins are not considered to avoid the possibility of confusion. (For greater detail regarding the normal anatomic relation and variations, references are made to selected comprehensive monographs and other works on the subject in "Suggested Readings" at the end of this chapter.)

Arterial Supply

A discussion of the cerebrovascular system must begin with the aortic arch, which is where the major vessels originate. The aortic arch has three major branches—the brachiocephalic trunk, the left common carotid artery, and the left subclavian artery (Fig. 15–1). The brachiocephalic trunk is about 4 to 5 cm long at the upper border of the right sternoclavicular articulation and bifurcates into the right subclavian and right common carotid arteries. The left common carotid artery originates at the highest point of the aortic arch. It ascends to the left sternoclavicular joint, where it enters the neck. The common carotid arteries are unequal in length, with the left being 4 to 5 cm longer than the right. The carotid line, which begins at the sternoclavicular joint and terminates midway between the angle of the mandible and the mastoid process of the temporal bone, defines the course of the carotid artery.[2] At the cranial edge of the thyroid cartilage, the common carotid arteries divide terminally into two main branches—the internal and external carotid arteries. At its bifurcation, there is a dilation of the terminal portion of the common carotid artery and the base of the internal carotid artery; this dilated portion is called the carotid sinus.

INTERNAL CAROTID ARTERY

The internal carotid artery has no named branches in its cervical region. It supplies chiefly the frontal, parietal, and temporal lobes of the brain and orbital structures. It accompanies the internal jugular vein to the base of the skull and enters the carotid canal in the petrous portion of the temporal bone. The internal carotid artery ascends to the peak of the pyramid, curves forward and then medially, and courses laterally to the sphenoidal structures (S5).[1] The artery then enters the cavernous sinus and passes next to the sella turcica (S4). It ascends, passes through the dural roof of the sinus under the base of the anterior clinoid process (S3), and then courses backward, passing under the optic nerve. At this point, the artery lies in the subarachnoid space (S2). It then ascends, dividing into the anterior and middle cerebral arteries (S1). The curving portions of the internal carotid artery, designated S2, S3, and S4, were called the carotid siphon by Moniz (Fig. 15–2). The ophthalmic artery originates at point S3 of the carotid siphon. Two other arteries arise as branches of the carotid siphon—the anterior choroidal and posterior communicating arteries.

The two main terminal branches of the internal carotid artery are the anterior cerebral and middle cerebral arteries. The anterior cerebral artery is the smaller of the two main branches. It continues from the bifurcation of the internal carotid as the medial branch, entering the longitudinal fissure of the cerebrum. (The longitudinal fissure

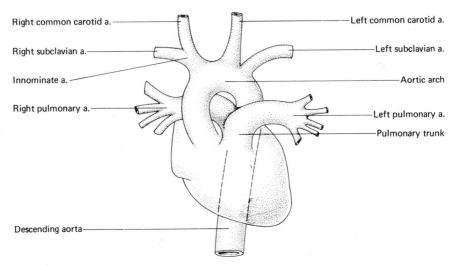

Figure 15–1. Schematic of the aortic arch and its major branches.

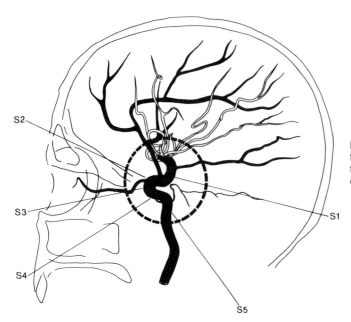

Figure 15–2. Schematic of the lateral view of the skull with arteries showing the course of the internal carotid artery. The portion in the circle is termed the carotid siphon.

separates the right and left cerebral hemispheres.) At this point, the two anterior cerebral arteries are near one another and are joined by the anterior communicating artery. This is the shortest of the cerebral arteries and connects the arterial systems of both hemispheres. It is generally thought that the anterior cerebral artery runs to the origin of the callosomarginal artery.[1] From this point, it is called the pericallosal artery.

The largest branch of the internal carotid artery is the middle cerebral artery. It courses laterally and is considered a direct continuation of the internal carotid artery. The middle cerebral artery appears to have many coils and loops as a result of the fetal growth of the cerebral hemisphere. During fetal development, the middle cerebral artery and its branches course smoothly over the insula, the central lobe of a cerebral hemisphere, which is also called the island of Reil. With further fetal evolution, the insula sinks deeply into the cerebral hemisphere, giving the middle cerebral artery and its branches a coiled appearance in this area. This occurs when the branches of the middle cerebral artery course superiorly in the sylvian fissure until they rise to the top of the island of Reil. From this point, they course laterally and inferiorly to the opening of the sylvian fissure and become dispersed in the cerebral hemispheres.

The island of Reil is a triangular structure that can be delineated by the middle cerebral artery and its branches, which form the sylvian triangle (see Fig. 15–3). This is a very important anatomic landmark; it is usually affected by most mass lesions, and any shift will probably be demonstrated angiographically.

The middle cerebral artery gives off many branches that are usually named for the areas they supply. They have a fan-shaped appearance and can be best seen in the lateral projection. The last branch leaving the sylvian triangle denotes the sylvian point and is called the angular branch. The middle cerebral artery and its branches supply the sensory, auditory, and motor areas of the brain.

VERTEBROBASILAR SYSTEM

Another important arterial system that supplies the posteroinferior portion of the brain, brain stem, and cerebellum is the vertebrobasilar system (Fig. 15–4). The vertebral arteries originate as branches of the subclavian arteries. The left is longer than the right, because the right subclavian artery originates as a branch of the brachiocephalic artery. The vertebral arteries course through the cervical region and then through the foramen magnum into the skull. Running parallel to each other for a short distance, the vertebral arteries begin to converge and then unite to form the basilar artery.

The basilar artery begins at the lower border of the pons and terminally divides into the paired posterior cerebral arteries. In general, the basilar artery can be found traveling in the longitudinal groove at the front of the pons (Fig. 15–5). A short distance after the union of the vertebral arteries, the paired anteroinferior cerebellar arteries arise as branches of the basilar artery. There are numerous pontine branches (paramedian arteries) coursing perpendicularly into the pons. As their name implies, these branches supply the pons. The paired superior cerebellar arteries can be found just before the terminal bifurcation of the basilar artery. These supply the upper surface of the cerebellum. The posterior cerebral arteries supply the inferior and medial surfaces of the temporal and occipital lobes.

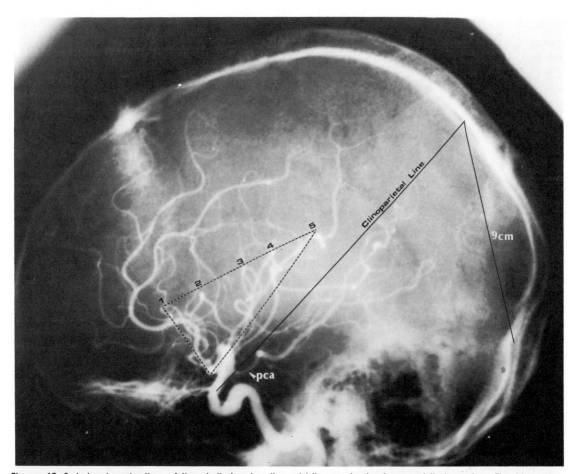

Figure 15–3. Lateral projection of the skull showing the middle cerebral artery and its branches. The triangular-shaped dotted line illustrates the sylvian triangle. The upper border or roof can be formed by drawing a line across the loops of the branches of the middle cerebral artery (numbered from 1 to 5 as they rise to the top of the sylvian fissure). Number 5 denotes the angular branch and the sylvian point. The floor of the sylvian triangle is shown by a dotted line drawn from the sylvian point to the genu (the area in which the middle cerebral artery bifurcates at its most lateral point). The anterior part of the sylvian triangle is demonstrated by connecting the anterior loop of the middle cerebral artery with the genu. (From Ramsey, R. G.: Neuroradiology with Computed Tomography, Philadelphia, W. B. Saunders, 1982.)

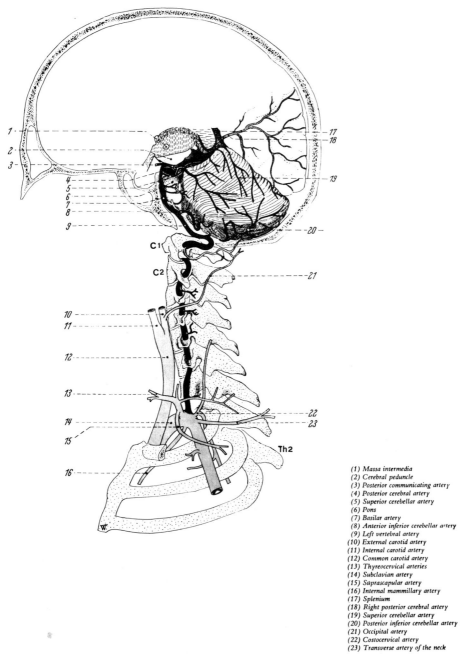

Figure 15–4. Schematic of the course of the arteries in the vertebrobasilar system. (From Krayenbuhl, H., and Yasargil, M.: Cerebral Angiography, 2nd ed., London, Butterworth Publishers, 1968.)

(1) Massa intermedia
(2) Cerebral peduncle
(3) Posterior communicating artery
(4) Posterior cerebral artery
(5) Superior cerebellar artery
(6) Pons
(7) Basilar artery
(8) Anterior inferior cerebellar artery
(9) Left vertebral artery
(10) External carotid artery
(11) Internal carotid artery
(12) Common carotid artery
(13) Thyreocervical arteries
(14) Subclavian artery
(15) Suprascapular artery
(16) Internal mammillary artery
(17) Splenium
(18) Right posterior cerebral artery
(19) Superior cerebellar artery
(20) Posterior inferior cerebellar artery
(21) Occipital artery
(22) Costocervical artery
(23) Transverse artery of the neck

CIRCLE OF WILLIS

Many cerebral arteries anastomose with each other on the surface of the brain. One major anastomosis, the circle of Willis (circulus arteriosus), is a union of the four major arteries supplying the brain (Fig. 15–6). This is not a direct union of the internal carotid and vertebral arteries but rather is formed by the major branches of these arteries. Through this anastomosis, an important means of collateral circulation is formed. In the event of obstruction of one of the arteries, circulation to the area may be continued

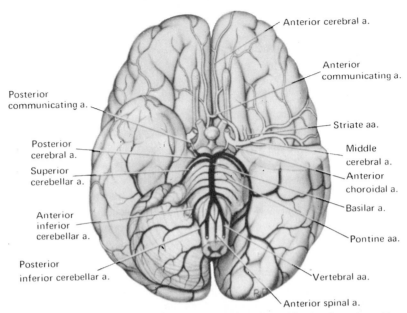

Figure 15–5. The inferior aspect of the brain showing the location of the basilar artery. (From Noback, C. R., and Demarest, R. J.: The Nervous System: Introduction and Review, New York, McGraw-Hill, 1972.)

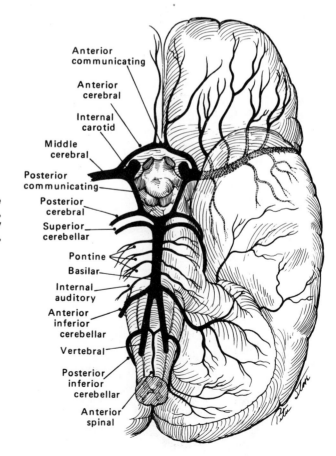

Figure 15–6. Schematic of the vessels that make up the circle of Willis. (From Langley, L. L., Telford, I. R., and Christensen, J. B.: Dynamic Anatomy and Physiology, 4th ed., New York, McGraw-Hill, 1974. © Copyright Mosby-Year Book, Inc.)

Table 15–1. SUMMARY OF MAJOR CEREBRAL AND CEREBELLAR VEINS

Type	Veins	Number	Termination
Superficial or external cerebral veins	Superior cerebral	8–10	Superior sagittal sinus
	Middle cerebral	1	Cavernous sinus
	Inferior cerebral	Numerous	Cavernous, petrosal, and transverse sinuses
	Basal	1	Great cerebral vein to straight sinus
Deep or internal veins	Internal cerebral	2	Join to form great cerebral vein that terminates in straight sinus
Cerebellar veins	Superior cerebellar	Numerous	Internal cerebral veins and straight sinus
	Inferior cerebellar	Numerous	Inferior petrosal, occipital, and sigmoid sinuses

through the circle of Willis. Each branch of the anastomosis has minute branches to the brain.

Venous Drainage

The venous drainage of the intracranial area can be considered in three segments—the cerebral veins, the dural sinuses, and the internal jugular.

Cerebral veins can be either superficial or deep-lying, inner veins. The superficial veins drain directly into the sinuses from the cortical region of the hemispheres and cerebellum. The inner, or deep, veins also empty into the sinuses, but they do so through a more circuitous route. The veins of the brain are thin walled and do not contain valves. A summary of the cortical and deep veins of the brain is given in Table 15–1.

The dural sinuses receive blood from the cerebral veins. These sinuses are simply dilated areas lined with endothelium continuous with that of the veins formed by a separation of the layers of the dura mater. The dural sinuses include the superior sagittal, inferior sagittal, occipital, right and left transverse, right and left sigmoid, straight, and cavernous sinuses (Fig. 15–7). The superior and inferior sagittal sinuses lie on the borders of the falx cerebri, the fold of the dura mater that separates the

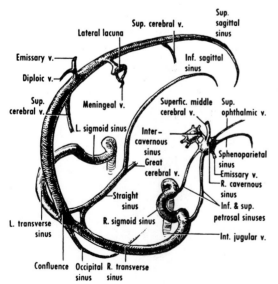

Figure 15–7. Schematic of the venous sinuses of the brain in the right lateral aspect. (From Gardner E., Gray, D. J., and O'Rahilly, R.: Anatomy, 4th ed., Philadelphia, W. B. Saunders, 1975.)

cerebral hemispheres. The straight sinus is located at the junction of the falx cerebri and the tentorium cerebelli, which forms a partition between the cerebrum and the cerebellum.

The torcular (confluence of sinuses) is the junction of the superior, sagittal, and occipital sinuses with the right and left transverse sinuses. It is near the internal occipital protuberance.[3]

The sigmoid sinuses are extensions of the transverse sinuses. They are located in a deep groove on the mastoid portion of the temporal bone and are contiguous with the internal jugular vein in the jugular foramen (Fig. 15–8).

The internal jugular segment begins with the sigmoid sinus in the jugular foramen. Its course can be represented on the surface of the body by a line from the lobe of the ear to the sternal end of the clavicle. The paired internal jugular veins join with the subclavian vein to form the innominate or brachiocephalic vein, which terminates in the superior vena cava. This segment receives blood from the dural sinuses and veins of the cranial cavity and the superficial veins of the face, and the neck.

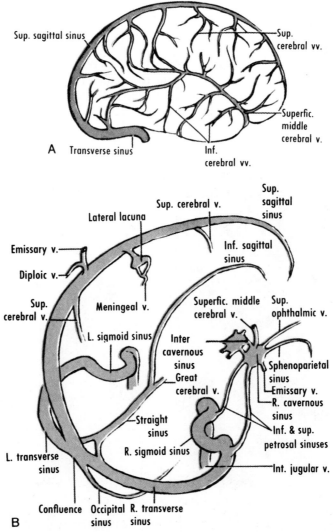

Figure 15–8. *(A)* Schematic drawing showing the cerebral veins as seen through the arachnoid after removal of the dura mater. *(B)* The venous sinus of the dura mater. (From O'Rahilly, R.: Basic Human Anatomy: A Regional Study of Human Structure, 3rd ed. Philadelphia, W. B. Saunders, 1983, p. 380, p. 388.)

INDICATIONS AND CONTRAINDICATIONS

Cerebral angiography is indicated only after a thorough clinical neurological examination, which includes routine skull radiography. Much of the diagnostic investigation of pathology of the brain is being relegated to computed tomography and magnetic resonance imaging, especially in identifying intracranial saccular aneurysms and carotid artery disease in the neck. The proportion of cerebral angiograms performed has declined, and it is no longer considered a primary diagnostic tool for cerebral pathology. However, the study will remain important in interventional neuroradiology and presurgical mapping.

Cerebral angiography can be used in the differential diagnosis of cerebrovascular disease for the differentiation of various intracerebral hematomas and vascular lesions and in the diagnosis and localization of intracranial tumors. These pathological conditions can also be demonstrated by magnetic resonance imaging and computed tomography; however, correlation with conventional or digital subtraction angiography cerebral studies should be made to confirm diagnosis (Fig. 15–9).

Cerebral angiography is an important tool in the differential diagnosis of cerebrovascular disease; in the differentiation of various intracerebral hematomas, vascular lesions, and intracranial aneurysms; and in the diagnosis and localization of intracranial tumors. It can also be indicated as an evaluative procedure after intracranial surgery or for diagnosis of postsurgical complications.

Contraindications for cerebral angiography include contrast media sensitivity, advanced arteriosclerosis, extremely ill or comatose patients, severe hypertension, or severe subarachnoid or intracerebral hemorrhaging. The examination can be hazardous and generally contraindicated in very old patients.

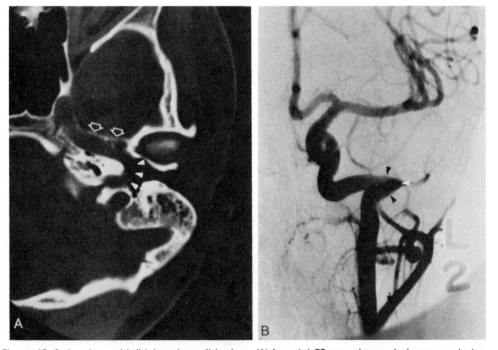

Figure 15–9. An aberrant left internal carotid artery. *(A)* An axial CT scan shows what appears to be a vascular structure coursing through the middle ear cavity (arrowheads) and then entering the carotid canal (arrows). *(B)* An anteroposterior view of a left common carotid angiogram confirms that this is an aberrant loop (arrowheads) of the internal carotid artery. (From Putman, C., and Ravin, C.: Textbook of Diagnostic Imaging, Vol. 1, Philadelphia, W. B. Saunders, 1988, p. 286.)

CONTRAST MEDIA

Any of the water-soluble iodine compounds can be used as a contrast agent for cerebral angiography. Depending on hospital protocol, the medium can be either ionic or nonionic. Suggested volumes for the various procedural methods are given in Tables 3–2 and 3–3. Specific volumes and flow rates vary according to institutional and physician preferences.

PROCEDURE

The procedural methods for injection of the contrast material are percutaneous (direct puncture) or catheter based (Fig. 15–10*A* and *B*). Each of these techniques has advantages and disadvantages (Table 15–2). The number of approaches available indicates that any one method would not be satisfactory for all cases. The technique chosen depends on the information desired and the personal preference of the physician performing the procedure. A brief discussion of the direct puncture method follows. The catheterization procedure for angiographic procedures is discussed in Chapter 9.

Direct Puncture Technique

The patient should be placed in a comfortable position on the radiographic table. As in all routine radiography, the procedure should be explained to the patient. This may be done by the physician; however, a short explanation of the positions you will ask the patient to assume and the sensations encountered when the contrast agent is injected is usually appreciated and should secure the patient's full cooperation.

The neck is shaved and surgically prepared, and the area is draped with sterile towels. The procedure is usually performed using local anesthesia; however, under certain conditions, general anesthesia may be required.

The patient's head is retroflexed during the puncture, with the amount varying

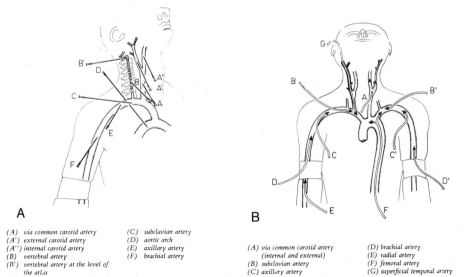

A

(A)	via common carotid artery	(C)	subclavian artery
(A')	external carotid artery	(D)	aortic arch
(A'')	internal carotid artery	(E)	axillary artery
(B)	vertebral artery	(F)	brachial artery
(B')	vertebral artery at the level of the atlas		

B

(A)	via common carotid artery (internal and external)	(D)	brachial artery
(B)	subclavian artery	(E)	radial artery
(C)	axillary artery	(F)	femoral artery
		(G)	superficial temporal artery

Figure 15–10. Schematics of the percutaneous *(A)* and catheter *(B)* methods for injection of contrast material. (From Krayenbuhl, H., and Yasargil, M.: Cerebral Angiography, 2nd ed., London, Butterworth Publishers, 1968.)

Table 15–2. ADVANTAGES AND DISADVANTAGES OF DIRECT PUNCTURE
AND CATHETER TECHNIQUES

Technique	Advantages	Disadvantages
Catheterization	Reduction in amount of contrast agent required	Thrombosis formation
	Minimized injection into surrounding tissue	Possible impairment of blood flow in extremities when additional catheterization is required for bilateral demonstration
	Greater mobility of the head for positioning	
	Blood flow measurements can be performed	More time required for procedure
	Higher contrast films	
	Catheter can remain in vessel for longer periods	
Direct puncture	Less time required	Lack of mobility of head
	Less strain on circulatory system	Superimposition of bilateral anatomy in nonselective direct puncture studies
	Reduction in possibility of thrombosis formation	
		Larger amount of contrast needed to reduce dilution

depending on the artery punctured. Direct puncture of the vertebral artery requires greater retroflexion than puncture of the common carotid. For common carotid puncture, the artery is palpated and fixed into position with one hand while the needle is inserted with the other. Pulsating arterial flow through the needle indicates successful placement. When the artery has been entered, the needle is flushed with saline solution to test the system. If the saline solution flows without resistance the cannulation is satisfactory, and the injection can be made.

Direct puncture of the vertebral artery is similar to the technique used for entering the common carotid artery, except the patient's head is extended farther back so the intertransverse foramina are opened as fully as possible. The common carotid artery is first displaced and fixed in place with one hand; the needle is then inserted through an intervertebral foramen into the vertebral artery. When successful insertion has been accomplished, the needle is flushed with saline solution to test for the free flow of fluid. When this is completed, the examination can proceed.

If selective injection of one of the carotid arteries is to be performed, successful entrance into the correct vessel should be proven by one of two methods. The first method involves injecting a small amount of contrast agent and asking the patient if a momentary burning sensation is experienced. A burning sensation at the chin indicates injection into the external carotid artery, whereas a burning sensation felt behind the eye indicates that the internal carotid artery has been entered. The second method is to inject a solution of methylene blue. If the corner of the mouth becomes discolored, the needle is in the external carotid artery; if the forehead region becomes discolored, the needle is in the internal carotid artery.

EQUIPMENT

Cerebral angiographic technique requires the use of very short exposure times when rapid serial film changers are used. Exposure times of 1/30 to 1/15 s are usually used. These short times require radiographic generators capable of both high- and low-capacity requirements. The 500-mA station is used with these exposure times. Principles of good radiographic technique must be applied to produce films of high contrast. The skull should be immobilized and positioned as close to the film as possible to minimize distortion and improve detail.

The kilovoltage used should be just sufficient for penetration of the skull. Use of higher kilovoltage with filtration usually compromises the contrast obtained.

The use of an image intensification system is helpful during technique requiring catheter placement and is, of course, a necessity when cineradiographic cerebrovascular studies are performed.

Cerebral angiography requires a serial film changer to record the passage of the contrast material through the cerebrovascular system. Naturally, the more sophisticated the film changing system, the more information that will be available from the examination. Any variety of serial film changer may be used. Film changers may be used as single-plane or biplane systems, each of which has advantages and disadvantages. When available, a biplane system should be used for cerebral angiography and is considered the method of choice.

When film changers are used as a biplane system, the lateral source-image distance must be increased to 48 or 72 in to compensate for the enlargement of the skull caused by the increased object-image distance. The change in source-image distance also necessitates an increase in the exposure factors.

Programming of the interval between films is usually dependent on the type of system used and the information required of the examination. For a differential diagnosis, the arterial, capillary, and venous phases of cerebral circulation must be demonstrated. Each phase is approximately 2 s apart. The exact time between phases is dependent on the circulation time of the contrast agent, which can vary from patient to patient and can be affected by any pathology present.

With rapid serial film changers, various time intervals can be programmed to demonstrate each phase in detail. The programming should be discussed with the physician performing the procedure to determine the interval that yields the greatest amount of information with the least amount of exposure to the patient.

Automatic injection devices are commonly used in angiography that uses catheterization techniques. In general, hand injections are the rule for direct puncture techniques because increased resistance can be readily felt should the needle become dislodged, and the injection can be terminated rapidly.

The amount of contrast media injected varies with the type of study being performed. The flow rates can range from 2 to 15 ml/s depending on the type of study and the physician's preference.

Table 15–3. EQUIPMENT IN A TYPICAL STERILE CEREBRAL ANGIOGRAPHY TRAY*

Equipment	Amount and/or Size
Needle	1 (25 × ⅝ in)
Needle	1 (22 × 1 in)
Needle	1 (20 × 1½ in)
Needle	1 (18 × 1½ in)
Needles	2 (17 × 2 in)
Luer-Lok control syringe	1 (10 ml)
Luer-Lok control syringe	1 (3 ml)
Luer-Lok syringe	1 (20 ml)
Syringe	1 (2 ml)
Topper sponges	24 (4 × 4 in)
Towels	3
Monel cups	2
Emesis basin	1
Three-way stopcock	1
Sponge stick	1

*Wrap in 36- × 36-in muslin, date, label, and autoclave 30 min. As a standard, two are kept in the x-ray department. Data from personal communication from Yeager, J., and Chief Technologist, Somerset Hospital, Somerville, NJ, 1973.

Needle or catheter insertions are done using sterile techniques. All necessary sterile equipment for cerebral angiography should be prepared ahead and assembled as a sterile tray. This should contain all necessary needles, syringes, drapes, towels, sponges, and receptacles. The equipment to be included in a typical cerebral angiography tray is shown in Table 15–3.

Other equipment that should be available during cerebral angiography includes the following:

1. A head binder or adhesive tape for immobilization of the patient's head
2. Additional sterile catheters and needles in the event of malfunction
3. Various radiation protection devices to ensure a minimum radiation dose to the patient and personnel involved in the procedure
4. An emergency drug cart and oxygen supply to treat possible reactions resulting from the procedure or contrast agent

PATIENT POSITIONING

Relatively few positions are used for recording the events of cerebral angiography. Usually, only anteroposterior and supine lateral views are taken; however, additional views may be requested in certain circumstances.

ANTEROPOSTERIOR VIEW. The anteroposterior view used varies slightly depending on whether a carotid or vertebral arteriogram is being performed. It is necessary to adjust the tube angle specifically for each procedure to demonstrate the desired anatomy in the best way. A caudal tube angle of 15° is used to demonstrate the anatomy during carotid arteriography (Fig. 15–11), whereas a 25° angle is needed during vertebral angiography (Fig. 15–12).

In each case, the patient is supine, with the head positioned over the rapid sequence changer. A support board should be used under the patient's head and shoulders to keep the head from touching the changer. This is done to avoid any motion distortion caused by the rapid sequence changer. The skull must be positioned symmetrically, that is, the median plane of the skull must be perpendicular to the film plane to avoid distortion of the anatomy. The chin should be depressed to place the orbitomeatal baseline perpendicular to the film. The tube is then adjusted to the proper caudal angle. The central ray is directed through the frontal bone and external auditory meatus to the center of the film. The field size should be collimated to the size of the head to minimize the production of scattered radiation.

LATERAL VIEW. Patient positioning for the routine lateral view is almost identical for both carotid and vertebral angiography. The only difference in the two procedures is the location of the central ray. During carotid angiography, the central ray is directed horizontally at a point approximately 2.5 cm anterior to and 2.5 cm above the external auditory meatus. Vertebral angiography requires that the central ray be directed 2.5 cm posterior to the external auditory meatus (Fig. 15–13).

For the lateral position, the skull must be positioned symmetrically with the orbitomeatal baseline perpendicular to the tabletop. The head should be immobilized to minimize motion. As in the anteroposterior view, the field size should be collimated to just cover the head.

Occasionally, certain pathological conditions require specialized views to delineate the anatomy. The most common of these is suspected aneurysms, which can be demonstrated best by using the supine oblique view. In cases in which subdural hematoma is suspected, a tangential projection may be used for delineation.

SUPINE OBLIQUE VIEW. The supine oblique view is accomplished by rotating the patient's head from 30 to 60° away from the injected side. The central ray is directed

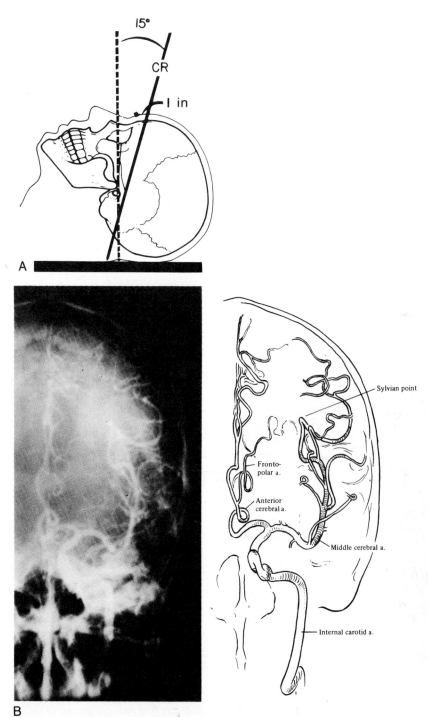

Figure 15–11. The standard anteroposterior view for carotid arteriography. *(A)* Schematic of the anteroposterior view for carotid arteriography; *(B)* radiograph and labeled tracing of an anteroposterior carotid anteriogram. *(A* from Selman, J.: Skull Radiography, Springfield, IL., Charles C Thomas, 1966; *B* from Toole, J. F., and Patel, A. N.: Cerebrovascular Disorders, 2nd ed., New York, McGraw-Hill, 1974.)

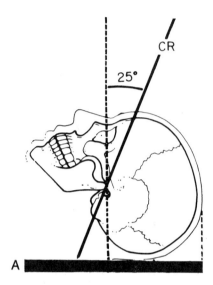

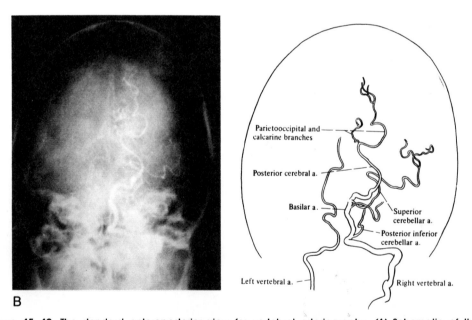

Figure 15–12. The standard anteroposterior view for vertebral arteriography. *(A)* Schematic of the anteroposterior view for vertebral arteriography; *(B)* radiograph and labeled tracing of an anteroposterior vertebral arteriogram. (*A* from Selman, J.: Skull Radiography, Springfield, IL., Charles C Thomas, 1966; *B* from Toole, J. F., and Patel, A. N.: Cerebrovascular Disorders, 2nd ed., New York, McGraw-Hill, 1974.)

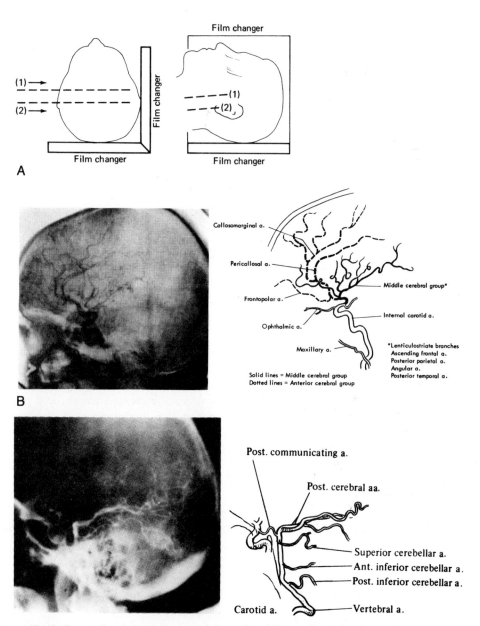

Figure 15–13. The routine lateral view. *(A)* Schematic of the routine lateral view for carotid *(1)* and vertebral *(2)* arteriography; *(B)* radiograph and labeled tracing of a routine lateral carotid arteriogram; *(C)* radiograph and labeled tracing of a routine lateral vertebral arteriogram. (*B* and *C* from Toole, J. F., and Patel, A. N.: Cerebrovascular Disorders, 2nd ed., New York, McGraw-Hill, 1974.)

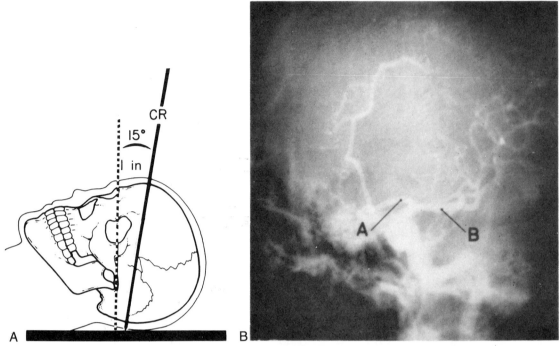

Figure 15–14. The supine oblique view. *(A)* Schematic of the supine oblique view; *(B)* radiograph showing the anterior cerebral **(A)** and middle cerebral **(B)** arteries. (From Selman, J.: Skull Radiography, Springfield, IL., Charles C Thomas, 1966.)

through a point approximately 2.5 cm above the supraorbital margin to the midpoint of the film at a caudal angle of from 15 to 20° (Fig. 15–14). Arterial aneurysms in the area of the anterior communicating artery are well delineated with this view.

TRANSORBITAL PROJECTION. Another supine oblique view, the transorbital projection, is used to demonstrate arterial aneurysms in the first portion of the middle cerebral artery.[4] The median plane of the skull is rotated approximately 10° toward the injected side. The central ray is then directed cephalad, through the center of the orbit, at an angle of 5° to the center of the film (Fig. 15–15). In all cases, the radiographic field size should be collimated to cover the size of the head.

TANGENTIAL PROJECTION. In some instances, it may be necessary to demonstrate a subdural hematoma specifically. This may be accomplished by rotating the median plane of the skull approximately 20° away from the injected side when the hematoma

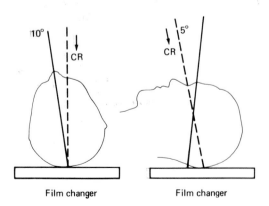

Figure 15–15. Schematic of the positioning for the transorbital oblique view.

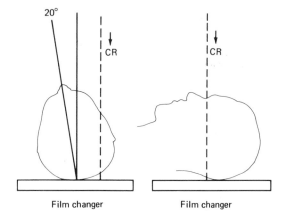

Figure 15–16. Schematic of the positioning for the optional tangential view.

is toward the posterior of the skull and 10° toward the injected side for hematomas located in the anterior of the skull. The central ray is directed tangentially to the suspected region at right angles to the film (Fig. 15–16).

For a summary of cerebral angiographic positioning, see Table 15–4.

Table 15–4. SUMMARY OF CEREBRAL ANGIOGRAPHY POSITIONING

Procedure	Projection	Position	Central Ray	Anatomy
Carotid angiography	Anteroposterior	OMBL* perpendicular to film, median plane perpendicular to film	15° caudal to enter 2.5 cm above glabella	Frontal view of anterior and middle cerebral arteries
	Lateral	OMBL perpendicular to table, median plane parallel to film	Horizontally directed at right angles to film to enter 2.5 cm anterior to and 2.5 cm above external auditory meatus	Lateral view of anterior and middle cerebral arteries and their branches, carotid siphon
	Supine oblique	Median plane 30–60° away from injected side	15° caudal to enter 2.5 cm above supraorbital margin	Anterior and middle cerebral arteries and anterior communicating artery can be delineated with lower angles
	Transorbital	OMBL perpendicular to film, median plane 10° toward injected side	5° cephalad to pass through center of orbit	Anterior and middle cerebral arteries, carotid siphon
	Tangential	OMBL perpendicular to film, median plane 20° away from or 10° toward injected side	Perpendicular to film to pass tangentially to region of interest	Subdural hematoma
Vertebral angiography	Anteroposterior	OMBL perpendicular to film, median plane perpendicular to film	25° caudal in median plane, entering at frontal bone and passing through external auditory meatus	Vertebrobasilar system
	Lateral	OMBL perpendicular to table, median plane parallel to film	Horizontally directed at right angles to film to enter 2.5 cm posterior to external auditory meatus	Lateral view to vertebrobasilar system

*OMBL: orbitomeatal baseline.

REFERENCES

1. Krayenbuhl, H.: Cerebral Angiography in Clinic and Practice. New York, Thieme-Stratton, 1982.
2. Woodburne, R. T.: Essentials of Human Anatomy, 7th ed. New York, Oxford University Press, 1983.
3. Gardner, E., Gray, D. J., and O'Rahilly, R.: Anatomy: A Regional Study of Human Structure, 4th ed. Philadelphia, W. B. Saunders, 1975.
4. Schobinger, R. A., and Ruzicka, F. F., Jr.: Vascular Roentgenology. New York, Macmillan, 1964.

SUGGESTED READINGS

Ballinger, P. W.: Merrill's Atlas of Radiographic Positions and Radiologic Procedures, 7th ed. St. Louis, C. V. Mosby, 1991.

Bryan, G. J.: Diagnostic Radiography, 3rd ed. Baltimore, Williams & Wilkins, 1977.

Crirjak, S., et al.: Significance of balloon catheter selective and superselective angiography in the diagnosis of cerebral vascular malformations, Acta Neurochir. (Vienna), 58:85, 1981.

Ecker, A.: The Normal Cerebral Angiogram, Springfield, IL, Charles C Thomas, 1951.

Ellis, H.: Clinical Anatomy, Oxford, Blackwell Scientific Publications, 1972.

Gentry, L. R., et al.: Prospective comparative study of intermediate field MR and CT in the evaluation of closed head trauma, Am. J. Roentgenol., 150:673, 1988.

Greitz, T., and Lindren, E.: In Abrams, H. L. (ed.), Angiography, Vol 1, Boston, Little, Brown, Co., 1961.

Hesselink, J. R., Dowd, C. F., and Healy, M. E.: MR imaging of brain contusions: A comparative study with CT, Am. J. Roentgenol., 150:1133, 1988.

Kappos, L., et al.: Magnetic resonance imaging in the evaluation of treatment in multiple sclerosis, Neuroradiology, 30:299, 1988.

Meschan, I.: Radiographic Positioning and Related Anatomy, 2nd ed. Philadelphia, W. B. Saunders, 1978.

Minimi, S.: Spinal arteriovenous malformation: MR imaging, Radiology, 169:109, 1988.

Olivecrona, H.: Complications of cerebral angiography, Neuroradiology, 14:175, 1977.

Quencer, R. M.: Neuroimaging and head injuries: Where we've been—where we're going, Am. J. Roentgenol., 150:13, 1988.

Ramsey, R. G.: Neuroradiology with Computed Tomography. Philadelphia, W. B. Saunders, 1981.

Selman, J.: Skull Radiography. Springfield, IL, Charles C Thomas, 1966.

Skalpe, I. O.: Complications in cerebral angiography with iohexol (Omnipaque) and meglumine metrizoate (Isopaque Cerebral), Neuroradiology, 30:69, 1988.

Thijssen, H. O. M., et al.: Comparison of brachiocephalic angiography and IVDSA in the same group of patients, Neuroradiology, 30:91, 1988.

Thron, A., and Voigt, K.: Rotational cerebral angiography: Procedure and value, Am. J. Nucl. Reson., 4:289–291, 1983.

Touho, H., et al.: Transbrachial artery approach for selective cerebral angiography in outpatients. Am. J. Nucl. Reson., 9:334, 1988.

Weinstein, M. A., et al.: Intra-arterial digital subtraction angiography of the head and neck, Radiology, 147:717, 1983.

sixteen

Central Nervous System Radiography

ANATOMIC CONSIDERATIONS
Brain
    Ventricular System
    Subarachnoid Cisternae
Spinal Cord
MYELOGRAPHY
Indications and Contraindications
Patient Preparation
Contrast Media
Procedure
    Lumbar Puncture Method
    Cisternal Puncture Method
    Sacral Hiatus Puncture Method
    Computed Tomography of the Spine
    Magnetic Resonance Imaging of the Spine

Equipment
Patient Positioning
    Opaque Lumbar Myelography
    Opaque Thoracic Myelography
    Opaque Cervical Myelography
PNEUMOENCEPHALOGRAPHY AND VENTRICULOGRAPHY
Contrast Media
Procedure
    Pneumoencephalography
    Ventriculography
Patient Positioning
    Pneumoencephalography
    Ventriculography
MAGNETIC RESONANCE IMAGING OF THE BRAIN

Radiography of the structures of the central nervous system has undergone a number of major changes over the past 10 years. Newer modalities such as computed tomography (CT) and magnetic resonance imaging (MRI) have replaced invasive studies such as pneumoencephalography, ventriculography, and, to some extent, myelography.

Myelography is the radiographic demonstration of the central nervous system structures located within the spinal canal. The procedure is accomplished easily through direct instillation of a contrast agent into the subarachnoid space. This technique can demonstrate various abnormalities of the spinal cord and spinal canal.

Pneumoencephalography and ventriculography are radiographic studies that were used to demonstrate the ventricular system of the brain. The ventricles are cavities within the brain that normally contain spinal fluid. These studies require that a suitable contrast agent be introduced into the ventricles to visualize anatomic details. The discussion of these procedures is limited; for a more detailed discussion, refer to an earlier edition of this text.

ANATOMIC CONSIDERATIONS

The nervous system can be separated into two major divisions—the peripheral and the central nervous systems. The central nervous system consists of the brain and the spinal cord. The central nervous system processes information to and from the peripheral nervous system and is the control center for the body.

Brain

The brain is the portion of the central nervous system found in the cranial cavity. The brain comprises the pons, medulla, mesencephalon, diencephalon, cerebellum, and cerebrum.

The pons, medulla, mesencephalon, and diencephalon are the components of the brain stem. The function of the brain stem is to provide some motor, sensory, and reflex functions. The spinal cord extends from the medulla oblongata and is considered to begin at the level of the foramen magnum.

The cerebellum is also called the hindbrain and is located in the posterior cranial fossa behind the brain stem. It also consists of two hemispheres separated by a groove. The middle section of the cerebellum, the vermis, is the connection between its hemispheres. The main function of the cerebellum is to coordinate voluntary muscular activity.

The cerebrum is the largest and uppermost portion of the brain. It is divided into right and left hemispheres by a central groove, the sulcus, and is connected at the bottom of the groove by the corpus callosum. The surface of the cerebrum is convoluted and lobed. The cerebrum is composed of an outer cerebral cortex (gray matter) and an inner portion, or semiovale (white matter). The cerebrum provides the sensory, motor, and integrative functions associated with the body's mental and physical activities. It is this portion of the brain that generates the electric waves that are monitored and recorded with an electroencephalograph.

VENTRICULAR SYSTEM

The ventricular system is a series of spaces or cavities located within the hemispheres of the brain. The system consists of four cerebral ventricles—two lateral ventricles and two other ventricles called the third and the fourth ventricles (Fig. 16–1). It is in the ventricles and subarachnoid space surrounding the brain and spinal cord that the cerebrospinal fluid circulates. The term "circulate" when applied to cerebrospinal fluid should not be compared with "circulation" as it applies to the blood. Cerebrospinal fluid is a complex substance containing various components, including water, electrolytes, and proteins. These substances are produced or absorbed in varying amounts over all the subarachnoid space. This is the basis for the circulation of the spinal fluid. The cerebrospinal fluid flows from areas of greatest production to areas of greatest absorption, but it is not true circulation. However, the spinal fluid does move through the subarachnoid system by this production-absorption process.

LATERAL VENTRICLES. There are two lateral ventricles, each located within one cerebral hemisphere. Each lateral ventricle has five divisions—anterior (frontal) horn, body, trigone (isthmus or atrium), posterior (occipital) horn, and inferior (temporal) horn. Each lateral ventricle connects on each side with the third ventricle by a narrow channel known as the interventricular foramen of Monro. The anterior (frontal) horns are usually found in the frontal lobes of the brain hemispheres.

The second division, the body, is located inferior to the corpus callosum (a bundle of fibers that connect the cerebral hemispheres) and superior to the thalamus. This division of the lateral ventricles lies between the anterior portion of the trigone and the area immediately posterior to the interventricular foramen of Monro.

The trigone is the area joined by the three posterior divisions of the ventricular system—the body and the posterior (occipital) and inferior (temporal) horns—to form a common cavity.

The posterior (occipital) horns usually exhibit asymmetry. They are formed approximately midway through the period of fetal development, and in the adult they vary in size. The posterior horns extend from the trigone into the occipital lobe of the cerebral hemispheres.

The inferior (temporal) horns extend anteriorly and inferiorly from the trigone. They are located in the temporal lobe of the cerebral hemisphere.

THIRD VENTRICLE. The third ventricle is bounded by the thalami superiorly and laterally and by the hypothalamus inferiorly and anteriorly. The superoanterior portion of the third ventricle supports the interventricular foramen of Monro, which connects to the lateral ventricles. In the posteroinferior portion of the third ventricle is found the aqueduct of Sylvius, by which the third ventricle communicates with the fourth ventricle below. The third ventricle is a narrow slitlike cavity located in the midline of the skull.

FOURTH VENTRICLE. The aqueduct of Sylvius is located in the midbrain. It begins at the third ventricle and extends downward, where it widens posteriorly and laterally to form the fourth ventricle. This cavity narrows below to become contiguous with the central canal of the spinal cord. The lateral portions of the ventricle are extended on each side for a variable distance, forming the lateral recesses. The lateral recesses open through openings called the foramina of Luschka into the pontine and anterior portion of the cerebellomedullary cisternae.[1] The fourth ventricle also connects with the subarachnoid of the cisterna magna (cerebellomedullary cisterna) through an opening called the foramen of Magendie.

SUBARACHNOID CISTERNAE

The brain, like the spinal cord, is covered by three membranes, or meninges; the pia mater and arachnoid are called the "leptomeninges."[2] It is between these two mem-

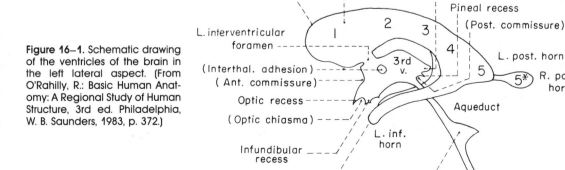

Figure 16–1. Schematic drawing of the ventricles of the brain in the left lateral aspect. (From O'Rahilly, R.: Basic Human Anatomy: A Regional Study of Human Structure, 3rd ed. Philadelphia, W. B. Saunders, 1983, p. 372.)

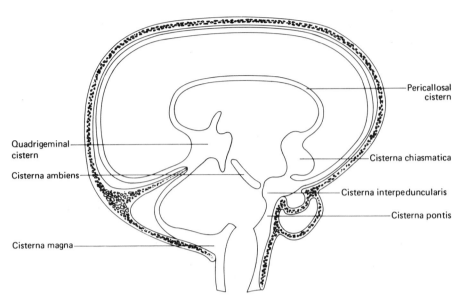

Figure 16–2. Schematic of the subarachnoid cisternae.

branes that the subarachnoid space is found. The arachnoid membrane follows the contour of the dura mater, whereas the pia mater follows the surface contours of the brain.

In some areas of the brain, the subarachnoid space enlarges the subarachnoid cisternae (Fig. 16–2). The cisterna magna is the most important of these from the radiographer's point of view. It is here that a needle can be inserted through the posterior atlanto-occipital membrane and the contrast agent injected. This procedure is called cisternal puncture. The cisterna magna extends down to merge with the spinal subarachnoid space. It is triangular in shape and contains approximately 5 to 10 ml of cerebrospinal fluid. The apex of the cisterna magna points toward the vallecula. This is the portion of the subarachnoid space that lies between the fourth ventricle and cisterna magna. It can be seen that air injected into the spinal subarachnoid space must pass through the cisterna magna and vallecula before entering the ventricular system. It is important that the flexion of the head be accurately maintained to prevent air from entering other subarachnoid spaces rather than the ventricular system. Further discussion of the subarachnoid cisternae is not presented here.

Spinal Cord

The vertebral canal tends to be triangular, relatively large in the cervical and lumbar regions, and small and ovoid in the thoracic region (Fig. 16–3). It contains the spinal cord and its meninges, spinal nerves and vessels, and the epidural space, which is located between the wall of the vertebral canal and the dura mater; this contains fat, venous plexi, and nerves that supply the meninges, intervertebral disks, and ligaments.

All of these structures are important in that any aberrations may cause encroachment on the vertebral canal. The spinal cord lies loosely within the vertebral canal and extends from the foramen magnum to the lower border of the first lumbar vertebra. At this point, it tapers into the conus medullaris, from which the filum terminale extends to the coccyx. It averages 45 cm (18 in) in length.

The spinal cord is enclosed by three layers continuous with those of the brain—the dura mater, or outer covering; arachnoid; and pia mater (Fig. 16–4). These are called the meninges.

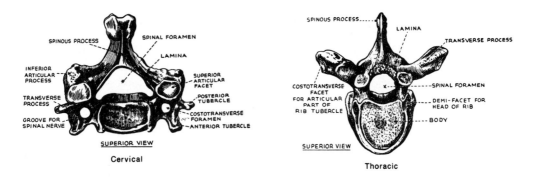

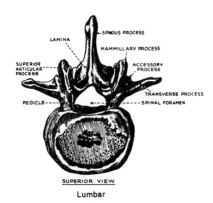

Figure 16–3. Representative individual vertebrae from the cervical, thoracic, and lumbar regions showing the differences in the size and shape of the vertebral canal. (From Meschan, I.: Synopsis of Radiological Anatomy, rev. ed., Philadelphia, W. B. Saunders, 1980.)

The spinal dura mater is a heavy elastic sheath extending from its attachments with the margins of the foramen magnum to the level of the second sacral vertebra. At this point, the dura mater tapers into a covering for the filum terminale of the spinal cord. A space exists between the wall of the vertebral canal and the dura mater; this is called the epidural space. This space contains semifluid fat and many small veins. Between the dura mater and arachnoid layers is a potential subdural space. The meningeal layers contact each other, with a film of fluid separating them.

The spinal arachnoid is continuous with the cerebral arachnoid layer that covers the brain. It is a delicate membrane that follows the dura mater to its termination at the second sacral vertebra. Between the arachnoid and pia mater is the subarachnoid space.

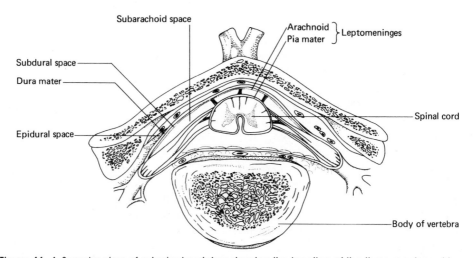

Figure 16–4. Superior view of a typical vertebra showing the location of the three meningeal layers.

This space is bathed in spinal fluid and is in direct communication with the ventricles of the brain and its surrounding spaces. The subarachnoid space is larger around the spinal cord than in the brain. It extends to the level of the second sacral vertebra. The spinal cord ends at the upper level of the lumbar spine and the subarachnoid space continues to the second sacral segment, making an ideal location for spinal fluid withdrawal or contrast media injection.[3] The nerve roots are seldom damaged because of their flexibility in this area.

The spinal pia mater is the innermost membrane that invests the spinal cord. It is a thin layer that contains some blood vessels. The pia mater extends into the filum terminale and terminates within it, blending into the periosteum at the posterior of the first coccygeal segment. The pia mater and arachnoid are occasionally referred to as one layer. When this is the case, they are called the pia arachnoid layer, or the leptomeninges.[4]

MYELOGRAPHY

Indications and Contraindications

Subarachnoid myelography is a safe procedure that can be used to visualize the subarachnoid space around the spinal cord. It is indicated when accurate diagnosis of anatomic abnormalities or pathological processes of the spinal cord and spinal canal is required. Some specific indications for subarachnoid myelography are encroachment of intervertebral disks, space-occupying lesions, degenerative diseases of the central nervous system, malformation of the spinal cord, and syringomyelia.

Epidural myelography is indicated when a demonstration of encroachment defects caused by tumors or herniated intervertebral disks into the lower thoracic and lumbar regions of the spinal canal is necessary.

Myelography is contraindicated when the patient exhibits signs of increased intracranial pressure.

Patient Preparation

In many cases, myelography can be done as an ambulatory procedure. When the examination is scheduled, the patient should be instructed not to take medication for at least 24 h and increase fluid intake before the examination. It is also recommended that they not eat solid food before the study; the length of the fast is variable depending on the protocol of the institution.

When the patient arrives, the procedure should be explained, and a consent form should be negotiated. The patient should be questioned concerning allergies, prior contrast agent reactions, results of any recent myelograms, and whether the patient is prone to seizures. Vital signs should be taken at this time to establish a baseline for monitoring during the procedure. The information from the history should be transmitted to the physician before the study begins. If the patient is to receive any medication before the examination, it should be administered by the physician or the special procedure nurse.

The radiographic room should be set up before the patient is brought in. All equipment should be tested, and the supplies necessary for the injection should be placed within easy reach. The patient should be gowned in preparation for the study. The injection site should be shaved; when the physician arrives, the site should be surgically prepared.

During the procedure, the patient should be monitored for changes and any unusual symptoms or complaints. If specimen samples are required, care must be taken to preserve the sterile environment. Samples should be readied for laboratory analysis as soon as possible. The procedure will be determined by the protocols developed by the medical laboratory department and must be carefully followed. Any complications or reactions should be noted on the patient's chart; the individual responsible for the charting will vary depending on the hospital protocol.

At the end of the myelogram, the patient should be told of the objective symptoms resulting from the procedure, which can include headache and pain at the injection site or in the lumbar area. The patient should be instructed to remain on bed rest for 8 to 24 h with the head slightly elevated. The patient should be instructed to alert the physician to any unusual symptoms that may occur, such as stiff neck, fever, seizures, or paralysis. If the patient appears normal, he or she may be released upon the physician's order.

Contrast Media

Myelography can be done with either positive or negative contrast agents. The procedural differences are in manipulating the contrast agent within the subarachnoid space. Negative contrast agents are lighter than spinal fluid and will rise to the highest available portion of the spinal canal. Positive contrast agents are heavier than spinal fluid and will flow with the effect of gravity, that is, if the patient is raised to a standing position, the contrast agent will flow toward the lower spine, or if the patient is placed in the Trendelenburg position, the contrast agent will flow toward the cervical region.

The negative contrast material most often used is air. When a myelogram is done with a negative contrast agent, it is usually called a pneumomyelogram. Negative contrast agents are readily absorbed by body tissues, so their removal is unnecessary. They have found widespread usage for cervical and thoracic myelography.

Positive contrast agents can be subdivided into those that are oily and those that are water soluble. The oily contrast agents are most commonly used for myelography because the water-soluble substances cause irritation to the spinal pia mater and arachnoid membranes. However, the water-soluble contrast agents give excellent visualization of the nerve roots and have the added advantage of being readily absorbed from the subarachnoid space. The major disadvantage of the use of water-soluble agents is the pain caused by the intrathecal injection during myelography. Spinal anesthesia must be given to offset the pain, thus limiting the procedure to the lumbar area.

The nonionic water-soluble contrast agents can generally be administered to patients without any premedication, and usually do not produce the type of irritation caused by the use of ionic water-soluble media. The nonionic contrast agents generally have an osmolarity similar to that of cerebrospinal fluid. They are somewhat hyperbaric and can be positioned by gravity in a similar manner to Pantopaque (iophendylate). They have the same advantages of the other ionic water-soluble contrast media and can reveal much diagnostic information regarding the nerve roots. Once the contrast agent is introduced, any movement of the patient should be minimized to prevent its dilution. The patient should be fully hydrated before its administration to minimize the possibility of side effects. One disadvantage to the use of water-soluble contrast agents is their rapid reabsorption rate. This process begins within 30 min of the injection, and the radiographs should be taken quickly to avoid loss of radiopacity.

The oily contrast agents have the disadvantage of very slow absorption by the body tissues; they have been demonstrated to persist years after the procedure has been done. This usually necessitates the removal of the contrast agent after the examination has been completed, but this is a minor consideration because many radiographers do not attempt to remove it at the conclusion of the examination.

Procedure

The two principal methods by which contrast media may be injected into the subarachnoid space are lumbar puncture and cisternal puncture. The former is used most often, whereas the latter is reserved for use when complete obstruction of the subarachnoid space has been determined.

LUMBAR PUNCTURE METHOD

This method provides a satisfactory injection point for most forms of subarachnoid myelography—cervical, thoracic, and lumbar. Depending on the contrast agent used, various postural maneuvers are required to distribute the material along the areas of interest.

The patient is placed in either a seated or lateral decubitus position for the injection. The skin is prepared and infiltrated with a suitable anesthetic agent. The needle and stylet are then inserted into the subarachnoid space. The stylet is removed, and an indication of successful entry is the free flow of spinal fluid from the needle.

The site of injection is the lower lumbar region, because this area reduces the possibility of trauma to the spinal cord (Fig. 16–5). It is important to note that during lumbar myelography the injection site is usually in the interspace between the second and third lumbar vertebrae, whereas for cervical and thoracic myelography the injection can be made lower (at the level of the L3–L4 or L4–L5 interspace). The lower lumbar region is usually the site of disease, and the higher injection point is required to minimize the possibility of needle deformities becoming confused with pathology.

When a successful lumbar puncture is made, a small sample of spinal fluid is collected for laboratory analysis. At this time, manometric pressure measurements may be made, and injection of the contrast medium can proceed. This is usually accomplished by withdrawing a small amount of spinal fluid and replacing it with an equal amount of contrast agent, with the total amount being dependent on the area of the spine under examination and the type of contrast agent used (positive or negative).

After instillation of the contrast agent, the stylet is replaced and the examination can proceed. The patient is rotated into the prone position and secured by means of a foot

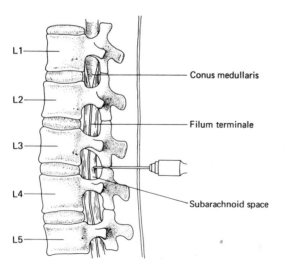

Figure 16–5. Lumbar region of the spine showing the location of the spinal structure. Spinal cord trauma is avoided at this level.

platform and shoulder harness; through the use of a tilting radiographic table, the contrast agent is distributed over the area of interest. If a positive contrast agent is used, the needle may be left in situ to facilitate removal of the contrast material. In some cases, the needle may be removed after the injection and a second puncture made to retrieve the contrast agent.

During myelography with a water-soluble contrast agent, the first radiograph is usually taken with the needle still in place. This is done to ensure that the needle is in the subarachnoid space and to record the puncture site radiographically to confirm or exclude the possibility of localized puncture bleeding. Once the initial radiograph has been completed satisfactorily, the needle is removed. Because the water-soluble iodine compounds are readily absorbed by the body, there is no need to remove the contrast agent after the examination is complete.

CISTERNAL PUNCTURE METHOD

When it is impossible to perform a lumbar puncture for the injection of contrast material, a cisternal puncture can be performed. The injection is made into the cisterna magna or cerebellomedullary cisterna (Fig. 16–6). The patient's scalp is shaved and prepared surgically, and a local anesthetic is given. A special needle is then inserted between the occipital bone and the atlas, passing through the atlanto-occipital membrane and advancing about 1 to 2 cm until spinal fluid appears. This procedure must be carefully performed to avoid trauma to the medulla. It is generally reserved for use when there is obstruction of the lumbar region of the spinal canal. Other indications for use of this method include lumbar epidural abscess, spondylitis, and infection of the dermal tissue of the lumbar region.

SACRAL HIATUS PUNCTURE METHOD

The above injection methods may be used for all forms of subarachnoid myelography. Epidural myelography, however, requires a special injection method for introducing the contrast agent into the extradural space. This may be called the sacral hiatus puncture method because of the location of needle insertion (Fig. 16–7). The procedure may be performed on an outpatient basis and has the added advantage that the contrast media is readily absorbed and excreted by the kidneys.

The patient is placed in the prone position between a footrest and shoulder harness. A small pad is placed under the lower abdomen to present the sacrum at the proper angle for needle insertion. The area is surgically prepared and infiltrated with local anesthetic. The needle is then inserted into the epidural space through the sacral hiatus. The needle position is confirmed radiographically, and 5 ml of anesthetic solution is injected. The angiographic table is then placed in a 30° Trendelenburg position, 20 ml of contrast agent is injected, the needle is withdrawn, and the puncture site is covered. Finally, the table is returned to its original position, and radiographs are made.[5]

COMPUTED TOMOGRAPHY OF THE SPINE

Postmyelography CT is becoming an important adjunct to the diagnosis of spinal cord pathology. The study is generally used to confirm a localized pathological process that may or may not have been demonstrated by large-field myelography. If follow-up CT is indicated, the myelogram is usually obtained with a water-soluble iodinated contrast media. This type of contrast agent provides improved resolution of the structures within the spinal canal. Figure 16–8 illustrates the images of the spinal cord and subarachnoid space as demonstrated by CT.

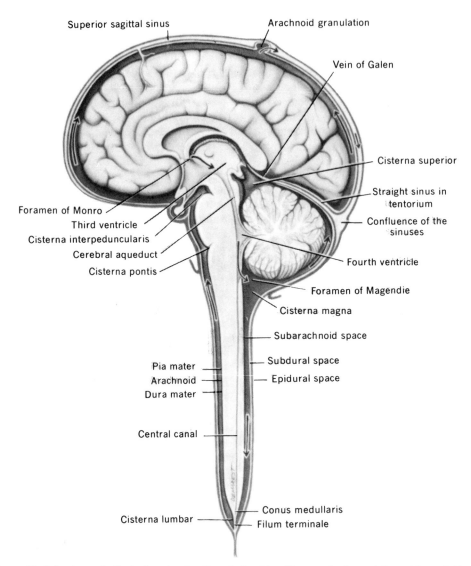

Figure 16–6. A schematic illustration showing the relationship of the cerebellomedullary cisterna (cisterna magna) to the other structures within the skull. (From Noback, C. R., and Demarest, R. J.: The Human Nervous System, New York, McGraw-Hill, 1967.)

MAGNETIC RESONANCE IMAGING OF THE SPINE

MRI is also used to image abnormalities of the spine and spinal cord. The development of surface coils that increase the signal-to-noise ratio and the use of various motion-compensating techniques to overcome the artifacts produced by the motion of the cerebrospinal fluid have made possible higher-quality images of vertebral anatomy. MRI is becoming the primary imaging modality for diagnosis of thoracic and lumbar spine pathology. The procedure is noninvasive and provides excellent soft tissue detail. Figure 16–9 shows some MR images of the spine.

Equipment

Myelography can be performed in any diagnostic radiographic room equipped with a tilting radiographic table and fluoroscopic unit. The radiographic table should be able

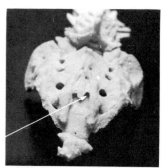

Figure 16–7. Dry bone specimen of the sacrum showing the location of the sacral hiatus (arrow). (Original photograph by A. Joaquim.)

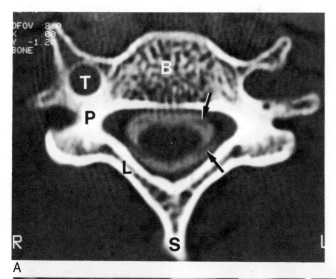

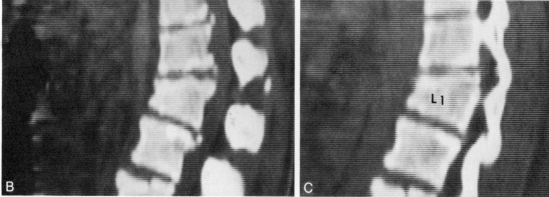

Figure 16–8. *(A)* Axial CT image of a typical cervical vertebra showing the dorsal and ventral nerve rootlet (arrows) emerging from the spinal cord, body (B), transverse foramen (T), pedicle (P), lamina (L), and spinous process (S). *(B)* A midsagittal reformation of an axial CT of the lumbar spine. (*A* from Putman C., and Ravin, C.: Textbook of Diagnostic Imaging. Philadelphia, W. B. Saunders, 1988, p. 316. *B* from Putman, C., and Ravin, C., p. 356.)

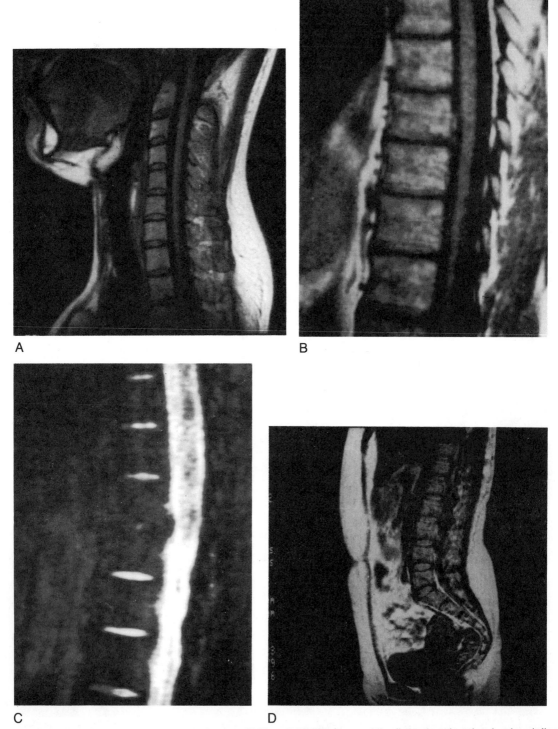

Figure 16–9. *(A)* MRI of the normal cervical spine. *(B)* T1 and *(C)* T2 images of the thoracic spine showing herniation of the intervertebral disk. The T2-weighted image demonstrates the impression made by the intervertebral disk on the spinal cord. *(D)* T1-weighted MRI of the lumbar spine. (From Partain, C., et al.: Magnetic Resonance Imaging, 2nd ed., Philadelphia, W. B. Saunders, 1988.)

to tilt in both directions to provide the positions required to move the contrast agent within the subarachnoid space. It should also be equipped with a footrest and shoulder harness to support the patient during the movement of the contrast material. Image intensification with television monitoring facilitates the fluoroscopic portion of the examination.

A sterile spinal tap tray should be available for use during myelography. Table 16–1 lists the equipment found in a typical sterile spinal tray.

Because cross-table lateral views with a horizontal beam are usually performed, some type of cassette support should be available to hold the grid cassette at right angles to the x-ray team.

Patient Positioning

After injection of the contrast agent, the radiographic table is moved through various positions while the flow of contrast is monitored fluoroscopically. Spot films or cineradiography may be performed during this portion of the examination. Because myelography can be performed with either positive or negative contrast agents, the various postural maneuvers necessary for the distribution of the contrast agent will differ. Of course, this is a result of the physical properties of the contrast agent. Both the postural maneuvers and fluoroscopic portion of the procedure vary considerably with the type of contrast agent (positive or negative) used and with the area of the spinal cord under examination; because they are under the direct control of the radiographer performing the procedure, a detailed description is not given in this text. However, the various radiographic positions required at the conclusion of the fluoroscopic portion of the procedure are discussed. Because positive contrast myelography is performed more often, positioning relevant to this method is presented.

In general, most radiographs are taken with a horizontal beam directed across the table at a grid cassette. Occasionally, the vertical beam projections may be requested by the physician. The anatomy demonstrated will vary with the region under examination.

OPAQUE LUMBAR MYELOGRAPHY

In this region, four views may be taken, three of which are performed with a horizontal beam.

Cross-Table Lateral View. In this view, the patient is prone. A 10- × 12-in (25-

Table 16–1. EQUIPMENT IN A TYPICAL STERILE MYELOGRAPHY TRAY

Equipment	Amount and/or Size
Spinal manometer	1
Three-way stopcock (not Luer-Lok)	1
Luer-Lok syringe	1 (2 ml)
Luer-Lok syringe	1 (5 ml)
Luer-Lok syringe	1 (10 ml)
Medicine glass	1
Hemostat	1
Towel	1
Applicators	3 (6 in)
Gauge needles	1 each (No. 18 and No. 22)
Needle	1 (⅝ in, No. 25 gauge)
Topper sponges	12 (3 × 3 in)
Specimen tubes with black rubber corks	3
Surgical drape	1

× 30-cm) grid cassette is supported on the side of the patient opposite the table. The exact level of the cassette is determined by the radiographer performing the examination. The central ray is directed across the table to the midpoint of the cassette. The structures demonstrated are lateral views of the vertebral bodies, intervertebral spaces of the lumbar vertebrae, and lumbar subarachnoid space (Fig. 16–10).

A variation of this basic position can be done to demonstrate the lowest portion of the lumbar subarachnoid space. The patient is in the same position as in the previous view; however, the radiographic table is raised into a semiupright position that allows the positive contrast agent to drop to the lowest portion of the subarachnoid space. A cross-table lateral view is performed, with the cassette centered to the level of the L5–S1 interspace.

CROSS-TABLE OBLIQUE VIEW. The patient is placed in a 45° right or left anterior oblique position. A 10- × 12-in (25- × 30-cm) grid cassette is supported next to the patient, centered at about the level of the L4–L5 interspace (Fig. 16–11). The central ray is directed horizontally (across the table) at a right angle to the midpoint of the cassette. Collimation to the field size or area of interest is essential for good detail. This view demonstrates the lumbar subarachnoid space in an oblique projection.

CROSS-TABLE LATERAL DECUBITUS VIEW. The patient is turned into a true lateral position with the knees and hips flexed (Fig. 16–12). A 14- × 17-in (35- × 42.5-cm) grid cassette is placed against the patient's abdomen to include the entire lumbar area. (If the needle has been removed, the cassette may be placed against the patient's back.)

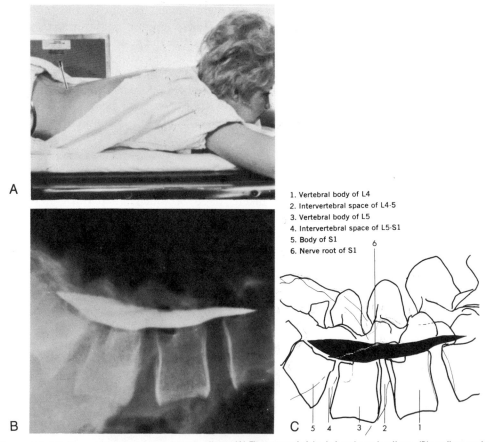

1. Vertebral body of L4
2. Intervertebral space of L4-5
3. Vertebral body of L5
4. Intervertebral space of L5-S1
5. Body of S1
6. Nerve root of S1

A

B

C

Figure 16–10. The cross-table lateral projection; *(A)* The cross-table lateral projection; *(B)* radiograph; *(C)* labeled tracing showing the contrast-column in the lumbar region. (From Radiography of the Spine, Wilmington, DE, E. I. du Pont de Nemours & Company, Inc., 1966. Out of print.)

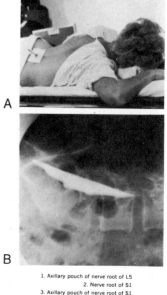

A

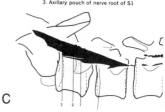

B

Figure 16–11. The cross-table oblique projection. *(A)* The cross-table oblique projection; *(B)* radiograph; *(C)* labeled tracing showing an oblique view of the lumbar region with the contrast column. (From Radiography of the Spine, Wilmington, DE, E. I. du Pont de Nemours & Company, Inc., 1966. Out of print.)

1. Axillary pouch of nerve root of L5
2. Nerve root of S1
3. Axillary pouch of nerve root of S1

C

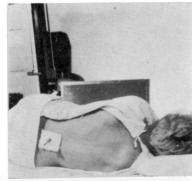

A

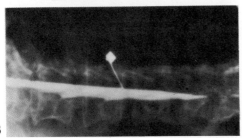

B

Figure 16–12. The cross-table lateral decubitus projection. *(A)* The cross-table lateral decubitus projection position; *(B)* a radiograph; *(C)* labeled tracing depicting the lumbar region with the needle *in situ*. (From Radiography of the Spine, Wilmington, DE, E. I. du Pont de Nemours & Company, Inc., 1966. Out of print.)

1. Nerve root of L4
2. Axillary pouch of nerve root of L4
3. Vertebral body of L5

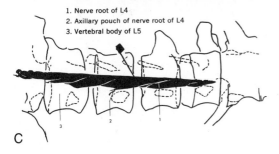

C

The central ray is directed at a right angle to the midpoint of the cassette. Collimation of the beam ensures maximum detail.

POSTEROANTERIOR VIEW WITH VERTICAL BEAM. For the frontal view, the patient is placed in the prone position and centered to the midline of the table. An 11- × 14-in (27.5- × 35-cm) cassette may be used, centered to the L4–L5 interspace. The central ray is directed at a right angle to the film. The Bucky should be used to maximize detail, and collimation should be to field size.

OPAQUE THORACIC MYELOGRAPHY

The additional overhead tube views required for thoracic myelography are essentially the same as for lumbar myelography. The major difference is in the cassette size used. For all views in the thoracic region, a 14- × 17-in (35- × 42.5-cm) cassette should be used. As in lumbar myelography, collimation is critical to maximize detail.

OPAQUE CERVICAL MYELOGRAPHY

In general, only cross-table lateral views with the overhead tube are taken during cervical myelography. Frontal views are usually not requested, because the patient's head must remain hyperextended. This is required to prevent the contrast material from entering the skull, because it cannot return to the cervical region.

In the routine cross-table lateral view, the lower cervical and upper thoracic regions are not well demonstrated. A specialized view is required to eliminate the superimposition of the shoulders—Twining's view or the swimmer's view.[6]

SWIMMER'S VIEW. The patient is placed in the prone position with the head hyperextended and the median sagittal plane perpendicular to the table. The arm

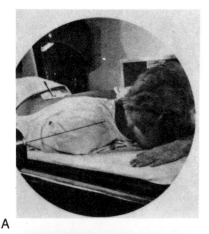

A

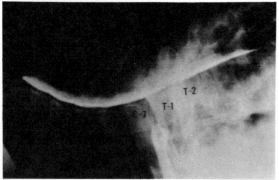

B

Figure 16–13. Swimmer's projection. *(A)* The patient positioned for the Swimmer's projection; *(B)* radiograph of the cervical region showing the contrast column. (From Radiography of the Spine, Wilmington, DE, E. I. du Pont de Nemours & Company, Inc., 1966. Out of print.)

Table 16–2. SUMMARY OF POSITIONING FOR OPAQUE MYELOGRAPHY

Region Examined	Projection	Patient Position	Central Ray	Anatomy
Cervical	Cross-table lateral	Patient prone, MSP* perpendicular to table, head hyperextended, arms at side	Horizontal transtable to enter at C3, perpendicular to center of grid cassette	C1—C6, posterior margin of foramen magnum, clivus, cervical subarachnoid space
	Swimmer's	Patient prone, MSP perpendicular to table, head hyperextended, one arm at side, other arm above head	Horizontal transtable to enter at C7, perpendicular to center of grid cassette	Lower cervical and upper thoracic regions
Thoracic	Cross-table lateral	Patient prone, arms raised	Horizontal transtable to enter at T7, perpendicular to center of grid cassette	Lateral view of thoracic subarachnoid space
	Cross-table lateral decubitus	Patient in right or left lateral position, arms raised	Horizontal transtable to enter at T7, perpendicular to center of grid cassette	Lateral decubitus view of thoracic subarachnoid space
Lumbar	Cross-table lateral	Patient prone, arms raised, table either horizontal or slightly upright	Horizontal transtable, perpendicular to center of grid cassette	Lateral lumbosacral region from L3–S1; with horizontal table, lateral view of lowest portion of subarachnoid space, vertebral bodies from L4 to coccyx
	Cross-table oblique	Right or left anterior oblique, arms raised	Horizontal transtable, perpendicular to midpoint of grid cassette	Oblique view of lumbar subarachnoid space
	Cross-table lateral	Right or left lateral position, arms raised, knees and hips flexed	Horizontal transtable, perpendicular to midpoint of grid cassette	Lateral decubitus view of lumbar subarachnoid space
	Posteroanterior	Prone position, arms flexed	Vertical beam to enter at L4–L5 interspace at right angles to film	Frontal view of lumbar subarachnoid space

*MSP: median sagittal plane.

closest to the tube is placed next to the patient, and the opposite hand is placed above the patient's head. This position is comparable to the body's position while swimming (Fig. 16–13). A 10- × 12-in (25- × 27.5-cm) grid cassette is supported next to the patient, centered at the level of the seventh cervical vertebra. The central ray is directed at a right angle to the cassette. The radiographic table should be tilted up slightly to pool the contrast agent in the desired area. Detail is maximized by collimating the field size.

A summary of the overhead tube positions for opaque myelography is presented in Table 16–2.

PNEUMOENCEPHALOGRAPHY AND VENTRICULOGRAPHY

Encephalography is the means by which the ventricular system of the brain was evaluated. Initial studies began in 1913 and developed as a diagnostic procedure through the 1950s. In 1963 through 1964, a specialized chair was developed that allowed the disbursement of contrast agent by rotating the patient as much as 360°. In 1974 through 1975, with the advent of CT, pneumoencephalography and pneumoventriculography were eliminated as viable diagnostic procedures in most institutions. With the recent development of MRI of the brain, these procedures have become obsolete and are no longer performed.

Contrast Media

Both positive and negative contrast agents were used for these procedures. The most often used negative contrast agent was air. Most available gases have been used, with varying results. Some were found to be absorbed too rapidly to provide visualization of all necessary positions. Oxygen and air were found to produce satisfactory results without rapid absorption.

The quantity of gas injected was variable depending on the type of procedure. Quantities as small as 5 ml and as large as 120 ml have been used (120 ml replaces almost all the cerebrospinal fluid). The average (normal) amount used was 15 to 20 ml, which is usually enough to visualize all of the necessary anatomy by using the various positions.

Some positive contrast agents have been used. Among these, iophendylate (Pantopaque, Myodil) was the most common. It was generally used during positive contrast ventriculography (approximately 1 to 2 ml was injected into the anterior horns and run downward).

Procedure

PNEUMOENCEPHALOGRAPHY

In pneumoencephalography, there were two methods by which the contrast agent was introduced into the ventricular system. The usual route was by lumbar puncture. The second method, cisternal injection.

LUMBAR PNEUMOENCEPHALOGRAPHY. The patient is maintained in a seated position for the lumbar injection. The puncture site is usually between the third and fourth lumbar vertebrae. This site is chosen to avoid trauma to the spinal cord. Spinal fluid samples can be taken and pressure measurements performed before the contrast agent is injected. The contrast agent is then introduced in small amounts after aspiration of approximately equal amounts of cerebrospinal fluid. Slightly less air is injected than the quantity of spinal fluid removed to compensate for its expansion. Various positions are used to distribute the contrast agent. Radiographs are taken after each maneuver to record the necessary anatomy.

CISTERNAL PNEUMOENCEPHALOGRAPHY. Cisternal puncture was indicated when a spinal subarachnoid block was present or in cases of lumbar epidural abscess, ankylotic spondylitis, or infection of the skin in the lumbar region. It was not as useful as lumbar pneumoencephalography because of the high risk involved and the inability to change the posture of the neck. The needle is inserted through the posterior atlanto-occipital membrane to enter the cisterna magna. Small amounts of contrast agent are introduced and equivalent amounts of spinal fluid are withdrawn until ventricular filling is achieved.

VENTRICULOGRAPHY

This procedure was indicated when lumbar and cisternal pneumoencephalography were contraindicated. It was a surgical procedure performed in an operating room. The procedure generally did not require a great amount of time. Two burr holes were made in the posterior parietal region, contrast material was injected directly into the anterior

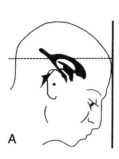

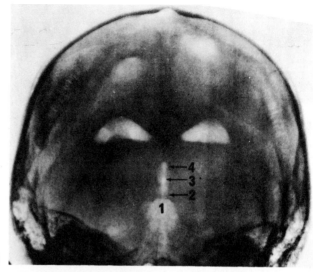

Figure 16–14. The erect frontal posteroanterior projection. *(A)* Schematic of the position of the skull; *(B)* radiograph of the erect posteroanterior projection showing the posterior part of the fourth ventricle *(1),* anterior part of the fourth ventricle *(2),* aqueduct of Sylvius *(3),* and third ventricle *(4).* (From Siemens Medical Systems, Inc. Elema AB.)

horn of the lateral ventricles, and the contrast agent was moved in the ventricular system by manipulation of the patient's head.

Patient Positioning

PNEUMOENCEPHALOGRAPHY

Because a minimal amount of contrast agent was generally introduced into the subarachnoid space, it was necessary to move the patient through various positions so that visualization of the entire ventricular system could be accomplished.

Figures 16–14 through 16–16 illustrate some of the projections used for pneumoencephalography. Table 16–3 is a summary of the positioning for a typical pneumoencephalogram.

VENTRICULOGRAPHY

In most cases, the positions required for ventriculography were the same as the brow-up supine and brow-down prone positions required for pneumoencephalography.

MAGNETIC RESONANCE IMAGING OF THE BRAIN

MRI has taken the lead in the diagnosis of a diverse group of intracranial abnormalities (Fig. 16–17). It has been successful in imaging congenital abnormalities as well as a variety of neoplastic disease processes and white matter lesions, especially those present in patients with multiple sclerosis. MRI is also useful in the diagnosis of hemorrhage, vascular anomalies, and cerebral infarction.

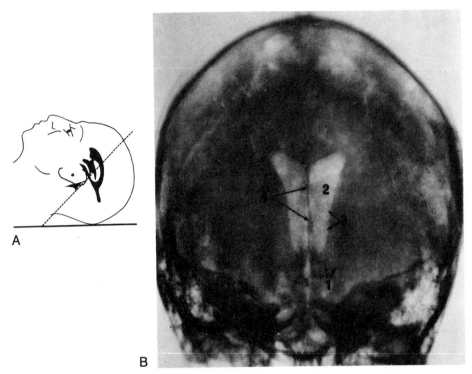

Figure 16–15. The brow-up half-axial anteroposterior projection. *(A)* Schematic of the skull position; *(B)* radiograph of the brow-up half-axial anteroposterior projection showing the anterior horn of the lateral ventricle *(1)*, body of the lateral ventricle *(2)*, indentation caused by the caudate nucleus *(3)*, and septum pellucidum *(4)*. (From Siemens Medical Systems, Inc.)

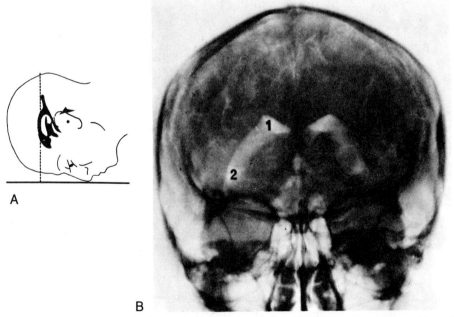

Figure 16–16. The brow-down frontal posteroanterior projection. *(A)* Schematic of the position of the skull; *(B)* radiograph of the brow-down frontal posteroanterior projection showing the body of the lateral ventricle *(1)* and posterior portion of the temporal horn *(2)*. (From Siemens Medical Systems, Inc.)

Table 16–3. PNEUMOENCEPHALOGRAPHIC POSITIONS

When Used	Projection	Position	Central Ray	Anatomy
During filling	Erect posteroanterior	OMBL* perpendicular to film; flexion variable	Perpendicular to film; exits at glabella	Third ventricle, aqueduct of Sylvius, fourth ventricle
	Erect lateral	Interorbital line perpendicular to film; same flexion as erect lateral	Perpendicular to film; enters 4 cm superior to external auditory meatus	Third ventricle, aqueduct of Sylvius, posterior horns of lateral ventricles, fourth ventricles
After filling	Brow-up straight anteroposterior	OMBL perpendicular to film; MSP perpendicular to film	Perpendicular to film; enters 2.5 cm superior to nasion	Anterior horns and bodies of lateral ventricles, third ventricles
	Brow-up half-axial anteroposterior (Towne)	OMBL perpendicular to film; MSP perpendicular to film	25° caudal angle; enters 5 cm superior to nasion	Anterior horns and bodies of lateral ventricles, third ventricles
	Brow-up lateral (cross-table)	Interorbital line perpendicular to film; MSP perpendicular to table	Perpendicular to film plane; enters 5 cm anterosuperior to external auditory meatus	Anterior horns and bodies of lateral ventricles, anterior third ventricle, foramen of Monro
	Brow-down straight posteroanterior	OMBL perpendicular to film; MSP perpendicular to film	Perpendicular to film plane; enters 2.5 cm above inion	Posterior horns, posterior bodies, portion of inferior horns of lateral ventricles
	Brow-down half-axial postero-anterior	OMBL perpendicular to film; MSP perpendicular to film	25–30° cephalic angle; enters 7.5 cm inferior to inion	Posterior horns of lateral ventricles
	Autotomographic erect lateral	Interorbital line perpendicular to film; patient slowly rotates head as if saying "no"	Perpendicular to film; enters 2.5 cm posterior to exterior auditory meatus	Aqueduct of Sylvius, third and fourth ventricles

*OMBL: orbitomeatal baseline; MSP: median sagittal plane.

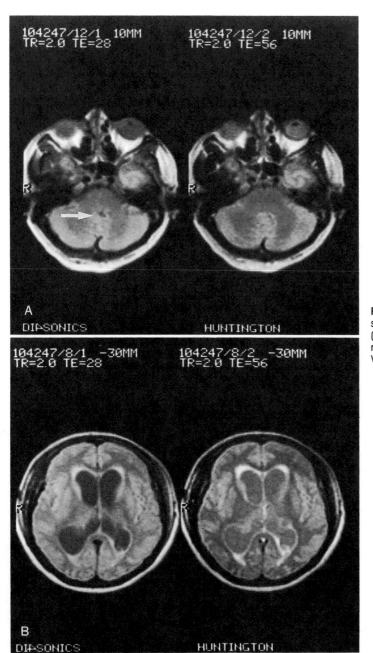

Figure 16–17. MR images of the brain showing secondary hydrocephalus. (From Partain, C., et al.: Magnetic Resonance Imaging, Vol. 1, Philadelphia, W. B. Saunders, 1988.)

REFERENCES

1. Wilson, M.: The Anatomical Foundation of Neuroradiology of the Brain, 2nd ed. Boston, Little, Brown, Co., 1972.
2. Steen, E. B., and Montague, A.: Anatomy and Physiology, Vol. 2. New York, Barnes and Noble, 1959.
3. Anthony, C. P., and Kolthoff, J.: Textbook of Anatomy and Physiology. St. Louis, C. V. Mosby, 1971.
4. Gardner, E., Gray, D. J., and O'Rahilly, R.: Anatomy: A Regional Study of Human Structure, 4th ed. Philadelphia, W. B. Saunders, 1975.
5. Ewart, J.: Epidural myelography, Radiography, *34*:93, 1968.
6. Pen-Tze Lin, J., Ramons, M., and Guzman, E.: Radiography of the Spine, Wilmington, DE, E. I. du Pont De Nemours & Co., 1966.

SUGGESTED READINGS

Bradley, W. G.: Pathophysiological correlates of signal alterations, in Brandt-Zawadski, M., and Norman, D. (eds.): Magnetic Resonance of the Central Nervous System. New York, Raven Press, 1987.

Brye, S.: Current views on the diagnostic value of pneumoencephalography, Ann. Univ. Maria Curie Sklodowska (Med.), *36*:19, 1981.

Campbell, C. B.: The value of autotomography in the demonstration of the midline ventricular system of the brain, Radiol. Technol., *41*:65, 1969.

Cohen, M. D., McGuire, W., Cory, D. A., et al.: MR appearance of blood and blood products: An in vitro study, Am. J. Roentgenol., *146*:1293, 1986.

Coolens, D., et al.: Cervical myelography and the lateral approach on a conventional examination table, J. Belg. Radiol., *69*:163–165, 1986.

Coughlin, J. R., et al.: Metrizamide myelography in conjoined lumbosacral nerve roots, J. Can. Assoc. Radiol., *34*:23, 1983.

DiChino, G., and Fischer, R. L.: Contrast radiography of the spinal cord, Arch. Neurol., *11*:125, 1964.

Dillon, W. P., Norman, D., Newton, T., et al.: Intradural spinal cord lesions: Gd-DTPA enhanced MR imaging, Radiology, *170*:229, 1989.

Eldevik, O. P., Nakken, K. O., and Haughton, V. M.: The effect of dehydration on the side effects of metrizamide myelography, Radiology, *129*:715, 1978.

Felmlee, J. P., and Ehman, R. L.: Spatial presaturation: A method for suppressing flow artifacts and improving depiction of vascular anatomy in MR imaging, Radiology, *164*:559, 1987.

Haughton, V. M.: MR imaging of the spine, Radiology, *166*:297, 1988.

Irstam, L.: Lumbar myelography with Amipaque, Spine, *3*:70, 1978.

Lutz, J. D., et al.: CT myelography of a fragment of a lumbar disk sequestered posterior to the thecal sac, Am. J. Nucl. Reson., *11*:610–611, 1990.

Meschan, I.: Synopsis of Radiologic Anatomy with Computed Tomography, Philadelphia, W. B. Saunders, 1980.

Robertson, G. E.: Pneumoencephalography, 2nd ed., Springfield, IL, Charles C Thomas, 1967.

Ross, J. S., Masaryk, T. J., Modic, M. T., et al.: Lumbar spine: Postoperative assessment with surface coil MR imaging, Radiology, *164*:851, 1987.

Tavares, J. M.: Neuroradiology: Past, present, future, Radiology, *175*:593–602, 1990.

Teplick, J. G., and Haskin, M. E.: Intravenous contrast enhanced CT of the postoperative lumbar spine, Am. J. Roentgenol., *143*:845, 1984.

Wright, C. J.: Epidurography, Radiography, *53*:131–132, 1987.

Valenti, R. M.: Lumbar myelography: Contrast agents used in the past, present and future, Radiol. Technol., *58*:493–496, 1987.

6 Other Special Procedures

seventeen

Hysterosalpingography

ANATOMIC CONSIDERATIONS

INDICATIONS AND
  CONTRAINDICATIONS

CONTRAST MEDIA

PATIENT PREPARATION

PROCEDURE

EQUIPMENT

PATIENT POSITIONING

This procedure involves radiography of the female reproductive system after instillation of a contrast agent. It is a procedure that requires sterile technique, and it is usually performed in a room equipped for specialized genitourinary radiography. Physicians as well as ancillary personnel are required to wear sterile gowns and operating room caps during the procedure. Hysterosalpingography is of value in sterility studies and is considered a safe and painless procedure.

ANATOMIC CONSIDERATIONS

The female reproductive organs are divided into external and internal groups. Hysterosalpingography involves mainly the internal group of reproductive organs—the ovaries, uterine tubes, uterus, and vagina (Fig. 17–1).

The ovaries produce the ova and the sex hormones. They are located near the lateral walls of the pelvis. Before pregnancy, the ovaries are approximately at the level of the anterior superior iliac spine lying lateral to the uterus. During pregnancy, however, the uterus rises into the abdomen, pulling the ovaries away from this general location. After pregnancy, they usually assume their original position.

The ovaries are almond-shaped, slightly flattened structures. Their size fluctuates, depending on patient age and stage of ovarian cycle. The average size is approximately 2.5 to 5 cm long, 2 cm wide, and 1 cm thick.

The ovaries are attached to the uterus by the ovarian ligament, which passes from the uterine end of the ovary to the body of the uterus. One of the ovarian fimbriae, which are fringed, branchlike structures, of the uterine tubes is usually attached at the tubal end of the ovary.

The uterine (fallopian) tubes, or oviducts, transmit the ova to the uterus. Spermatozoa are also transmitted by the uterine tubes from the uterus. Fertilization of the ovum usually occurs in the oviducts. The oviducts can be subdivided into three parts—the isthmus, ampulla, and infundibulum.[1] The isthmus is thick walled and narrow and is attached to the uterine wall. The ampulla is the longest and widest part of the oviduct. Its walls are relatively thin. The funnel-shaped infundibulum terminates in fimbriae. At this point, the oviduct is opened to the peritoneal cavity.

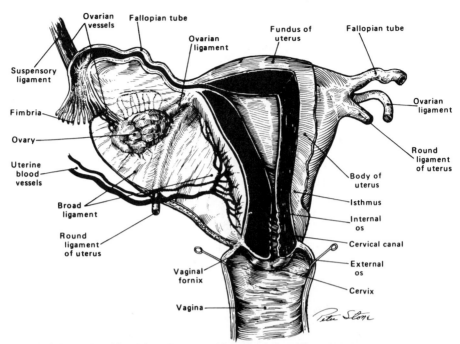

Figure 17–1. Schematic of the internal group of female organs. (From Langley, L. L., Telford, I. R., and Christensen, J. B.: Dynamic Anatomy and Physiology, 4th ed., New York, McGraw-Hill, 1974. © Copyright Mosby-Year Book, Inc.)

The uterus is a thick-walled, muscular organ lying within the pelvis. Its position changes with the degree of fullness of the bladder and rectum.[2] It can also be subdivided into several parts—the fundus, body, isthmus, and cervix (Fig. 17–2). The fundus is the rounded upper portion of the uterus. It is found above the line joining the entrance of the uterine tubes. The body of the uterus, a small triangular area between the uterine walls, extends down toward the isthmus. The body is the main portion of the uterus. Between the cervix and the body of the uterus lies the isthmus, a narrow, constricted, very short segment about 1 cm long. The cervix communicates with the vagina and can be divided into a supravaginal and a vaginal part. The vaginal portion extends into the vagina, whereas the supravaginal part extends up to the isthmus.[2]

The vagina is a muscular tube about 3 in (7.6 cm) long that forms the lower portion of the birth canal. It communicates with the uterus above, the cervix inside, and the vestibule of the vagina below.

INDICATIONS AND CONTRAINDICATIONS

Hysterosalpingography is a safe diagnostic and therapeutic tool in the diagnosis and treatment of the female genital organs. It has been used in the study of infertility to determine possible structural or functional defects not obvious by clinical examination. Many other abnormal gynecologic conditions have also been demonstrated by this procedure.

As a therapeutic tool, hysterosalpingography has been shown to be effective in some cases of infertility. The procedure has had success in restoring patency to occluded tubes, straightening kinks, stretching adhesions, and dilating narrowed tubes.

Other uses for the procedure are preoperative and postoperative evaluations of the genital organs; determination and location of ectopic, misplaced, or lost contraceptive devices; and determination of the cause for dysmenorrhea.

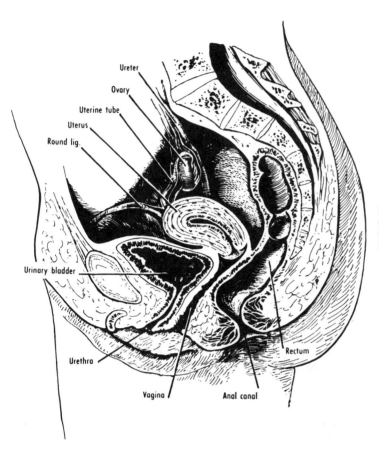

Figure 17–2. Schematic cross section of the uterus. (From Gardner, E., Gray, D. J., and O'Rahilly, R.: Anatomy, 4th ed., Philadelphia, W. B. Saunders, Company, 1975.)

The following list is a summary of the indications for hysterosalpingography:

Diagnosis
    Abnormal uterine bleeding
    Patency of fallopian tubes
    Congenital uterine anomalies
    Habitual abortion
    Amenorrhea
    Preoperative evaluation for localization
    Postoperative evaluation
    Locate ectopic or lost contraceptive devices
    Dysmenorrhea
    Pelvic masses
    Fistulae
    Cervical stenosis
    Malignancy
    Endometrial polyps
    Leiomyoma
Therapy
    Restore patency of fallopian tubes
    Stretch tubal adhesions
    Straighten kinks
    Dilate tubes

This is by no means a complete list because the indications for any specialized procedure increase as its possibilities and limitations are further evaluated.

Hysterosalpingography is contraindicated when an acute or subacute pelvic inflammation exists. In cases of vaginal or cervical infection accompanied by purulent discharge, the procedure is also contraindicated. The procedure is not advised during the immediate premenstrual or postmenstrual phase.

Active uterine bleeding also contraindicates hysterosalpingography. If the study were performed under these conditions, it would not be of diagnostic value, and there would always be the danger of seepage of the contrast medium into the general circulation.

Pregnancy is usually considered an absolute contraindication, except in special cases.

CONTRAST MEDIA

The contrast agents used to delineate anatomic structures during hysterosalpingography are divided into two groups—water soluble and oily. All are organic iodine compounds, and each group has its advantages. The water-soluble contrast agents are absorbed quickly and do not leave a residue within the genital tract; the iodized oils are extremely opaque and are well tolerated by the structures under study. The main disadvantage to the iodized oils is their persistence in the body cavities. Table 17–1 is a comparison of oily contrast media with water-soluble media.

The ideal contrast medium possesses the following characteristics:

1. Rapid absorption and excretion rates
2. Sufficient radiologic density
3. Adequate viscosity
4. Does not cause general or local reactions
5. Ability to delineate anatomic structures

In general, when iodized oils are used, 24-h delayed films are taken to demonstrate tubal patency. Table 17–2 is a summary of contrast media available for hysterosalpingography. The use of the low-osmolality contrast agents offers no significant advantage over the use of the ionic agents in hysterosalpingography.[3] Their use would not be

Table 17–1. COMPARISON OF OILY AND WATER-SOLUBLE CONTRAST MEDIA

Characteristic	Oily Medium	Water-Soluble Medium
Viscosity	High	Low to moderate
Radiopacity	Very good	Moderate to satisfactory
Absorption rate	Very slow; delayed for many months when large amounts are injected	Prompt excretion through kidneys; after 20–60 min in hydrosalpinx the medium is only slowly absorbed and may persist for 24–48 h
Toxicity	Not observed unless decomposed oil is used	Rare
Allergic reactions	Not observed	Occasionally observed
Peritoneal reactions	Only when large amounts are injected; not observed when small quantities are injected	Observed, mostly transient
Pain	Not observed when small amounts are injected under low pressure	Nearly always present; may be transient or persist for many hours
Dangers	Intravasation, pulmonary embolism	None

From Rozin, S.: Uterosalpingography in Gynecology, Springfield, IL, Charles C Thomas, 1965, p. 10.

Table 17–2. SUMMARY OF CONTRAST MEDIA FOR HYSTEROSALPINGOGRAPHY

Trade Name	Manufacturer	Iodine Content (%)	Water-Soluble	Oily
Ethiodol	E. I. Fougera	37		X
Hypaque 50%	Winthrop	30	X	
Hypaque-m 90%	Winthrop	46	X	
Lipiodol 40%	Savage	38–42		X
Lipiodol 28%	Savage	26.5–29.5		
Salpix	Ortho	27	X	
Sinografin	Squibb	38	X	
Renografin-60	Squibb	29	X	
Conray 60	Mallinckrodt	28	X	

justified in this study owing to the extreme cost difference between ionic and nonionic water-soluble contrast agents.

The total amount of contrast agent introduced is variable. Approximately 4 ml is required to fill a normal uterine cavity. An additional 4 ml may be required to visualize the fallopian tubes, and larger amounts may be used in some disease conditions.

The negative contrast medium, carbon dioxide, can be used after positive contrast hysterosalpingography to diagnose many gynecologic problems. Approximately 100 ml of carbon dioxide is introduced into the uterus after the removal of the positive-contrast agent. The carbon dioxide is usually absorbed within 25 to 30 min and causes a minimal amount of patient discomfort.

PATIENT PREPARATION

Before the day of the examination, the patient is instructed in the protocol for proper bowel cleansing. This includes taking a non–gas-forming laxative on the evening before the study. On the morning of the study, the patient takes cleansing enemas until the flow is clear. In some cases, restriction of intake is recommended.

The procedure is explained to the patient, and she is instructed to empty her bladder to prevent possible displacement of the uterus and fallopian tubes. The patient is requested to irrigate the vagina and cleanse the perineal region at this time.

Unless the patient is unusually apprehensive, premedication is not required. As with all contrast examinations, a history is taken. If the patient indicates an allergic history, notify the physician performing the study because premedication with steroids, an antihistamine, or both is indicated. The history should contain the date of the last menses. Hysterosalpingography should be done toward the end of the first week after menstruation and before the 12th day of the menstrual cycle to avoid radiation exposure to the oocyte, which becomes radiosensitive at this time. The patient's menstrual flow should have been completed for at least 3 days before the study to prevent intravasation of the contrast agent.

Hysterosalpingography is normally done as an outpatient procedure, and follow-up care is limited. Sometimes, the patient experiences some subjective transitory aftereffects and requires bed rest before leaving the department.

PROCEDURE

Hysterosalpingography can be performed in a radiographic/fluorographic room or a radiographic room equipped with a urologic table like that used for cystoscopy and retrograde pyelography. The patient assumes the lithotomy position, and the table is adjusted to a slight Trendelenburg position.

The cervix is exposed with a bivalved speculum, a specialized cannula is introduced into the cervical os, and the cannula is fixed in place. The main objective of the cannula is to occlude the cervical os to create a water-tight fit. The contrast medium is slowly injected, and radiographs are then taken.

Fractional injection of the contrast agent is usually practiced. Standard fractional routines are nonexistent because they vary with the individual patient. Films are taken after each fractional injection and evaluated before additional contrast material is introduced. The cannula remains in situ throughout the procedure to prevent backflow of contrast material into the vagina.

It is important to follow strict aseptic technique throughout the procedure to avoid the possibility of introducing infection into the peritoneal cavity.

If an oily contrast medium is used, the patient is required to return in 24 h for a delayed radiograph to show whether the contrast medium has reached the free peritoneal cavity or has been trapped by pathological fallopian tubes. If a water-soluble contrast medium is used, this is evident during the procedure.

EQUIPMENT

Hysterosalpingography requires a minimum of specialized equipment. The room must be equipped with a urology table to enable the patient to comfortably assume the lithotomy position. In some institutions, fluoroscopic control of hysterosalpingography is practiced. When fluoroscopy is used, it may be adapted for cineradiography to facilitate serial filming of the procedure. When an oil-soluble contrast medium is used, fluoroscopy can reduce the incidence of contrast medium intravasation into veins and lymph vessels, resulting in fewer cases of oil embolization.

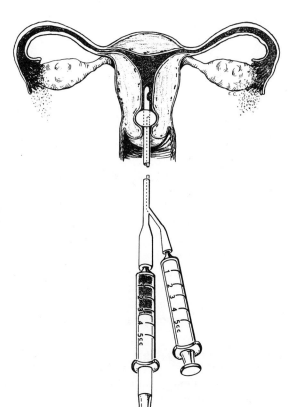

Figure 17–3. The balloon catheter occlusion technique for hysterosalpingography. (From Siegler, A.: Hysterosalpingography, New York, Harper & Row, 1967.)

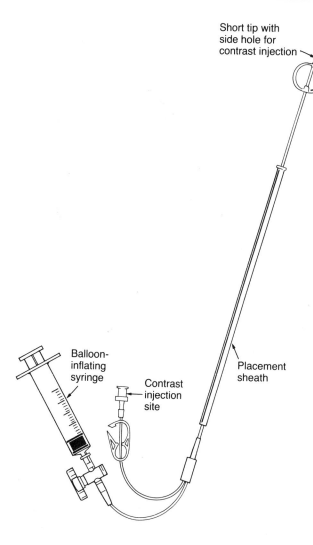

Short tip with
side hole for
contrast injection

Balloon-
inflating
syringe

Contrast
injection
site

Placement
sheath

Figure 17–4. Schematic illustration of the Ackrad H/S catheter set. The unit allows for an easier examination for both the patient and the physician and eliminates the need for the use of a tenaculum. It is available as a basic set or in a complete procedural tray. (From Ackrad Laboratories, Inc.)

A sterile tray should be prepared and available for the procedure. Items recommended for inclusion in the sterile tray include a vaginal speculum, dilators, sponge-holding forceps, uterine sound, tenacula, uterine cannula, sterile towels and drapes, and small sterile containers. Additional items may be added, depending on the specific technique used. If a catheter balloon occlusion technique is used, the specialized catheter and syringes should be added to the sterile tray (Fig. 17–3).

Many cannulae are available for hysterosalpingography, including the Malmstrom vacuum, Leech-Wilkinson, Jarcho, and Hayes-Provis cannulae. A No. 16 or 18 Foley catheter can also be used. The cannula seals the cervical os to prevent leakage of the contrast medium during the procedure. Cannulae differ only in their specific method of sealing the cervical os. Figure 17–4 shows the Ackrad H/S catheter set, which uses a 1.5- to 4-ml balloon to occlude the cervix.

Other items necessary for the examination include sterile gloves (various sizes), antiseptic cleansing solution for the outer vaginal area, contrast media, and face masks.

PATIENT POSITIONING

Almost all filming during hysterosalpingography is done with the patient in the anteroposterior position. Occasionally, other positions such as prone, oblique, and lateral positions may be requested if indicated by specific pathology.

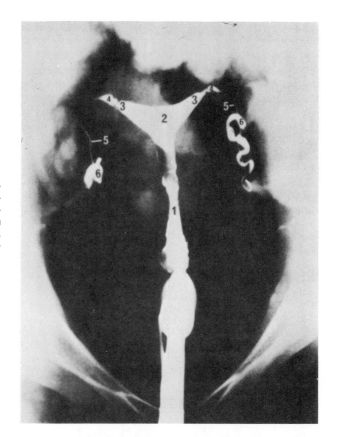

Figure 17–5. Radiograph of a normal hysterosalpingogram following pneumoperitoneum. *(1)* Cervical canal; *(2)* uterine cavity; *(3)* cornua; *(4)* intramural portion of the fallopian tubes; *(5)* fallopian tubes; *(6)* fimbriae. (From Potchen, E. J., Koehler, R. P., and Davis, D. O.: Principles of Diagnostic Radiology, New York, McGraw-Hill, 1971.)

Table 17–3. SUMMARY OF POSITIONS FOR HYSTEROSALPINGOGRAPHY

Projection	Patient Position	Central Ray	Anatomy
Anteroposterior	Patient in dorsal lithotomy position, centered to table; point approximately 2 in (5 cm) superior to symphysis pubis is centered to a transverse 10- × 12-in (25- × 30-cm) cassette	Directed at a right angle to film	Speculum in vagina, cannula inserted in cervix, uterine body cavity, uterine horns, fallopian tubes; spill of contrast medium into peritoneal cavity
Oblique (optional view)	Patient rotated into either right or left posterior oblique position; cassette centered to same location as above	Directed at a right angle to film	Oblique view of above anatomy used to demonstrate pathology not otherwise well shown
Lateral (optional view)	Patient in right or left lateral position; cassette centered to same location as above	Directed at a right angle to film	Lateral view of above anatomy used to demonstrate pathology not otherwise well shown, very rarely done
Prone (optional view)	Patient rotated into the prone position, centered to the table; point approximately 2 in (5 cm) superior to the symphysis pubis centered to a transverse 10- × 12-in (25- × 30-cm) cassette	Directed at a right angle to the film	Differentiates free peritoneal spill from loculated collections related to peritubal adhesions

The necessary anatomy can be easily recorded on a 10- × 12-in (25- × 30-cm) cassette. The patient should be in the supine position and adjusted so that a point approximately 2 in (5 cm) superior to the symphysis pubis is centered to the cassette. The central ray should be directed at right angles to the film.

If oblique views are required, the physician usually specifies the amount of obliquity necessary.

The filming procedure varies with each patient, ranging from one anteroposterior view to a sequential series attempting to demonstrate tubal patency, by the spill of contrast medium into the peritoneal cavity (Fig. 17–5). Accuracy is stressed because unnecessary radiation exposure to the gonads due to technical error is inexcusable.

Table 17–3 is a summary of positioning for hysterosalpingography.

REFERENCES

1. Woodburne, R. T.: Essentials of Human Anatomy, 7th ed. New York, Oxford University Press, 1983.
2. Gardner, E., Gray, D. J., and O'Rahilly, R.: Anatomy: A Regional Study of Human Structure, 4th ed. Philadelphia, W. B. Saunders, 1975.
3. Winfield, A. C.: Contrast media for hysterosalpingography: Water soluble materials are preferred, Radiol. Rep., 2:208, 1990.

SUGGESTED READINGS

Alper, M. M., Garner, P. R., Spence, J. E. H., and Quarrington, A. M.: Pregnancy rates after hysterosalpingography with oil and water soluble contrast media, Obstet. Gynecol., 68:7, 1986.

Avnet, N. L., and Elkin, M.: Hysterosalpingography, Radiol. Clin. North Am., 5:105, 1969.

Austin, R. M., Sacks, B. A., Nowell, M., and Feital, C.: Catheter hysterosalpingography, Radiology, 151:249, 1984.

Beyth, Y., Navot, D., and Lax, E.: A simple improvement in the technique of hysterosalpingography achieving optimal imaging and avoiding possible complications, Fertil. Steril., 44:543, 1985.

Burnhill, M. S., and Birnberg, C. H.: The size and shape of the uterine cavity determined by hysterography with an intrauterine contraceptive device as a marker, Int. J. Fertil., 11:187, 1966.

Ellison, J. M.: The McCallum suction sialographic cannula and technique, Radiography, 35:177, 1969.

Eschenbach, D. A.: Acute pelvic inflammatory disease, Urol. Clin. North Am., 11:65, 1984.

Friedman, P. J., and Pine, H. L.: Radiographic localization of the ectopic intrauterine contraceptive device, Obstet. Gynecol., 27:814, 1966.

Green, T. H., Jr.: Gynecology: Essentials of Clinical Practice, 3rd ed. Boston, Little, Brown, Co., 1977.

Karasick, S.: Contrast media for hysterosalpingography: Oil soluble materials are preferred, Radiol. Rep., 2:204–207, 1990.

Malmstrom, T.: A vacuum uterine cannula, Obstet. Gynecol., 18:773, 1961.

Moore, D. R.: Pain associated with hysterosalpingography: Ethiodol versus Salpix media, Fertil. Steril., 38:629, 1982.

Ries, G., et al.: Values and possibilities for the improvement of hysterosalpingography (English abstract), R. O. E. F. O., 138:197, 1983.

White, W. E., and Denton, M.: Therapeutic dividends of hysterosalpingography, J. Med. Assoc. State Ala., 29:86, 1959.

Wilson, R. B., and Massee, J. S.: Sequential gas-oil-gas procedure in the therapy of infertility, Fertil. Steril., 13:366, 1966.

Winfield, A. C.: Contrast media for hysterosalpingography: Water soluble materials preferred, Radiol. Rep., 2:205–209, 1990.

eighteen

Lymphangiography

ANATOMIC CONSIDERATIONS
Lymph Vessels
Lymph Nodes
INDICATIONS AND
    CONTRAINDICATIONS
CONTRAST MEDIA

PATIENT PREPARATIOIN
PROCEDURE
EQUIPMENT
PATIENT POSITIONING

The lymphatic system is considered part of the circulatory system. It serves as a filtering center for bacteria, carbon particles, and malignant cells. It manufactures lymphocytes and monocytes (white blood cells, the corpuscular constituents of blood) and serves to return certain substances to the bloodstream, such as electrolytes, water, and colloidal materiai.

Lymph is the substance that is transported by the lymphatic circulation. It is absorbed by the lymphatic capillaries and is usually clear and colorless. Its chemical composition closely resembles that of blood plasma. Lymph is not pumped through the system but rather moves as a result of differences in capillary pressure, peristalsis, respiratory movements, cardiac activity, massage, and muscular activity. Changes in arterial pressure do not affect the movement of lymph; however, the flow is increased by increases in venous pressure. Lymph is continuously being produced from tissue fluid by filtration.

The lymphatic system serves as a supplement to the capillaries and veins. It is considered a connection between the blood and tissue fluid.

Lymphangiography is the radiographic investigation and demonstration of the lymphatic system. This procedure has been abandoned by many institutions as the method of choice for imaging the lymphatic system. It is an invasive procedure that is accompanied by a moderate amount of complications. It is somewhat painful for the patient, usually takes several hours to perform, and requires a high degree of technical skill.[1] Computed tomography (CT) and ultrasonography have been used successfully to stage tumors of the lymphatic system and have become the methods of choice. Magnetic resonance imaging (MRI) and, more recently, radioisotope lymphangiography (lymphoscintography) are undergoing investigation as possible tools for the diagnosis of lymphatic tumors.

The use of lymphangiography is primarily limited to oncologic centers and large research and teaching institutions where the higher volume of cases and expertise justifies its use as a diagnostic tool. It's greatest value has been in the diagnosis of neoplastic involvement in nonenlarged lymph nodes, and it is the procedure of choice for the diagnosis and staging of Hodgkin's lymphoma and testicular tumors. Despite its limitations for the diagnosis of pathology in the renal and hepatic nodes and the poor opacification of high para-aortic and mesenteric nodes, it remains a useful diagnostic procedure.

ANATOMIC CONSIDERATIONS

The lymph vascular system, which is summarized in Table 18–1, consists primarily of the lymph vessels and lymph nodes. The main lymphoid organs of the body are the spleen, tonsils, and thymus gland.

Lymph Vessels

The lymph capillaries are located within the tissues. They are unevenly distributed throughout the body and are centered primarily in areas with a rich blood supply. As in the blood vascular system, the lymph capillaries unite to form larger vessels, which are known as lymphatics.

The lymphatics are collecting vessels. They are similar to the veins in structure and contain valves to ensure that the lymph flows only toward the heart. They are divided into superficial and deep lymphatic vessels, and they usually run parallel to the veins. The superficial lymphatics are found just beneath the skin; the deep lymphatic vessels are larger and fewer than the superficial lymphatics and usually accompany the deep veins.

Lymphatic vessels originating in the villi of the small intestine are called lacteals. They usually continue as the lymphatic vessels of the intestinal wall and mesentery. The lacteals absorb the hydrolyzed fats produced by fat digestion and give the lymph a whitish color. Lymph in this state is called chyle.

From the lymphatic vessels, the lymph drains into one of the two lymphatic ducts. The right lymphatic duct is a short vessel that empties into the right subclavian vein. It drains the lymph from vessels originating on the right sides of the head, neck, right upper extremity, liver, and right thoracic cavity, including the right lung and the right side of the heart.

Lymphatic vessels from the lower extremities, pelvic viscera, and abdomen drain into a dilation called the cisterna chyli, which is located at about L1 or L2. The superior portion of the cisterna chyli narrows to form the thoracic duct. The thoracic duct, or left lymphatic, travels up in front of the vertebral bodies. It passes through the aortic hiatus in the diaphragm to the thoracic cavity. At about the level of the fifth or sixth thoracic vertebra, the thoracic duct crosses obliquely to the left. It ascends to the neck, where it arches to terminate in the left subclavian vein (Fig. 18–1).

The points of drainage of the right and left lymphatic ducts are variable. For example,

Table 18–1. LYMPH VASCULAR SYSTEM

System	Constitutes
Lymph vessels	Lymph capillaries
	Superficial lymphatic vessel
	Deep lymphatic vessel
	Lacteals
	Cisterna chyli
	Thoracic duct
	Right lymphatic duct
Lymph nodes	Masses of lymphoid tissue situated throughout the body, both singly and in groups

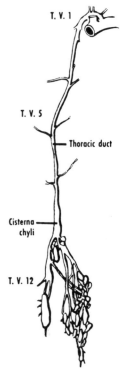

T. V. 1

T. V. 5

Thoracic duct

Cisterna chyli

T. V. 12

Figure 18-1. Schematic showing drainage of the lymphatic into the cisterna chyli and thoracic duct. (From Gardner, E., Gray, D. J., and O'Rahilly, R.: Anatomy, 4th ed., Philadelphia, W. B. Saunders, 1975.)

the thoracic duct may actually terminate in the left jugular vein or at the junction of the left jugular and left subclavian veins. The lymphatic drainage will, however, ultimately find its way into the innominate (brachiocephalic) veins.

Lymph Nodes

Lymph nodes are round or oval bodies that vary in size and are located in the path of lymphatics. They are composed of lymphoid tissue surrounded by a capsule of connective tissue (Fig. 18–2). Lymph nodes are situated throughout the body, usually in groups or chains; however, single lymph nodes are occasionally found.

Lymph nodes are grouped by the areas of the body that they drain (Fig. 18–3). A group of lymph nodes is present on the back of the head and neck.

Superficial and deep lymph nodes are found in the upper extremity. There are relatively few nodes in the superficial system. In general, three groups of nodes are of interest in the upper extremity—a small group located at the medial epicondyle, which drains the hand and forearm; a larger group at the axilla; and a subclavicular or medial group under the pectoral muscles.

The lower extremities also have superficial and deep groups of nodes—the popliteal group in the space behind the knee, the anterior tibial nodes, and the inguinal nodes, the largest area.

In the abdomen and thoracic cavity, the lymph nodes are divided into the parietal node, which is situated behind the peritoneum in the abdomen and in the thoracic wall of the thorax, and the visceral node, which is associated with the organs located within the abdomen or thoracic cavity.

The pelvis contains three main groups of lymph nodes—external iliac, hypogastric, and common iliac nodes. All of these drain into the thoracic duct through the cisterna chyli.

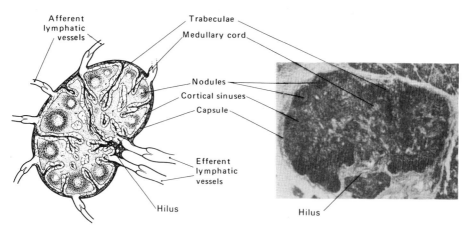

Figure 18–2. Schematic and photomicrograph of a lymph node. (From Langley, L. L., Telford, I. R., and Christensen, J. B.: Dynamic Anatomy and Physiology, 4th ed., New York, McGraw-Hill, 1974. © Copyright Mosby-Year Book, Inc.)

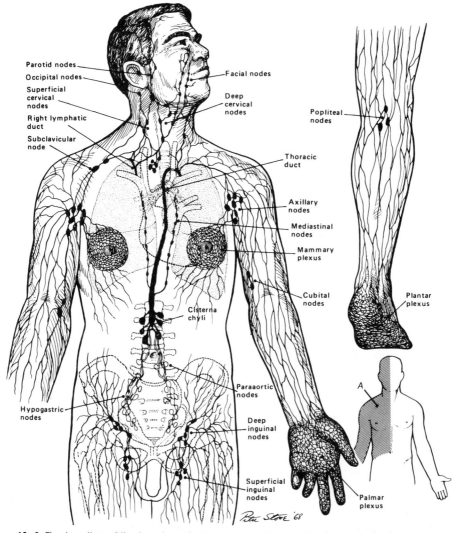

Figure 18–3. The location of the lymph nodes in the human body. The shaded area *(A)* corresponds to drainage into the right lymphatic duct, whereas the rest of the body drains into the left lymphatic or, as it is sometimes called, thoracic duct. (From Langley, L. L., Telford, I. R., and Christensen, J. B.: Dynamic Anatomy and Physiology, 4th ed., New York, McGraw-Hill, 1974. © Copyright Mosby-Year Book, Inc.)

INDICATIONS AND CONTRAINDICATIONS

Lymphangiography is indicated for patients who exhibit unexplainable peripheral swellings, in cases of suspected carcinoma, for postsurgical evaluation of nodal dissection, and in evaluating the effects of chemotherapy on treated nodes. Specifically, the procedure is requested for cancer of the reproductive organs (both male and female), Hodgkin's disease, and prostatic carcinoma and as a follow-up to normal or equivocal CT findings in suspected cases of non-Hodgkin's lymphoma. Lymphangiography is also performed when information concerning the patency of the deep lymphatic trunks is required. CT is the method of choice for non-Hodgkin's lymphomas and pelvic malignancies at the level of the thoracolumbar junction.

This procedure is contraindicated in patients with a known sensitivity to iodine. Patients with advanced pulmonary diseases should not have the procedure done. The lungs receive the overflow of iodized oil from the procedure; therefore, if active disease is present, complications can occur. Exposure to large amounts of radiation, to either the lungs or the area to be examined, is a contraindication to lymphangiography. Radiation decreases the filtration rate of the lungs, creating the possibility of fatal complications resulting from oil emboli.[2] Interruption of the lymphatic system by surgery and suspected obstruction caused by advanced disease are also considered relative contraindications. Because the procedure requires cannulation of delicate lymphatic vessels, patients who exhibit marked tremors are not good candidates for the study.

CONTRAST MEDIA

Lymphangiography requires that a suitable contrast agent be injected into a lymphatic vessel. The most common method is direct injection into a lymphatic of an extremity. These vessels are similar in appearance to the small veins, and differentiation is difficult without the aid of an indicator dye. The substance used for this purpose must be selectively absorbed by the lymphatic vessels and provide a visual contrast with the surrounding tissue without subsequent staining of the field. It must also be nontoxic to the lymphatic or surrounding tissue.

Blue is the dye color that provides the best contrast. There are many blue dyes marketed today, not all of which are suitable for use in lymphangiography. Table 18–2 lists the commonly used indicator dyes for this procedure.

Various dyes have different absorption rates into the lymphatics. The process may be hastened by gentle massage over the injection site or by allowing the patient to walk for a short period.

Table 18–2. COMMONLY USED INDICATOR DYES FOR LYMPHANGIOGRAPHY

Dye	Color Index*	Catalog Number	Size (g)	Manufacturer
Direct Blue 1 (Chicago Blue 6B)	24410	CX0685	25	EM Science
Direct Blue 53 (Evans Blue)	23860	EX0975	10 25	EM Science
Brilliant Blue FCF (Erioglaucine)	42090	EX0120	25	EM Science
Alphazurine 2G (Patent Blue)	42045	PX0070	25	EM Science

*The color index is necessary when requesting indicator dyes from the manufacturer because many dyes contain mixtures of isomers that affect the effectiveness of the dye as an indicator for lymphangiography.

Oil-based organic iodine compounds are used as contrast agents for lymphangiography. Water-soluble contrast media are occasionally used; however, these irritate the lymphatic vessels and cause the patient some discomfort. The discomfort will manifest itself by a burning sensation along the extremity as the contrast column advances. In addition to the discomfort to the patient, the water-soluble media have the disadvantage of diffusing through the lymphatic vessels 5 to 10 min after the start of the injection.

Some of the more common agents currently in use are Ethiodol and Lipiodol Ultra Fluid. These are organic combinations of iodine with ethyl esters of the fatty acids of poppy seed oil. The unused portion of contrast agent should be discarded because the iodine is liberated from the compound by oxygen.

The oil-based compounds can remain in the lymphatic system for as short as several days to as long as 2 years. This can be an advantage by allowing the monitoring of the tumor's response to the treatment; the follow-up is easily accomplished with abdominal and pelvic radiographs. This is a relatively inexpensive method compared with the use of CT as a follow-up procedure.

PATIENT PREPARATION

Before the day of the procedure, the patient should be acquainted with the procedure and told that the test requires 2 days for completion. Approximately 4 to 5 h is spent in the department for the first segment of the procedure, which consists of isolation of the vessel, cannulation, and injection of the contrast agent. On the second day, the patient is required to return for additional filming. The patient should also be told that temporary skin and urine discoloration occurs as a result of the vital indicator dye and disappears over time. The patient should be urged to bring something to occupy his or her time, such as reading material.

Depending on the route of injection, the patient's feet or hands should be cleansed and shaved. For comfort, the patient is urged to empty the bladder before the procedure begins. The area to be cannulated is then surgically cleansed and draped.

Although reactions are rare, the patient should be monitored during the procedure for any subjective or objective symptoms. The majority of reactions are those caused by hypersensitivity to the contrast agent, oil embolism, and local infection at the site of injection.

After the procedure, the incisions are sutured and bandaged, and the patient is given general instructions regarding incision care. There also is the possibility that the patient may experience a transient mild fever and cough during the night after the procedure.

PROCEDURE

The most common method of introducing contrast agent into a lymphatic channel is by direct injection after surgical exposure of a suitable vessel.

The patient is placed on the radiographic table in a supine position. The area to be injected is surgically "prepped" and then infiltrated with indicator dye and a local anesthetic. This can be accomplished by separate injections, or by a single injection into which the substances have been combined. The dye is then given time to diffuse into the lymphatic vessels, which should take from 15 to 20 min. The lymphatic channels will appear as bluish-green stripes.

A small incision (approximately 3 cm) is made, and a suitable lymphatic vessel is isolated. A small hemostat is passed under the chosen vessel, and by opening and closing the hemostat, the vessel is dissected from the surrounding tissue (Fig. 18–4).

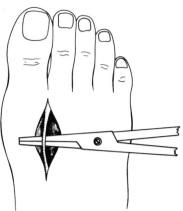

Figure 18–4. Incision made on the dorsum of the foot to isolate a lymphatic channel for cannulation.

Before cannulation of the lymphatic can proceed, the vessel must be dilated to facilitate insertion of the needle. This is accomplished by placing two pieces of 4-0 black silk suture thread around the lymphatic, which makes it possible to obstruct the flow of lymph in the vessel. Massage the area distal to the incision while the proximal thread is secured. The threads also immobilize the vessel during cannulation (Fig. 18–5).

When the vessel is sufficiently distended, the threads are secured with the index finger and thumb, and the cannulation can be accomplished. Once the needle is in place in the lymphatic channel, it must be secured by tying the proximal suture around the lymphatic vessel and needle tip.

Free passage of fluid in the vessel must be verified by injecting some tiny air bubbles through the cannula. Their movement indicates that the fluid will pass freely through the vessel.

The tubing attached to the needle is looped and fastened to the skin with an adhesive bandage. Another bandage is placed over the needle at the incision site. This ensures that the needle will not be accidentally torn from the vessel during the injection.

The tubing is then connected to the syringe containing the contrast agent. This is placed into the injection device, and the infusion is begun. The injection pressure should be regulated so that the contrast agent is delivered in no less than 1.25 h. The amount of contrast medium injected should be from 5 to 10 ml for each lower extremity and one half this amount if injection is made via the upper extremity.

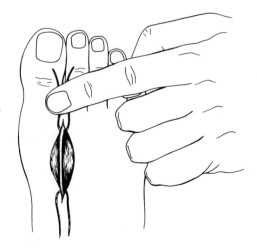

Figure 18–5. Incision and suture thread used to immobilize the lymphatic channel for cannulation.

EQUIPMENT

Lymphangiography does not require specialized x-ray equipment; it can be done in a general diagnostic room if a special procedure suite is not available. The initial phase involving isolation of the lymph vessel and its cannulation does not have to be carried out in a radiographic room.

An automatic injection device of some type is required to facilitate infusion of the contrast medium into the lymphatic vessel because the low and constant pressure required to move the contrast medium through the vessel are impossible to maintain over the period of the injection.

A sterile tray containing an assortment of syringes, sponges, glassware, and needles should be prepared for use during the procedure. The contents of a typical lymphangiogram tray are listed in Table 18–3.

Standard sterile supplies available with the sterile tray include surgical masks, gloves, and basins. Scrub suits should be worn to avoid possible staining of clothing with the indicator dye.

The cannulation set can be prepared during the procedure or purchased as a sterile disposable set (Fig. 18–6). In most institutions, it has become routine to use the sterile disposable set rather than the homemade variety.

The specialized cannulator available for lymphangiography is called the Tegtmeyer lymph duct cannulator. It is a simple device that facilitates accurate cannulation of a lymphatic channel. The cannulation process using this device is shown in Figure 18–7.

Additional necessary equipment includes an adjustable lamp to provide adequate lighting of the surgical area and an adjustable stool to provide a comfortable working position during the tedious cannulation procedure.

PATIENT POSITIONING

The views most often taken for lymphangiography are anteroposterior, lateral, and posterior oblique (Fig. 18–8). Scout views are taken during infusion of the contrast agent to monitor its progress through the lymphatic system. When the infusion is completed, the needle is removed, the incision is sutured, and the wound is dressed. Radiographs are taken of the pelvis, abdomen, and chest as soon as possible after closure of the incision. These early flow films are important for the demonstration of

Table 18–3. CONTENTS OF TYPICAL STERILE LYMPHANGIOGRAM TRAY

Item	Amount and/or Size
Luer-Lok syringe	2 (20 ml)
Luer-Lok syringe	3 (10 ml)
Syringe	1 (2 ml)
Marked medicine glasses	3
Gauze sponges	8 (3 × 3 in)
Gauze sponges	12 (4 × 4 in)
Small surgical drape	1
Towels	4
Scalpel handle and blade	1
Needle	1 (5/8 in, 25 gauge)
Needle	1 (1½ in, 18 gauge)
Small hemostat	1
Skin rake	1
Vein dissector	1
4-0 black silk	2 (12-in pieces)
Small scissors	1
Autoclave tape	4 (6-in strips)

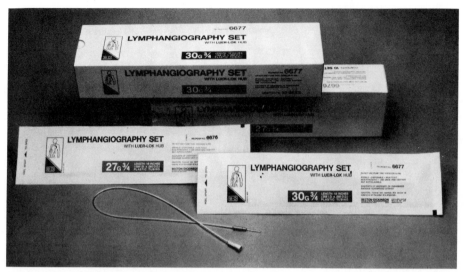

Figure 18–6. The sterile disposable lymphangiography set. (From Becton Dickinson and Company.)

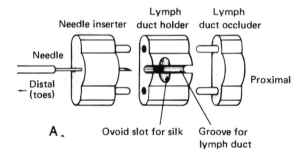

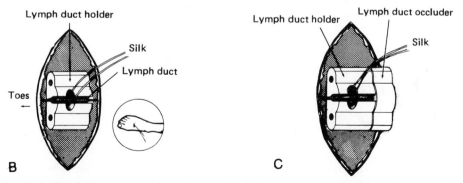

Figure 18–7. The Tegtmeyer lymph duct cannulator for lymphangiography. *(A)* The lymph duct cannulation set. *(B)* After the vessel is isolated, the lymph duct holder is placed under it with the vessel in the cannulator groove. The ovoid slot must be closest to the toes. *(C)* A piece of 4-0 silk is looped around the vessel and positioned in the ovoid slot. A loose overhand knot is placed in the silk.

Illustration continued on following page

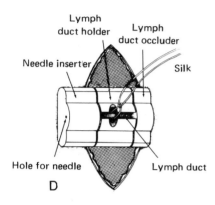

D

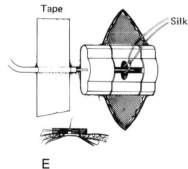

E

Figure 18–7 *Continued (D)* The lymph duct occluder has been inserted and the foot is milked to cause the vessel to dilate and fill the groove in the holder. When this is accomplished, the needle inserter is put into place. This effectively holds the distended vessel for cannulation. *(E)* A 27- or 30-gauge needle attached by tubing to a saline-filled syringe is advanced through the needle inserted into the dilated vessel. A small amount of saline solution is injected to further dilate the vessel. The needle is advanced past the ovoid slot, and the silk suture is tightened over it. *(F)* The cannulator is affixed to the skin by adhesive tape. The lymph duct occluder is removed, and the injection can proceed. (From NAMICO U.S.A. Corporation.)

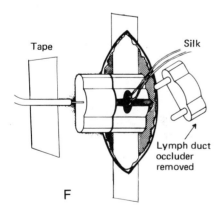

F

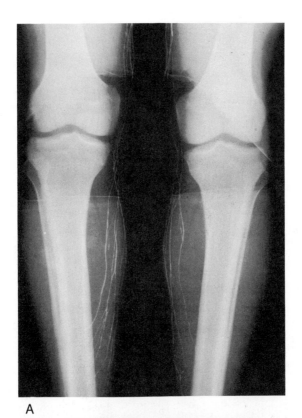

A

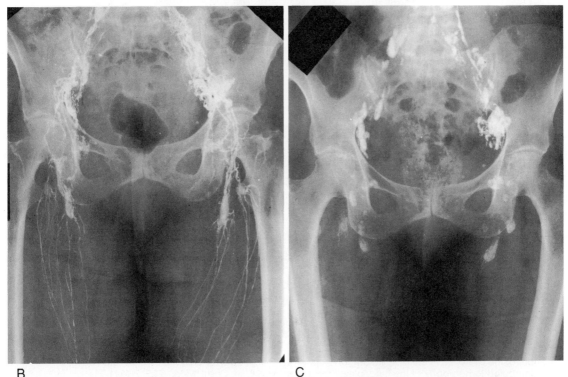

B   C

Figure 18–8. Representative radiographs from a lymphangiographic study. (A) Normal leg lymphatics along course of greater saphenous vein; (B) contrast medium in dye and inguinal lymph vessels at end of injection; (C) film taken about 24 h later showing that lymph nodes in inguinal and iliac regions have become opacified.

Illustration continued on following page

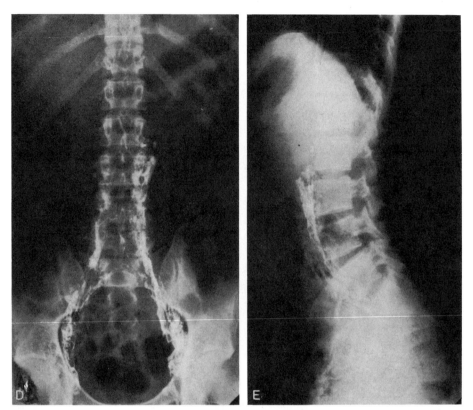

Figure 18–8 *Continued (D)* and *(E)* lymphatic vessels converge at level of L2 to form cisterna chyli. (From Juergens, J. L., Spittell, J. A., Jr., Fairbairn, J. F., II: Allen-Barker-Hines Peripheral Vascular Diseases, 5th ed., Philadelphia, W. B. Saunders, 1980. Copyright Mayo Clinic, Rochester, MN.)

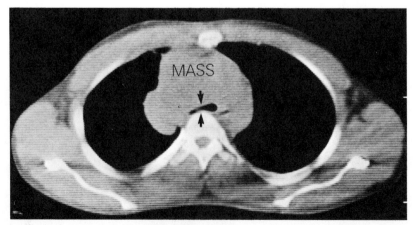

Figure 18–9. A large mediastinal lymphoma demonstrated compressing the patient's airway. This is an example of the use of CT in thoracic staging of lymphoma. (From Pugatch, R. D., Munn, C. S., and Faling, L. J.: Computed tomography of the lung, pleura, and chest wall. Clin. Chest. Med., 5:267, 1984.)

Table 18–4. SUMMARY OF POSITIONS FOR LYMPHOGRAPHY

Type of Study	Projection	Patient Position	Central Ray	Anatomy
Lower extremity lymphography (pedal lymphangiography)	Anteroposterior	Patient supine, centered to table, cassette positioned under area of interest: ankle and lower leg, pelvis, abdomen, chest (Bucky)	Vertical beam to center of film to pass through area of interest	Lymphatic channels during lymphangiography phase; lymph nodes during lymphadenography phase
	Posterior oblique	Patient placed in either left or right 45° posterior oblique position, centered to table, cassette under area of interest: pelvis, abdomen		
	Lateral	Patient placed in true lateral recumbent position, centered to table, cassette under area of interest: abdomen, chest (Bucky)		
Upper extremity lymphography (brachiolympho-graphy)	Anteroposterior	Patient supine, area of interest centered to cassette: forearm, upper arm, axillary region, supraclavicular region, chest	Vertical beam to pass through area of interest (collimate to film size)	Either radial or ulnar group of vessels, depending on site of injection; brachial trunks and cubital nodes; axillary lymphatic system
	Posterior oblique	Patient in left or right posterior oblique position (25°), cassette center to area of interest: axillary region, supraclavicular region		
	Lateral	Area of interest centered to cassette: forearm, upper arm		

neoplastic disease processes. Delayed films of the same areas at 24 h, and occasionally at 48 to 72 h, show the emptying of the vessels and better demonstrate the lymph nodes. The lymphatic channels in the patient with a normal flow pattern should not retain the contrast agent after 24 h. The delayed phase of the study is called lymphadenography. This portion of the procedure outlines the lymph nodes rather than the lymphatic channels.

Other techniques that may be used to more accurately demonstrate the lymphatic system in certain areas are magnification radiography, lymphoscintography, MRI, CT, and ultrasonography. (See "Suggested Readings" at the end of the chapter for more information regarding these techniques.)

Table 18–4 is a summary of patient positioning for lymphography. Figure 18–9 illustrates compression of the bronchi against the spine.

REFERENCES

1. Dixon, A. K.: The current practice of lymphography: A survey in the age of computed tomography, Clin. Radiol., 36:287–290, 1985.

2. Kuisk, H.: Technique of Lymphography and Principles of Interpretation. St. Louis, Warren H. Green, 1971.

SUGGESTED READINGS

COMPUTED TOMOGRAPHY

Lien, H. H., Kolbenstvedt, A., Talle, K., et al.: Comparison of computed tomography, lymphography, and phlebography in 200 consecutive patients with regard to retroperitoneal metastases from testicular tumor, Radiology, *146*:129–132, 1983.

Pera, A., Capek, M., and Shirkhoda, A.: Lymphangiography and CT in the follow up of patients with lymphoma, Radiology, *164*:631–633, 1987.

Strijk, S. P.: Lymphography and abdominal computed tomography in the staging of non-Hodgkin lymphoma, Acta Radiol. [Diagn.], *28*:263–269, 1987.

Vercamer, R., Janssens, J., Usewils, R., et al.: Computed tomography and lymphography in the presurgical staging of early carcinoma of the uterine cervix, Cancer, *60*:1745–1750, 1987.

INDICATOR DYES

Lillie, R. D.: Conn's Biological Stains, 9th ed., Baltimore, Williams & Wilkins, 1977.

Threefoot, S. A.: Some chemical, physical and biological characteristics of dyes used to visualize lymphatics, J. Appl. Physiol., *15*:925, 1960.

LYMPHOGRAPHY

Abrams, H. L. (ed.): Angiography: Vascular and Interventional Radiology, 3rd ed. Boston, Little, Brown & Co., 1983.

Altman, D., Shaver, W., and Viamonte, M., Jr.: Lymphangiography in children, Am. J. Dis. Child., *104*:335, 1962.

Halm, A.: Lymphography and supplementary procedures, X-Ray Focus, *13*:32, 1973.

Newfang, K. F., et al.: Conventional roentgen diagnosis of mediastinal lymphadenopathy: Part 1, Lymphology, *15*:132, 1983.

Staton, R.: Lymphography, Radiol. Technol., *55*:233–238, 1984.

Weiner, S. A., Lee, J. K. T., Kao, M. S., et al.: The role of lymphangiography in vulvar carcinoma, Am. J. Obstet. Gynecol., *154*:1073–1075, 1986.

LYMPHOSCINTOGRAPHY

Ege, G.: Lymphoscintography—techniques and applications in the management of breast carcinoma, Semin. Nucl. Med., *13*:26–34, 1983.

Feigen, M., Crocker, E. F., Read, J., et al.: The value of lymphoscintography, lymphangiography, and computer tomography scanning in the preoperative assessment of lymph nodes involved by pelvic malignant conditions, Surg. Gynecol. Obstet., *165*:107–110, 1987.

Gloviczki, P., et al.: Noninvasive evaluation of the swollen extremity: Experiences with 190 lymphoscintigraphic examinations, J. Vasc. Surg., *9*:683–689, 1989.

Golueke, P., Montgomery, R. A., Petronis, J., Minken, S., Perler, B. A., and Williams, G. M.: Lymphoscintography to confirm the clinical diagnosis of lymphedema, J. Vasc. Surg., *10*:306–312, 1989.

Intenzo, C. M., Desai, A. G., Kim, S. S., Park, C. H., and Merli, G. J.: Lymphedema of the lower extremities: Evaluation by microcolloidal imaging, Clin. Nucl. Med., *14*:107–110, 1989.

MAGNETIC RESONANCE IMAGING

Dooms, G. C., and Hricak, H.: Radiologic imaging modalities, including magnetic resonance, for evaluating lymph nodes, West J. Med., *144*:49–57, 1986.

nineteen

Bronchography

ANATOMIC CONSIDERATIONS
Right Lung
Left Lung
INDICATIONS AND
   CONTRAINDICATIONS
CONTRAST MEDIA
PATIENT PREPARATION

PROCEDURE
Catheter Insertion Method
Percutaneous Transtracheal Puncture
   of Intercricothyroid Membrane
Aspiration Bronchography
EQUIPMENT
PATIENT POSITIONING

Bronchography is the radiographic study of the lower respiratory tract. The examination is primarily concerned with the bronchial tree. The contrast medium is introduced into the lung, and the anatomy of the bronchial tree is recorded radiographically through the use of various patient positions.

Bronchography is not as widely practiced as a generalized diagnostic procedure today. Computed tomography and the use of fiberoptic bronchoscopy as diagnostic tools have limited the use of the procedure. Bronchography, however, remains the definitive procedure for bronchiectasis and is used in patients being assessed for surgery where computed tomography has demonstrated limited pathology.[1]

In considering the anatomy of the lower respiratory tract, the major anatomic features and location of the trachea and lungs are presented. The description of the bronchial tree is confined primarily to the bronchopulmonary segments.

ANATOMIC CONSIDERATIONS

The lower respiratory tract consists of the trachea, bronchi, and lungs. The lungs are located in the pleural cavity and are the primary organs of respiration. They communicate with the external environment through the trachea and upper respiratory tract.

The trachea, a tube-shaped continuation of the larynx, begins at the level of the sixth cervical vertebra. It extends down through the neck and into the superior mediastinum and ends at the upper border of the fifth to eighth thoracic vertebrae. The trachea contains approximately 20 U-shaped cartilaginous rings. These enable the trachea to maintain its tube shape. The last cartilaginous ring of the trachea forms the carina, which lies between the openings of the two main bronchi.[2]

The main bronchi are the connections between the trachea and lungs. The right main bronchus is more vertical than the left and is also shorter and wider than its counterpart. The left main bronchus is longer and narrower than the right. It passes under the arch of the aorta and courses laterally to enter the hilum of the left lung at the level of the sixth thoracic vertebra.

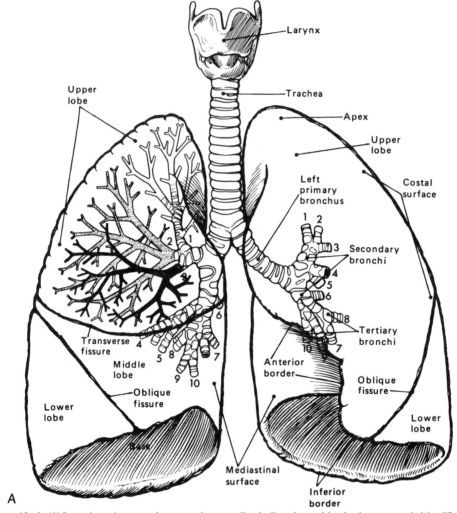

Figure 19–1. *(A)* Bronchopulmonary tree; numbers on the tertiary bronchi refer to segments identified in the bronchopulmonary segments *(B)*. (From Langley, L. L., Telford, I. R., and Christensen, J. B.: Dynamic Anatomy and Physiology, 4th ed., New York, McGraw-Hill, 1974. © Copyright Mosby-Year Book, Inc.)

Lateral branches are given off from each of these main bronchi called the lobar bronchi. Branches of the lobar bronchi along with branches of the pulmonary artery and vein subdivide the lobes of the lungs into the bronchopulmonary segments.

The lungs are located in the pleural cavity. They are basically cone shaped and consist of an apex, base, two surfaces, and three borders (Fig. 19–1).

Right Lung

The right lung is shorter and wider than the left because the liver, which occupies the upper abdominal cavity, somewhat compresses the right lung. Three lobes—the right upper, right middle, and right lower—compose the right lung. Each lobar bronchus gives off branches to the right bronchopulmonary segments. The right lung contains 10 segmental bronchi (Fig. 19–2). Three segmental bronchi serve the upper lobe, two serve the middle, and five serve the lower.

The right main bronchus subdivides into two main branches, one above and the other

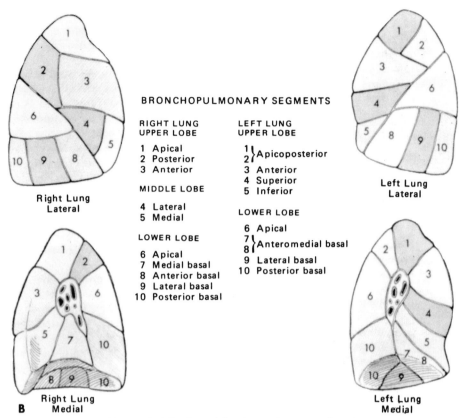

BRONCHOPULMONARY SEGMENTS

RIGHT LUNG
UPPER LOBE

1 Apical
2 Posterior
3 Anterior

MIDDLE LOBE

4 Lateral
5 Medial

LOWER LOBE

6 Apical
7 Medial basal
8 Anterior basal
9 Lateral basal
10 Posterior basal

LEFT LUNG
UPPER LOBE

1 ⎫
2 ⎬ Apicoposterior
3 Anterior
4 Superior
5 Inferior

LOWER LOBE

6 Apical
7 ⎫
8 ⎬ Anteromedial basal
9 Lateral basal
10 Posterior basal

Right Lung
Lateral

Left Lung
Lateral

Right Lung
B   Medial

Left Lung
Medial

Figure 19–1 Continued *See legend on opposite page.*

below the right pulmonary artery. These are the right upper lobe bronchus and the continuation of the main stem. The right upper lobe bronchus serves the upper lobe of the right lung. It gives off three segmental bronchi—the apical, posterior, and anterior. The continuation of the main stem subdivides into a middle lobe bronchus, serving the right middle lobe, and a lower lobe bronchus, serving the right lower lobe. The right middle lobe bronchus divides into two segmental branches—the medial and lateral. The right lower lobe bronchus supports the superior, medial basal, anterior basal, posterior basal, and lateral basal branches.

Left Lung

The left lung is longer than the right; however, because the heart is located toward the left side of the thorax, the left lung has less volume than the right. The left lung comprises two lobes, the left upper and left lower. The two lobar bronchi subdivide to form the segmental bronchi of the left lung. There are eight segmental branches in the left lung, with four serving the left upper lobe and four serving the left lower lobe (Fig. 19–3).

The left main bronchus subdivides into the left upper lobe and left lower lobe bronchi.

The left upper lobe bronchus divides into an upper and a lower division. These divisions supply the left upper lobe and lingula, respectively. The lingula is the portion of the left lung that corresponds to the middle lobe of the right lung. The upper division of the left upper lobe bronchus supports two segmental branches—the apicoposterior

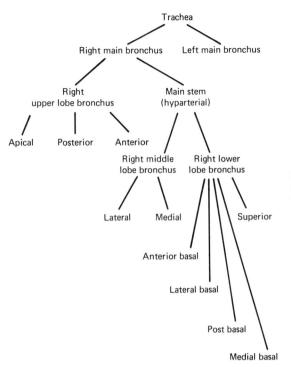

Figure 19–2. Flow chart summarizing the 10 bronchopulmonary segments of the right lung and their relations with their respective main bronchi.

and anterior. The lower division of the left upper lobe bronchus also divides into two segmental branches—the superior and inferior branches.

The left lower lobe bronchus, which supplies the inferior lobe of the left lung, is almost identical to its counterpart on the right side, with one exception—the medial basal branch arises as an offshoot of the anterior basal branch rather than as a direct branch of the left lower lobe bronchus. This gives the left lower lobe bronchus a total of four segmental branches—the superior, anterior basal, posterior basal, and lateral basal.

Beyond the 18 bronchopulmonary segments are a multitude of finer branches called secondary bronchi, bronchioles, and terminal bronchi, in order of occurrence. These

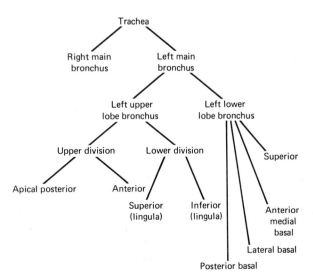

Figure 19–3. Flow chart summarizing the bronchopulmonary segments of the left lung and their relations with their respective main bronchi.

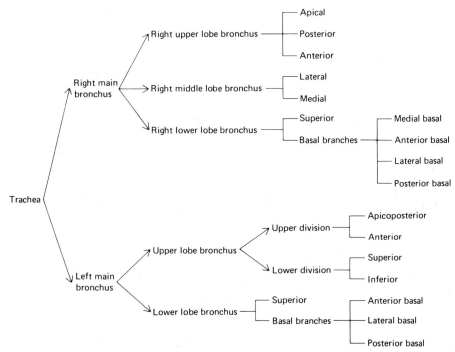

Figure 19-4. Flow chart summarizing the entire bronchopulmonary system.

ultimately terminate in alveolar sacs that are lined by the alveoli, the functional units of the lungs.

A summary of the anatomy of the bronchial tree is given in Figure 19–4.

INDICATIONS AND CONTRAINDICATIONS

Bronchography yields a great amount of diagnostic information without undue risk to the patient. The procedure has been used to diagnose diseases of the bronchopulmonary tree to clarify various nonspecific clinical findings. Bronchography is indicated primarily for the diagnosis of bronchiectasis. It was the method of choice for bronchial obstruction, fistulas, chronic bronchitis, and hemoptysis, and the identification of a variety of pulmonary lesions.[3, 4] However, fiberoptic bronchoscopy has supplanted bronchography in the diagnosis of most pulmonary pathology. Fiberoptic bronchoscopy has the advantage of also allowing simultaneously the biopsy of lung tissue and observation of the anatomy and pathology. The major indication for the use of bronchography is suspected bronchiectasis when the results of computed tomography demonstrate limited pathology.

In patients exhibiting high fever, asthma, severe hypertension, cardiac failure caused by valvular abnormalities, or severe generalized weakness, the procedure is contraindicated.[5] It is well to remember also that the instillation of contrast agent into the lung will cause diminished pulmonary function for a period of time. Dyspnea may occur immediately after the procedure, and require the administration of oxygen.

Reactions may also occur because of a sensitivity to the anesthetic agent or contrast medium; manifestations include fever, headache, nausea, vomiting, urticaria, allergic dermatitis, pneumonia, and fatal anaphylaxis.[6]

CONTRAST MEDIA

There are various contrast agents currently in use for bronchography. The choice is primarily one of physician preference and patient sensitivity to iodine compounds. Bronchographic contrast media may be divided into two major groups—those that contain iodine and those that do not. Iodine-containing contrast agents are of two types—aqueous iodine compounds and iodized oils.

The use of aqueous iodine compounds has certain advantages. These compounds are rapidly excreted by the kidneys and rapidly absorbed from the bronchi into the bloodstream. The rapid absorption and excretion of this type of contrast agent can also be a decided disadvantage in that filming must be accomplished rapidly and accurately. Because they are water soluble, the contrast agents can be diluted by the bronchial secretions, resulting in a decrease of tissue contrast. The aqueous agents are also more irritating to the tracheobronchial mucosa than are the oily compounds.

The oil-based iodine compounds, although widely used, are not without disadvantages. These compounds are slowly absorbed into the blood and can cause lipoid pneumonia and granulomatous reactions. They are not miscible with bronchial secretions, which can produce an inaccurate picture of the shape of the bronchi. Also, smaller bronchi may be obstructed, causing accumulations of bronchial secretions with subsequent fever.

The contrast media in the oil-based category are usually preparations of iodized poppy seed oil or suspensions of propyliodone in peanut oil. This group has had the most widespread use as contrast agents for bronchography.

PATIENT PREPARATION

Bronchography requires a minimum of preprocedural patient preparation. The patient should be instructed to restrict intake of solid foods to minimize the possibility of aspiration of foreign material during the procedure. In most cases, the patient has local anesthetic applied to the laryngotracheal area before the contrast agent is injected.

If a percutaneous method of introduction is used, the procedure is done on an inpatient basis, and the patient is sedated before arriving at the department. Normal aseptic technique should be practiced during this type of study.

In all cases, a possibility of reaction to the contrast agent exists, and standard precautions should be taken.

PROCEDURE

There are various methods that can be used to introduce the contrast agent into the bronchial tree. The method of choice rests with the physician performing the examination. The following is a list of methods for the introduction of contrast media:

Transglottic catheter insertion
Supraglottic catheter insertion
Percutaneous puncture of the intercricothyroid membranes
Aerosol bronchography
Transnasal catheter insertion
Aspiration bronchography
Use of the bronchoscope during bronchoscopy

Bronchography can be done as a selective or nonselective procedure, depending on the information desired. Regardless of the method chosen, bronchography is usually done as a unilateral examination. There are several reasons for this, including super-imposition of the bilateral anatomy and increased disturbance of pulmonary function caused by the bilateral introduction of the contrast agent.

The most commonly used technique for introduction of the contrast agent is the transglottic catheter method, which enables either selective or nonselective bronchography to be performed.

Three procedural methods are presented in this chapter—catheter insertion, percutaneous transtracheal puncture, and aspiration bronchography. They are generally discussed; not all of the patient maneuvers used to distribute the contrast agent into the various segments of the bronchial tree are presented.

Catheter Insertion Method

This method involves the introduction of a catheter into the bronchial tree by several routes. The most commonly used are the transglottal and transnasal routes. In all cases, anesthesia must be administered locally so that the pharyngeal and cough reflexes are suppressed. This is accomplished by spraying a suitable anesthetic agent onto the larynx and vocal cords and into the trachea. When the anesthesia has been successfully administered, the catheter is introduced. The catheter tip is positioned by fluoroscopy, and for nonselective methods, the tip should not be placed lower than the tracheal bifurcation, preferably above the carina. The contrast agent can then be slowly introduced into the bronchial tree. Various maneuvers are applied to the patient to distribute the contrast agent throughout the lung. Once this is accomplished, the radiographs are taken.

With this method, a lung biopsy can be performed by introducing a specialized controllable brush attached to a guide wire. This "bronchial brush" can be manipulated into the desired bronchus, and any lesion can be brush biopsied.[7]

Percutaneous Transtracheal Puncture of Intercricothyroid Membrane

The patient is sedated 1 h before the procedure is performed. On arrival in the department, the patient is placed on the radiographic table, and the head is hyperextended. This can be done by placing a small pillow under the shoulders. The patient's neck is then "prepped" and draped. A suitable anesthetic agent is administered locally to the area, the cricothyroid membrane is punctured, and after anesthetizing the trachea to suppress the cough reflex, a 17-gauge Teflon needle is introduced. The contrast agent is then introduced through the needle.

Selective bronchography is also performed with this method by the insertion of premeasured guides and catheters, which can then be manipulated into the desired areas under fluoroscopic control.

Aspiration Bronchography

This method of bronchography requires the least amount of specialized instrumentation. It uses the normal respiratory mechanism to disperse the contrast agent throughout the lung.

The patient is placed in the seated position, slightly tilted toward the side to be visualized. The tongue is then grasped with a gauze pad and pulled forward firmly but gently. A few milliliters of anesthetic agent are allowed to flow over the tongue, which usually stimulates the cough reflex. Coughing helps to disperse the anesthesia and should not be suppressed. The tongue must be released during the coughing. Both sides must be anesthetized, even if unilateral bronchography is to be performed. After the anesthesia has been successfully administered, the contrast agent is introduced in the manner previously described for introduction of the anesthetic agent. When the contrast agent has been introduced, adequate filling should be confirmed fluoroscopically. When filling has been confirmed, the examination can proceed.

It is necessary to use the shortest possible exposure time to record the contrast-filled lungs because immobilization of the patient for long periods is not recommended.

The contrast agent must be removed at the conclusion of the examination. This is done in all procedural methods by postural drainage and the normal cough mechanism. The patient is instructed not to take any food or drink by mouth for at least 2 h to avoid the possibility of aspirating substances into the tracheobronchial tree.

EQUIPMENT

Bronchography does not require much specialized equipment. The examination may be done in any radiographic room equipped with an image intensifier and a spot filming device. It is necessary to monitor placement of the catheter.

Contents of the bronchogram tray vary with the method used to introduce the contrast agent into the lungs. A typical bronchogram tray includes the items shown in Table 19–1. The items in the bronchogram tray also vary with the preference of the physician performing the study. If more than one method is used at an institution, a single bronchogram tray can be prepared that includes the necessary specialized equipment required for each different technique. Consequently, one standard tray could contain materials for several different techniques.

An emergency cart should also be available in the radiographic room. Complications may arise from use of the anesthetic agent (hypersensitivity reactions), the contrast medium (e.g., fever, headache, nausea, vomiting, hypersensitivity to iodine, impaired pulmonary function), and the method of injection or the procedure itself (e.g., airway obstruction, hemorrhage, spread of infection, or extranasation of contrast medium or air after transtracheal puncture). Preparations should be made for all these complications in case any occur during the course of the examination.

Table 19–1. CONTENTS OF A TYPICAL BRONCHOGRAM TRAY

Item	Amount and/or Size
Atomizer containing anesthetic agent	1
Curved laryngeal cannula for injection of anesthetic agent	1
Gauze pads	15–20 (4 × 4 in)
Curved forceps (large)	1
Syringe for anesthetic	1 (10 ml)
Syringe for contrast agent	1 (20 ml)
Syringe for skin anesthetic	1 (2 ml)
Syringe for percutaneous puncture technique	1 (5 ml)
Tongue depressor	1
Needles for use in syringes listed above	Assorted
Specialized intercricothyroid needle	1
Small containers	Several
Specialized intratracheal catheters	Various

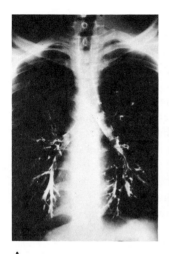
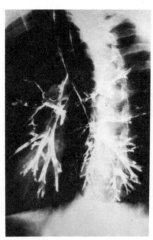
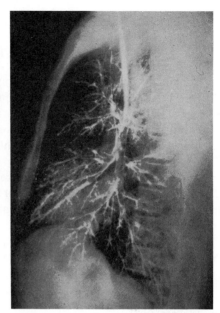

A   B

Figure 19–5. Selected radiographs showing routine bronchographic films. *(A)* Anteroposterior projection; *(B)* anterior oblique projection; *(C)* lateral projection. (Original photographs in *A* and *B* by author; *C* from Lehman, J. S., and Crellin, J. A.: Medical Radiology and Photography, *31.* Heidelberg, Springer-Verlag, 1955.)

C

Table 19–2. SUMMARY OF POSITIONS FOR BRONCHOGRAPHY

Projection	Patient Position	Central Ray	Anatomy
Posteroanterior	Patient erect, facing film holder, median sagittal plane to center of cassette, acromion process 3 in (7.5 cm) below top of cassette, chin resting on cassette holder, shoulders rolled forward, hands on hips; exposure on inspiration	Directed horizontally and at right angle to center of cassette, 72-in (180-cm) SID*	Anterior view of mediastinum and its structures, contrast-filled tracheobronchial tree in anterior view
Anterior oblique (right or left)	Patient erect, facing film holder; rotate filled side approximately 35° away from cassette, center on point midway between lateral margin of chest wall and vertebral column of side being examined; arm of filled side is abducted with elbow flexed, hand resting on top of film holder; exposure on inspiration	Directed horizontally and at right angle to center of cassette, 72-in (180-cm) SID	Contrast-filled right bronchial tree (left anterior oblique); contrast-filled left bronchial tree (right anterior oblique)
Lateral	Patient erect, with side to be examined against film holder, arms above head, patient centered to cassette; adjust to true lateral position	Directed horizontally and at right angle to center of film, 72-in (180-cm) SID	Contrast-filled bronchial tree (unilateral bronchogram), lateral view of both contrast-filled lungs superimposed (bilateral bronchogram)

*SID; source-image distance.

PATIENT POSITIONING

The bronchographic procedure is usually monitored by fluoroscopy. As the contrast agent is introduced into the lung, the radiologist may wish to make spot radiographs during the filling procedure. Fluoroscopy permits the examiner to observe the physiological function of the bronchial tree. After completion of the fluoroscopic portion of the examination, conventional radiography is required.

Three basic views are required during this phase of the examination—the postero-anterior, anterior oblique, and lateral. These views are positioned in the same manner as conventional chest positions; however, it is essential that the filming be done accurately and rapidly. The radiographs are taken in the erect position with a standard 72-in source-image distance.

Recumbent views are occasionally required. These are usually necessary during the filling of contrast medium in the first stage of a bilateral bronchogram and include anteroposterior recumbent, posterior oblique, and lateral of the side that was injected first.

Filming routines vary with the particular physician performing the procedure. Figure 19–5 illustrates a normal bronchogram. Table 19–2 is a summary of patient positions for bronchography.

REFERENCES

1. Munro, N. C., Cooke, J. C., Currie, D. C., Strickland, B., and Cole, P. J.: Comparison of thin section computed tomography with bronchography for identifying bronchiectatic segments in patients with chronic sputum production, Thorax, *45*:139, 1990.
2. Woodburne, R. T.: Essentials of Human Anatomy, 7th ed. New York, Oxford University Press, 1983.
3. Shanks, S. C., and Kerley, P.: A Textbook of X-ray Diagnosis, 4th ed. Vol. 1, Philadelphia, W. B. Saunders, 1972.
4. Fraser, R. G.: Bronchography 1972 (editorial), J. Can. Radiol., *23*:236, 1972.
5. Zsebok, Z. B.: Technic of Roentgenologic Investigations, Budapest, Akademiai Kiado, 1969.
6. Weigen, J. F., and Thomas, S. F.: Complications of Diagnostic Radiology. Springfield, IL, Charles C Thomas, 1973.
7. Wilson, J., and Estridge, M.: Bronchial brush biopsy with a controllable brush, Am. J. Roentgenol., *109*:471, 1970.

SUGGESTED READINGS

Cooke, J. C., Currie, D. C., Morgan, A. D., et al.: Role of computed tomography in the diagnosis of bronchiectasis, Thorax, *42*:272–277, 1987.

Friedman, P. J.: Radiology of the superior segment of the lower lobe: A regional perspective introducing the B6 bronchus sign, Radiology, *144*:15, 1982.

Gamsu, G., Thurlbeck, W. M., Macklem, P. T., and Fraser, R. G.: Peripheral bronchographic morphology in the normal human lung, Invest. Radiol., *25*:392–401, 1990.

Jenkins, P., et al.: Selective bronchography using the fibreoptic bronchoscope, Br. J. Dis. Chest, *76*:88, 1982.

Joharjy, I. A., Bashi, S. A., and Abdulah, A. K.: Value of medium thickness CT in the diagnosis of bronchiectasis, Am. J. Roentgenol., *149*:1133–1137, 1987.

Lang, E. V., and Friedman, P. J.: The anterior wall stripe of the left lower lobe bronchus on the lateral chest radiograph: CT correlative study, Am. J. Roentgenol., *154*:33–39, 1990.

Limper, A. H., and Prakash, U. B.: Tracheobron-chial foreign bodies in adults, Ann. Intern. Med., *112*:604–609, 1990.

Llamas, R., et al.: Experimental bronchography by tantalum insufflation, Dis. Chest, *56*:75, 1969.

McGuirt, W. F., Holmes, K. D., Feehs, R., and Browne, J. D.: Tracheobronchial foreign bodies, Laryngoscope, *98*:615–618, 1988.

Nadel, J. A., et al.: Powdered tantalum: A new contrast medium for roentgenographic examination of human airways, N. Engl. J. Med., *283*:281, 1970.

Nelson, S. W., Christoforidis, A. J., and Pratt, P. C.: Further experience with barium sulfate as a bronchographic contrast medium, Am. J. Roentgenol., *92*:595, 1964.

Strickland, B., Brennan, J., and Denison, D. M.: Computed tomography in diffuse lung disease: Improving the image, Clin. Radiol., *37*:335–338, 1986.

Webb, W. R., et al.: Computed tomography of the left retrobronchial stripe, J. Comput. Assist. Tomogr., *7*:65, 1983.

twenty

Arthrography

ANATOMIC CONSIDERATIONS
INDICATIONS AND
    CONTRAINDICATIONS
CONTRAST MEDIA

PROCEDURE
EQUIPMENT
PATIENT POSITIONING

Radiography of joint space and its surrounding structures is called arthrography. The many joints in the human body vary in structure and arrangement. They are freely movable (diarthrosis), slightly movable (amphiarthrosis), or immovable (synarthrosis). All joints are junctions between bones or between cartilage and bone.

Joints can be grouped by structural feature into three groups—fibrous, cartilaginous, and synovial. Fibrous and cartilaginous joints permit very little movement, if any. Synovial joints, on the other hand, permit free movement of the articulating bones. Arthrography is exclusively concerned with this last group of bones. Figure 20–1 shows the joints exhibiting diarthrosis (free movement) and synarthrosis (fibrous and cartilaginous).

ANATOMIC CONSIDERATIONS

Synovial joints are classified according to axis of movement, as follows:

GLIDING OR PLANE JOINT. This type permits a sliding of one surface on the other.

HINGE JOINT. This type allows movement in only one plane. The movements of this joint are flexion and extension.

PIVOT JOINT. This type of joint permits rotational movement around a pivot in one axis.

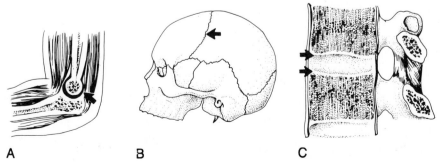

A   B   C

Figure 20–1. Diarthrotic and synarthrotic joints. *(A)* Synovial joint; *(B)* fibrous joint; *(C)* cartilaginous joint.

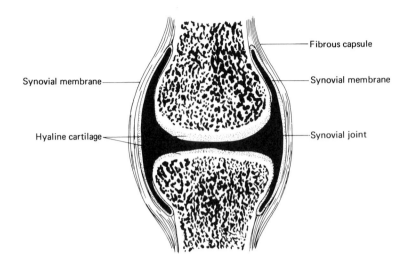

Figure 20–2. Schematic of a synovial joint; shown are its major features.

ELLIPSOIDAL OR CONDYLAR JOINT. In this type, an oval head or condyle articulates with an elliptic cavity. This joint exhibits movements of flexion, extension, adduction, abduction, and circumduction.

SADDLE JOINT. This type is similar to ellipsoidal or condyloid joints in its movements. Structurally, its articular surfaces are convex in one direction and concave in the other, at right angles to each other.

BALL-AND-SOCKET JOINT. This type is formed by a concave socket that receives a ball-shaped head. It permits movement in three axes—flexion, extension, adduction, abduction, and rotation.

A summary of the various individual synovial joints and their types and movements is presented in Table 20–1.

Synovial joints take their name from the fluid contained within the joint space (Fig. 20–2). Synovial fluid is a clear viscous fluid that serves primarily as a lubricant to facilitate joint movement. This fluid, along with the specialized articular surfaces and intra-articular structures (the menisci, disks, and fat pads), allows for almost frictionless movement of the joint surfaces. The coefficient of friction during joint movement is less than that of ice sliding on ice.[1]

Synovial fluid resembles the white of an egg in consistency, and it nourishes the hyaline cartilage lining the articular surfaces. The synovial fluid is produced by the synovial membrane, the inner lining of the joint capsule.

The synovial joint space is enclosed in a fibrous layer called the joint capsule. The fibers composing the joint capsule are arranged in irregular bundles that make them sensitive to any tension from the joint. Nerve endings are also located within the joint capsule; they pass impulses to the spinal cord and brain to transmit information regarding position and movement of the joint. The joint capsule attaches to the articulating bones just beyond the joint space uniting the bones of the joint.

The inner surface of the fibrous joint capsule is lined with a connective tissue called the synovial membrane. This membrane covers all of the structures within the joint except the hyaline articular cartilage, menisci, and intra-articular disks. It produces the synovial fluid that lubricates the joint surfaces.

Hyaline articular cartilage is located on the bearing surfaces of the bones composing the joint. It does not contain nerve endings or blood vessels. Nutrients are supplied to the cartilage by the synovial fluid and the capillaries adjacent to the bone marrow.

The intra-articular joint structures include the menisci, fat pads, synovial folds, and intra-articular disks. These intra-articular structures aid in providing efficient lubrication of the articular surfaces.

Table 20–1. DESCRIPTION OF INDIVIDUAL JOINTS

Joint	Articulating Bones	Type	Movements
Atlantoepistropheal	Anterior arch of atlas rotates about dens of axis (epistropheus)	Diarthrotic (pivot type)	Pivoting or partial rotation of head
Vertebral*	Between bodies of vertebrae	Synarthrotic cartilaginous; amphiarthrotic by other system of classification	Slight movement between any two vertebrae but considerable motility for column as whole
	Between articular processes	Diarthrotic (gliding)	
Clavicular Sternoclavicular	Medial end of clavicle with manubrium of sternum; only joint between upper extremity and trunk	Diarthrotic (gliding)	Gliding; weak joint that may be injured comparatively easily
Acromioclavicular	Distal end of clavicle with acromion of scapula	Diarthrotic (gliding)	Gliding; elevation, depression, protraction, and retraction
Thoracic	Heads of ribs with bodies of vertebrae	Diarthrotic (gliding)	Gliding
	Tubercles of ribs with transverse processes of vertebrae	Diarthrotic (gliding)	Gliding
Shoulder	Head of humerus in glenoid cavity of scapula	Diarthrotic (ball-and-socket type)	Flexion, extension, abduction, adduction, rotation, and circumduction of upper arm; one of most freely movable of joints
Elbow	Trochlea of humerus with semilunar notch of ulna; head of radius with capitulum of humerus	Diarthrotic (hinge type)	Flexion and extension
	Head of radius in radial notch of ulna	Diarthrotic (pivot type)	Supination and pronation of lower arm and hand; rotation of lower arm on upper, as in using screwdriver
Wrist	Scaphoid, lunate, and triquetral bones articulate with radius and articular disk	Diarthrotic (condyloid)	Flexion, extension, abduction, and adduction of hand
Carpal	Between various carpals	Diarthrotic (gliding)	Gliding
Hand	Proximal end of first metacarpal with trapezium	Diarthrotic (saddle)	Flexion, extension, abduction, adduction, and circumduction of thumb and opposition to fingers; motility of this joint accounts for dexterity of human hand compared with animal forepaw

Table continued on following page

Table 20–1. DESCRIPTION OF INDIVIDUAL JOINTS *Continued*

Joint	Articulating Bones	Type	Movements
	Distal end of metacarpals with proximal end of phalanges	Diarthrotic (hinge)	Flexion, extension, limited abduction, and adduction of finger
	Between phalanges	Diarthrotic (hinge)	Flexion and extension of finger sections
Sacroiliac	Between sacrum and two ilia	Diarthrotic (gliding); joint cavity mostly obliterated after middle life	None or slight (e.g., during late months of pregnancy and during delivery)
Symphysis pubis	Between two pubic bones	Synarthrotic (or amphiarthrotic), cartilaginous	Slight, particularly during pregnancy and delivery
Hip	Head of femur in acetabulum of os coxa	Diarthrotic (ball-and-socket type)	Flexion, extension, abduction, adduction, rotation, and circumduction
Knee	Between distal end of femur and proximal end of tibia; largest joint in body	Diarthrotic (hinge type)	Flexion and extension; slight rotation of tibia
Tibiofibular	Head of fibula with lateral condyle of tibia	Diarthrotic (gliding type)	Gliding
Ankle	Distal ends of tibia and fibula with talus	Diarthrotic (hinge type)	Flexion (dorsiflexion) and extension (plantar flexion)
Foot	Between tarsals	Diarthrotic (gliding)	Gliding; inversion and eversion
	Between metatarsals and phalanges	Diarthrotic (hinge type)	Flexion, extension, slight abduction, and adduction
	Between phalanges	Diarthrotic (hinge type)	Flexion and extension

*Vertebrae are not easily dislocated. They are securely held by the following ligaments—anterior and posterior longitudinal ligaments (between anterior and posterior surfaces of bodies of vertebrae); supraspinous ligaments, called ligamentum nuchae in cervical region (between tops of spinous processes); interspinous ligaments (between sides of spinous processes); and ligamentum flavum (between laminae).

Ligaments may also be present within the joint space, as well as in the joint capsule. The accessory ligaments limit motion in undesirable directions and function as sense organs of motion and position.

Because joints constitute a mechanical system, wear and tear can be expected even though friction has been greatly reduced, and this usually results in the destruction of the hyaline articular cartilage. Other factors culminating in deterioration of the joints are trauma and disease.

INDICATIONS AND CONTRAINDICATIONS

This procedure is used to obtain diagnostic information regarding the joints and surrounding soft tissues or cartilage. It has been used primarily in the investigation of the knee and shoulder joint; it has also shown its diagnostic value by demonstrating various diseases of the hip, elbow, ankle, and temporomandibular joints. Magnetic resonance imaging (MRI) has become the method of choice in the evaluation of arthrographic disorders. The use of surface coils has improved the signal-to-noise ratio, which has had a profound effect on image resolution.[2] MRI is used to study abnormalities in the knee, temporomandibular joint, hip, shoulder, wrist, and ankle.

Arthrography is a safe procedure that can be used to delineate the joint space and its surrounding structures, providing accurate diagnostic information concerning lesions of the menisci. It is indicated in cases of suspected injury to the meniscus of the joint, particularly tears. The procedure is also advised for the diagnosis of suspected capsular damage, rupture of the articular ligaments, arthritic deformities (specifically of the temporomandibular joint), congenital luxation of the hip joint, and the extent of damage resulting from traumatic injuries of the joint.

There are relatively few absolute contraindications to arthrography. Hypersensitivity to iodine is a relative contraindication to positive contrast arthrography.

CONTRAST MEDIA

Arthrography can be performed with a negative contrast agent, positive contrast agent, or both.

Pneumoarthrography uses air or other easily absorbed gases. One disadvantage to the use of negative contrast agents is that large amounts are usually necessary, and this produces a somewhat painful distention of the joint. The diagnostic accuracy of the "air" study is considerably less than that when the other two contrast methods are used. This diminished diagnostic accuracy results because there is relatively little difference in density between the joint anatomy and the contrast medium. A possible hazard of pneumoarthrography is air embolism, which occurs rarely but cannot be totally disregarded.

Positive contrast arthrography is performed with water-soluble contrast media because they are readily absorbed, are usually well tolerated, and are easily excreted by the body. They also produce arthrograms of greater diagnostic accuracy. The concentration of the positive contrast medium should be no more than 30%.

The double-contrast arthrogram combines the best of both methods to produce a highly accurate diagnostic study. With the use of both types of contrast media, smaller amounts of each can be used, thus providing a more comfortable study for the patient and reducing the possibility of air embolism.

PROCEDURE

The arthrographic procedure varies with the site to be studied. It is a simple procedure and is useful for the investigation of all encapsulated joints. The arthrographic procedure varies with the site to be studied. Arthrography, however, is, an invasive procedure and can pose certain risks for the patient. Among these risks is the potential for reaction to the contrast agent. This type of reaction is relatively uncommon, but its occurrence should not be discounted. The most common type of reaction to the procedure is the vasovagal reaction, which can be triggered by fright, pain, or trauma. It is usually accompanied by nausea, perspiration, and pallor. Other possible reactions include allergy to the anesthetic agent and inflammatory synovitis.

The joint most frequently examined by arthrography is the knee joint, so this technique is discussed. Radiographs may be taken by using either a vertical or horizontal x-ray beam or with the use of fluoroscopy and spot films. The horizontal beam method is generally used during double-contrast arthrography. With the use of a horizontal beam, smaller amounts of contrast agent can be used to produce a study that is more accurate and less uncomfortable to the patient. Arthrography should be carried out under strict aseptic conditions because infection of the joint can be a serious complication of the procedure. In single-contrast arthrography, the patient is placed in the supine position. The extremity under investigation can be placed in a special frame that widens the intrastructural spaces and allows the contrast agent to be distributed freely around the meniscus. Other positions for the injection may be used, depending on the physician's preference. Lindblom described a simple method that uses no specialized equipment.[3]

When the knee has been properly positioned to permit easy entrance into the joint cavity, the needle is inserted behind the patella (retropatellar) with the tip directed toward its articular surface. Approximately 2 to 4 ml of anesthetic agent is then introduced. Synovial fluid is withdrawn, followed by injection of the contrast agent. When this has been completed, the joint is actively moved to spread the contrast medium into the articular surface of the joint. On completion of this maneuver, radiographs are taken of each side of the joint.

The horizontal beam double-contrast technique is more complex because it is necessary to topographically identify anatomic landmarks with fluoroscopy before the injection.[4] With the use of a metal ruler, the radiographer draws a line on each side of the laterally placed knee to topographically locate each aspect of the tibial plateau. The extremity must be in maximal extension while this is being done. A specialized tunnel table is required to facilitate marking the lateral side of the knee. The identification of the landmarks is important for the closely coned radiographs that follow.

Double-contrast arthrography demonstrates the menisci to best advantage and is useful when injured menisci or articular ligament damage is suspected. With this method, the positive contrast medium coats the meniscus and then drains to the lowest point of the knee while the air rises, offering a contrast similar to that seen during a double-contrast study of the colon. In cases in which the meniscus is torn, a single-contrast study may obscure the pathology or fail to demonstrate it. Single-contrast studies are usually reserved for demonstrating loose particles in the joint.

On completion of the fluoroscopic identification of landmarks, the patient is placed in the supine position. The knee is washed and swabbed with an antiseptic solution. Under local anesthesia, the needle is introduced into the joint between the patella and the medial femoral condyle. Some synovial fluid is aspirated; then, both air and the positive-contrast medium are introduced. As before, the knee must be moved to properly distribute the contrast medium within the joint. The patient is then placed in the prone position, with a small support located under the distal femur and a small sandbag placed over the ankle to provide the necessary widening of the joint space. The radiographic recording begins.

The fluoroscopic method is the simplest method. The positioning for spot films is accomplished under direct fluoroscopy. Scout films and additional overhead radiographs are usually required to complete the fluoroscopic study; these additional views are usually specified by the physician. Occasionally, a view of the intercondyloid fossa is requested; however, a true lateral with 90° flexion of the knee for the cruciate ligaments is a standard view for this procedure.

Table 20–2 is a summary of the injection sites for some other joints usually studied by arthrography.

EQUIPMENT

The equipment necessary for arthrography is minimal. The procedure itself, especially the double-contrast technique, depends on the use of a fluoroscopic unit. Therefore, the radiographic room should be equipped with an image-intensified fluoroscopic unit.

Table 20–2. SUMMARY OF CONTRAST MEDIA INJECTION SITES

Joint	Injection Site	Amount of Contrast Medium (ml)
Lower extremity		
Ankle	Insertion made from ventral surface of ankle toward medial malleolus	4–6
Hip	Insertion made approximately 4 cm below inguinal ligament	5–8
Upper extremity		
Elbow	Insertion made from dorsal surface at height of radial capitulum	5–6
Shoulder	Insertion made approximately 2 cm lateral from acromioclavicular joint toward humerus	6–8
Temporomandibular joint	Two injections necessary because intra-articular disk separates joint into upper and lower parts; insertion made at point anterior to tragus directed toward the face to puncture upper cavity; lower cavity cannulated by directing needle caudally	1.0–1.5

From Zsebok, Z. B.: Technic of Roentgenologic Investigation, Budapest, Akaddemiai Kiado, 1969.

If the horizontal beam technique is used, a shielded cassette holder equipped with a window measuring 2.5 × 7 in (6.25 × 17.5 cm) can be used. This permits one series of six exposures to be made on a 7- × 17-in (17.5- × 42.5-cm) cassette. A small support of either radiolucent sponges or cotton approximately 5 in (12.5 cm) in diameter and 7 in (17.5 cm) in length is placed under the distal femur during the examination. Also required for the double-contrast arthrogram is the tunnel table for support of the extremity. This can be simply constructed and should measure 27 × 16 × 7.25 in (67.5 × 40 × 18.1 cm).[5] If the vertical beam method is used, a special extremity frame is required to widen the joint space during the procedure.

Because the injection must be carried out under aseptic conditions, a sterile tray is required (Table 20–3). In addition to the items listed in Table 20–3, the special procedure room should have available sterile disposable gloves, antiseptic solution, anesthetic, and contrast agents.

PATIENT POSITIONING

The positioning for knee arthrography is considered because this is the most often performed procedure. Regardless of the method chosen, scout films should always be taken. Four views—anteroposterior, internal and external 45° obliques, and true lateral—should be taken.

Table 20–3. CONTENTS OF TYPICAL ARTHROGRAM TRAY

Equipment	Amount, Type, and/or Size
Medicine cup	1
Forceps	1
Syringe	1 (5 ml, glass)
Syringes	2 (20 ml, glass)
Needle	1 (25 gauge)
Needles	2 (20 gauge)
Sterile towels	6
Sterile drape	1
Gauze pads	4 × 4 in

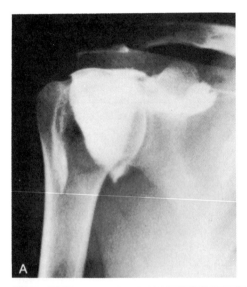

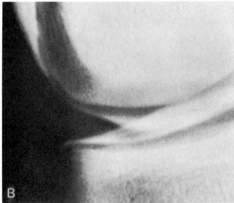

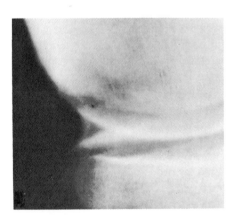

Figure 20–3. *(A)* Illustration of a conventional shoulder arthrographic image; *(B)* selected images from a conventional knee arthrogram showing a normal *(1)* and abnormal *(2)* meniscus;

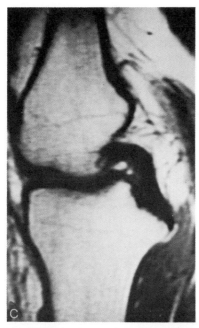
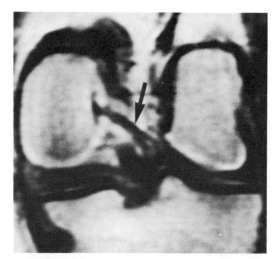

Figure 20–3 *Continued (C)* MR images of the normal knee in a lateral projection *(1)* and frontal projection *(2)*; the arrow denotes a normal right anterior cruciate ligament as it appears in the frontal projection. (From Putman, C., and Ravin, C.: Textbook of Diagnostic Imaging, Vol. 1, Philadelphia, W. B. Saunders, 1988.)

With the vertical beam method, five views are usually required. These are listed in the order in which they are taken—anteroposterior, supine external 45° oblique, supine internal 45° oblique, posteroanterior with knee flexed approximately 30°, and mediolateral with knee flexed 90°. These must be taken accurately and quickly, especially during positive contrast arthrography, because of the rapid absorption of the contrast agent.

The double-contrast arthrogram requires that two sets of six radiographs be made tangentially to the meniscus. After each exposure, the patient is rotated 25 to 30° from the prone through the lateral and finally to the supine position. Both the lateral and medial menisci are radiographed in this manner. If the series is begun with the patient in the prone position and the leg in a lateral anterior oblique position, the first two exposures will demonstrate the posterior portion of the medial meniscus, the third and fourth exposures will demonstrate the middle portion of the medial meniscus, and the last two exposures will demonstrate the anterior portion of the medial meniscus. At this point, the patient is in the supine position. The patient is then placed in the prone position again. However, for this series, the extremity being investigated is rested on the specialized tunnel table while the other leg is placed under the table. The same six exposures are made at 30° intervals from the prone to the supine. This set of radiographs demonstrates the posterior, middle, and anterior portions of the lateral meniscus.

The views taken during double-contrast arthrography should be closely but accurately collimated. Exposure times should be short, and the kVp should be as low as possible to produce good short scale contrast. Because positive contrast media are used, the radiographs must be completed rapidly as a result of the rapid absorption of the contrast medium and the subsequent loss of contrast.

Table 20–4 is a summary of the arthrographic positions for knee arthrography. Figure 20–3 shows some joint images that illustrate the results of both conventional arthrography and magnetic imaging techniques.

Table 20–4. SUMMARY OF POSITIONS FOR KNEE ARTHROGRAPHY

Projection	Patient Position	Central Ray	Anatomy
Scout films			
Anteroposterior	Patient supine, knee maximally extended and centered to an 8- × 10-in (20- × 25-cm) cassette	Angled approximately 6° caudad, to enter slightly below tip of patella	Preliminary views of knee joint before instillation of contrast medium show distal femur, proximal tibia and fibula, and patellar shadow
Internal oblique	Patient supine, knee joint extended, extremity rotated internally 45° and knee centered to an 8- × 10-in (20- × 25-cm) cassette	Angled approximately 6° caudad	
External oblique	Patient supine, knee joint extended, extremity rotated externally 45° and knee centered to an 8- × 10-in (20- × 25-cm) cassette	Angled approximately 3° cephalad	
Lateral	Patient comfortably positioned so that knee is in "true" lateral position in 90° flexion	Angled 3° cephalad	
Vertical beam technique			
Anteroposterior	Patient supine, knee maximally extended and centered to an 8- × 10-in (20- × 25-cm) cassette	Angled approximately 6–9° toward ankle	Anteroposterior view of contrast-filled knee joint
Supine external oblique	Patient supine, leg rotated 45° externally, knee centered to an 8- × 10-in (20- × 25-cm) cassette	Angled approximately 6° toward ankle	External oblique view of contrast-filled knee joint
Supine internal oblique	Patient supine, leg rotated 45° internally, knee centered to an 8- × 10-in (20- × 25-cm) cassette	Angled approximately 9° toward ankle	External oblique view of contrast-filled knee joint
Posteroanterior	Patient prone, knee flexed approximately 30° and centered to an 8- × 10-in (20- × 25-cm) cassette	Angled approximately 6° cephalad	Posteroanterior view of contrast-filled knee joint
Mediolateral	Patient supine and rotated toward affected side, knee flexed 90° and centered to an 8- × 10-in (20- × 25-cm) cassette	Angled 3–5° cephalad	Lateral view of contrast-filled knee joint
Horizontal beam technique			
Tangential	Medial meniscus: patient initially in prone position, extremity positioned in lateral anterior oblique position, six exposures made; after each exposure, patient rotated 30° until supine position achieved	Directed horizontally at right angles to a lead-shielded 7- × 17-in (17.5- × 42.5-cm) cassette; field size 2.5 × 7 in (6.25 × 17.5 cm)	Tangential views of medial meniscus
	Lateral meniscus: patient in prone position, extremity placed on tunnel table in anterior medial oblique position, six exposures made; after each exposure, patient rotated 30° until supine position achieved		Tangential views of lateral meniscus

REFERENCES

1. Gardner, E., Gray, D. J., and O'Rahilly, R.: Anatomy: A Regional Study of Human Structure, 4th ed. Philadelphia, W. B. Saunders, 1975.
2. Burk, D. L., Jr., Kanal, E., Brunberg, J. A., et al.: 1.5 T surface coil MRI of the knee, Am. J. Roentgenol., *147*:293, 1986.
3. Lindblom, K.: Arthrography of the knee, Acta Radiol., *27*:521, 1946.
4. Freiberger, R. H., Killoran, P. J., and Cardona, G.: Arthrography of the knee by double contrast method, Am. J. Roentgenol., *97*:736, 1966.
5. Schawelson, R. T.: Double contrast knee arthrography with horizontal beam, Radiol. Technol., *41*:98, 1969.

SUGGESTED READINGS

Apple, J. S., et al.: A comparison of Hexabrix and Renografin-60 in knee arthrography, Am. J. Roentgenol., *145*:139–142, 1985.
Crues, J. V., III, Mink, J., Levy, T. L., et al.: Meniscal tears of the knee: Accuracy of MR imaging, Radiology, *164*:445, 1987.
Ehman, R. L., Berquist, T. H., and McLeod, R. A.: MR imaging of the musculoskeletal system: A 5-year appraisal, Radiology, *166*:313, 1988.
Freiberger, R. H., Kaye, J. J., and Spiller, J.: Arthrography. New York, Appleton-Century-Crofts, 1979.
Gasparini, D., et al.: Shoulder arthrography, Rays, *10*:23–30, 1985.
Gerson, E. S., and Griffiths, H. J.: A simple marking device for knee arthrography, Am. J. Roentgenol., *127*:1057, 1976.
Goldberg, R. P., Hall, F. M., and Wyshak, G.: Pain in knee arthrography: Comparison of air versus CO_2 and reaspiration versus no reaspiration, Am. J. Roentgenol., *136*:377, 1981.
Hall, F. M.: Further pitfalls in knee arthrography, J. Can. Assoc. Radiol., *29*:179, 1978.
Hall, F. M.: Methodology in knee arthrography, Radiol. Clin. North Am., *19*:269, 1981.
Hall, F. M.: Pitfalls in knee arthrography, Radiology, *118*:55, 1976.
Hall, F. M., and Tegtmeyer, C. H.: Double and single contrast arthrography of the knee (letter to the editor), Radiology, *134*:796, 1980.
Herman, L. J., and Beltran, J.: Pitfalls in MR imaging of the knee, Radiology, *167*:775, 1988.
Kanal, E., Burk, D. L., Jr., Brunberg, J. A., et al.: Pediatric musculoskeletal magnetic resonance imaging, Radiol. Clin. North Am., *26*:211, 1988.
Lee, J. K., and Yao, L.: Stress fractures: MR imaging, Radiology, *169*:217, 1988.
Newberg, A. H.: The radiographic evaluation of shoulder and elbow pain in the athlete, Clin. Sports Med., *6*:785–809, 1987.
Pavlov, H., and Freiberger, R. H.: An easy method to demonstrate the cruciate ligaments by double contrast arthrography, Radiology, *126*:817, 1978.
Quinn, S. F., et al.: Digital subtraction wrist arthrography: Evaluation of the multiple compartment technique, Am. J. Roentgenol., *151*:1173–1174, 1988.
Rosenthal, D. I., et al.: Stressing the knee joint for arthrography, Radiology, *134*:250, 1980.
Westall, D. R.: Arthrography: A critical study of the technique and possible improvement of knee arthrograms, Radiol. Technol., *45*:311, 1974.
Zimmer, W. D., Berquist, T. H., McLeod, R. A., et al.: Magnetic resonance imaging of osteosarcomas: Comparison with computer tomography, Clin. Orthop., *208*:289, 1986.

twenty-one

Sialography

ANATOMIC CONSIDERATIONS
Parotid Glands
Submandibular Glands
Sublingual Glands
INDICATIONS AND
    CONTRAINDICATIONS
CONTRAST MEDIA
PATIENT PREPARATION

PROCEDURE
EQUIPMENT
PATIENT POSITIONING
Anteroposterior Projections
Posteroanterior Projections
Lateral Projections
Inferosuperior (Occlusal) Projection

The radiographic visualization of the salivary glands and ducts is called sialography. The evaluation of the salivary glands is most often accomplished with computed tomography or magnetic resonance imaging; however, sialography becomes the method of choice when a definitive diagnosis is required. It involves the introduction of a water-soluble contrast agent into the orifices of the salivary ducts. In most cases, this procedure requires a minimum of specialized equipment and can be performed in a regular radiographic or fluoroscopic room.

ANATOMIC CONSIDERATIONS

The salivary glands secrete saliva into the mouth. Saliva is a liquid that is approximately 99% water. The salivary glands secrete between 1000 and 2000 ml of saliva every day. Found in the saliva are basically two types of materials secreted by the salivary glands—mucus, a combination of mucin and water that is a very viscous substance used to lubricate food particles and maintain oral hygiene, and serous fluid, which contains the enzyme amylase, a substance that begins the digestive process of starches.

There are three pairs of salivary glands—the parotid glands, submandibular glands, and sublingual glands (Fig. 21–1).

Parotid Glands

These are the largest of the salivary glands, with each consisting of a superficial and a deep portion. The parotid glands lie anterior and somewhat inferior to the ear. The deep portion of the parotoid gland extends into the neck approximately 0.75 in below and behind the angle of the mandible. The parotid duct, also called Stensen's duct, is

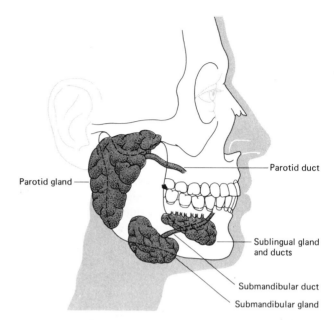

Figure 21–1. A schematic showing the location of the three pairs of salivary glands and their associated ducts. (From Solomon, E. P., and Davis, W. P.: Human Anatomy and Physiology, Philadelphia, Saunders College Publishing, 1983.)

between 5 and 7 cm long. It courses across and to the anterior margin of the masseter muscle where it turns medially, opening into the mouth opposite the second upper molar tooth. Occasionally, a small accessory lobe may be found, the socia parotidis.

Submandibular Glands

The submandibular glands, also called the submaxillary glands, lie medial to the body of the mandible, with each gland also composed of a superficial and a deep portion. The superficial portion is inferior and anterior to the angle of the mandible, where its posterior portion can be found next to the apex of the parotid gland. It extends anteriorly along the mandibular body. A small, deep portion of the gland curves around the posterior border of the mylohyoid muscle and extends into it. The submandibular duct, also called Wharton's duct, arises from this deep portion. It averages approximately 5 cm in length, passing anteriorly and medially to the mandible and opening at the sides of the base of the frenulum.

Sublingual Glands

These are the smallest of the three pairs of salivary glands. They are located under the mucosa of the mouth and form a longitudinal ridge at either side of the base of the tongue, the sublingual fold. The sublingual glands, unlike the parotid or submandibular glands, do not have a single duct. There are approximately 12 smaller sublingual ducts, the ducts of Rivinus, coming from the superior border of the gland to open at the sublingual fold. One or two of these ducts, Bartholin's ducts, may open into the submaxillary duct.

INDICATIONS AND CONTRAINDICATIONS

Sialography is used to demonstrate the relation of the salivary glands to their adjacent structures. It provides both diagnostic and preoperative information in cases of salivary gland pathology. Other indications for sialography are calculi, strictures of the ducts, sialectasia (dilation of a duct), fistulae, and demonstration of pleomorphic salivary gland tumors, commonly called mixed parotid tumors.

Contraindications for this procedure include severe inflammation of the salivary ducts and history of sensitivity to iodinated contrast media.

CONTRAST MEDIA

Two types of contrast media—water soluble and oily—are used to opacify the salivary glands. The final choice remains with the physician performing the procedure. Certain factors govern the use of a specific type of contrast medium for a particular procedure. Oily contrast media, such as Ethiodol, have a very slow excretion rate and can cause granulomatous tissue formation, which can be disadvantageous in cases in which complete removal of the contrast medium is impossible. Oily contrast media, however, provide a greater density in the ducts and parenchyma, which is necessary when tomography is used. For routine sialography, a water-soluble contrast medium, such as Renografin-60 or Renografin-76, is usually used. Table 21–1 gives a comparison of the types of contrast media and the indications for their use in sialography.

PATIENT PREPARATION

Sialography does not require specific preprocedural preparation by the patient. A history should be taken before the study to determine if the patient has allergies or has had prior reactions to iodinated contrast media. The patient should be monitored for signs of reaction during the examination. At the conclusion of the study, the patient is usually given a secretory stimulant to clear the contrast medium from the gland and ducts.

PROCEDURE

Scout films of the area of interest may or may not be taken. In cases of suspected sialolithiasis (salivary gland or salivary duct calculi), scout films are mandatory. In cases in which scout films are not taken, stones may be obliterated by the contrast medium, causing an inaccurate diagnosis to be made. The study may also be performed with fluoroscopic visualization and spot filming as well as with overhead radiographic projections.[1]

After scout films have been taken, the radiographer locates the orifices of the salivary ducts by having the patient express some saliva. The physician can either palpate the salivary gland or have the patient suck on a lemon slice. When the salivary duct is

Table 21–1. COMPARISON OF CONTRAST MEDIA USED FOR SIALOGRAPHY

Type	Example(s)	Indications for Use
Water soluble	Renografin-60 Renografin-76	Possible retention of contrast Presence of large ductal stones or strictures Possible extravasation Traumatic cannulation
Oily	Ethiodol	Tomography Greater density provided Visualization of ducts and parenchyma

located, it is dilated with standard double-ended blunt dilators or with lacrimal probes. After dilation of the orifice, the duct is cannulated. Several types of cannulae are available, but the use of a modified Abbott butterfly set has proved successful in most cases, especially when the patient has to be moved to another location for computed tomography sialography. The modification is accomplished by filing the beveled tip of the needle flat and smooth with a medium-fine metal file. The wings of the butterfly are then secured with a hemostat. This allows for ease of insertion of the cannula into the duct.[2] The cannula should be prefilled with the contrast medium to avoid injection of air bubbles.

After the duct has been successfully cannulated, the cannula is immobilized. When the modified butterfly setup is used, the patient is instructed to close the mouth. When a blunt-tipped or other type of cannula is used, a folded piece of sterile gauze is placed between the cannula and the tongue; the tubing is held in place by closing the mouth and lips around it. The tubing and syringe are taped to the shoulder or chest, and the contrast medium is then slowly injected. This is usually done with fluoroscopy and spot films. Overhead films and/or tomography may also be done at this time. Occasionally, delayed films may be requested to determine functional emptying of the gland. There are two major methods of injecting the contrast agent—manual and hydrostatic. Manual injection is accomplished as described above. The hydrostatic method uses gravity to introduce the contrast agent. The syringe barrel, with the plunger removed, is secured to an intravenous pole about 25 to 30 cm above the level of the salivary duct. Filling is accomplished slowly and is usually monitored with fluoroscopy.

This procedure may be used for parotid and submandibular sialography. Once Wharton's duct has been entered for sublingual sialography, the cannula should not be advanced too far. This allows the sublingual ducts located just behind the orifice to be filled. Sublingual sialography is not usually feasible because of the anatomic structure of the sublingual ductal system. In some patients, however, because of anatomic variations that provide access through Wharton's duct or, in rare cases, through a single sublingual duct anomaly, retrograde filling of the sublingual duct system is possible.[3]

EQUIPMENT

Sialography can be performed in any radiographic or fluoroscopic room. It is a procedure that does not require the use of automatic injection devices or rapid sequence film changers. Most supplies needed for this study can be found in any radiology department and assembled just before the examination or in the form of a prepackaged sialography setup. The system used will depend on the number of studies done.

The supplies required will vary according to the type of cannula preferred by the physician. A typical sialography setup is shown in Table 21–2.[2, 4] Additional necessary items are sterile disposable gloves, anesthetic (topical), and contrast agent of choice. The sterile setup will vary with the preference of the radiographer performing the

Table 21–2. CONTENTS OF TYPICAL SIALOGRAPHY TRAY

Equipment	Amount, Type, and/or Size
Syringe	1 (2½ or 3 ml)
Adhesive tape	1 roll (½ in)
Cotton swabs	2–3
Extension tubing	1 (size dependent on cannula used)
Gauze pads	10 (4 × 4)
Cannulae	4 (blunt-tipped, single sideport; 19, 21, 23, and 25 gauge)*
Cannulae	4 (modified butterfly setup; 19, 21, 23, and 25 gauge)*

*Size used depends on the duct size.

procedure, and it may be necessary to have two or more different types of setups to provide for the physician's preference.

PATIENT POSITIONING

In most cases, fluoroscopy is used to monitor the filling of the salivary glands with the contrast medium. The radiographer performing the procedure usually takes spot film radiographs in several different positions. Overhead radiography is then done to include lateral, anteroposterior, posteroanterior, tangential, and basal projections or specific combinations as required by the radiographer. Tomography or computed tomography may also be performed as part of the procedure. In cases of ductal obstruction or sialectasia, delayed films are requested to evaluate gland and duct functions.

Anteroposterior Projections

STANDARD ANTEROPOSTERIOR PROJECTION. In this projection, the patient is placed in either the supine recumbent or the erect position. The head is adjusted to a true anteroposterior position with the median sagittal plane perpendicular to the table. The patient's chin is depressed toward the chest to place the orbitomeatal baseline perpendicular to the film. The cassette should be centered just below the patient's mouth. The beam is collimated to the film size, and the central ray is directed perpendicular to the midpoint of the film. This projection is used primarily to demonstrate the parotid gland.

TANGENTIAL ANTEROPOSTERIOR PROJECTION. The patient is placed in either the supine recumbent or the erect position. The head is adjusted so that the canthomeatal line is at a right angle to the cassette. The patient's head is rotated slightly toward the affected side. The amount of rotation should be just enough to place the parotid gland at a right angle to the film. The angle of the mandible should be centered to the film. The central ray is directed at a right angle to the midpoint of the cassette.

Posteroanterior Projections

The positioning techniques for these projections produce views similar to those taken in the anteroposterior projections. The parotid gland lies approximately midway between the anterior and posterior aspects of the body, allowing for either anteroposterior or posteroanterior positioning of the patient.

STANDARD POSTEROANTERIOR PROJECTION. In this projection, the patient is placed in either the prone recumbent or the erect position. The nose and forehead are placed against the cassette. The patient's head is adjusted to a true posteroanterior position, with the orbitomeatal baseline at a right angle to the film. The cassette should be centered approximately 2½ in inferior to the gonion. The central ray should be directed at a right angle to the film.

TANGENTIAL POSTEROANTERIOR PROJECTION. The patient is placed in either the prone recumbent or the erect position with the chin and nose in contact with the cassette. The head is rotated so that the longitudinal axis of the mandibular body is perpendicular to the film. The vertical plane is centered so that it runs through the angle of the mandible to the center of the film. The central ray is directed at a right angle to the midpoint of the cassette.

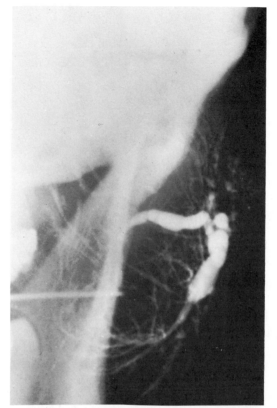

A

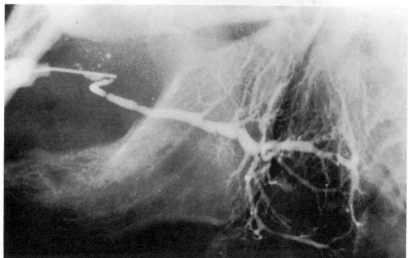

B

Figure 21–2. Representative sialographic radiographs. *(A)* Anteroposterior projection; *(B)* lateral projection.

Illustration continued on following page

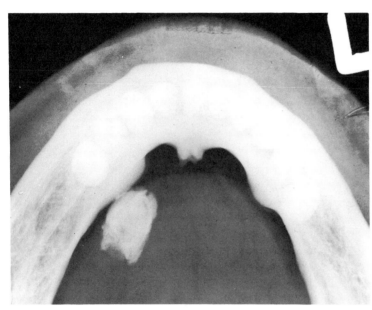

Figure 21–2 *Continued (C)* Occlusal projection. (From Rankow, R. M., and Polayes, I. M.: Diseases of the Salivary Glands, Philadelphia, W. B. Saunders, 1976.)

C

Lateral Projections

TRUE LATERAL PROJECTION. The patient is placed in the seated, erect, or semiprone position. The head is adjusted to a true lateral position. The median sagittal plane is parallel to the film. The neck should be slightly extended to prevent possible superimposition of the salivary glands with the cervical spine. The central ray is directed at a right angle to the midpoint of the film, entering at a point approximately 1 in anterior to the external auditory meatus.

MODIFIED LATERAL PROJECTION. The patient is placed in the seated, erect, or semiprone position with the affected side down. The head is adjusted to a true lateral position and rotated forward 15°. The skull is centered to a point approximately 1 in anterior to the external auditory meatus. The central ray is directed at a right angle to the midpoint of the film.

LATERAL OBLIQUE PROJECTION. With the patient in either an erect, seated, or semiprone position, the head is placed in a true lateral position and centered at the level of the external auditory meatus. The central ray is directed at an angle of 25° cephalad to the midpoint of the film.

Inferosuperior (Occlusal) Projection

The patient is placed in the supine position. The shoulders and thorax are supported by a pillow or folded sheets. The head is gently dropped into a submentovertical position, with the neck fully extended. The median sagittal plane should be perpendicular to the film. The transverse axis of the body is adjusted so that it is parallel with the table. An occlusal film is inserted into the patient's mouth. Placement of the packet depends on the gland to be radiographed. The packet should be inserted lengthwise when the submaxillary gland is opacified; when the sublingual glands are radiographed, the packet should be placed more anteriorly in the mouth and can be inserted crosswise. The central ray is directed at a right angle to the plane of the film.

Table 21–3 summarizes the positions used during sialography. Figure 21–2 illustrates some representative radiographs taken during sialography.

Table 21–3. SUMMARY OF POSITIONS FOR SIALOGRAPHY

Projection	Patient Position	Central Ray	Cassette Size	Anatomy
Lateral oblique	Semiprone or seated erect; head in true lateral position (MSP* parallel to cassette)	Tube angled 25° cephalad to enter inferior to and just behind angle of upper mandible	8 × 10 in (20 × 25 cm)	Parotid gland
Lateral (true)	Seated erect or semiprone; head in true lateral position (MSP parallel to cassette); neck slightly extended	Directed perpendicular to midpoint of film	8 × 10 in (20 × 25 cm)	Submaxillary gland
Lateral (modified)	Seated erect or semiprone; head in modified lateral position (MSP rotated forward approximately 15°)	Directed perpendicular to midpoint of film	8 × 10 in (20 × 25 cm)	Parotid gland
Inferosuperior occlusal	Supine with shoulders and thorax supported; head in submentovertical position (fully extended); transverse axis of body parallel to table	Directed perpendicular to plane of occlusal packet	Occlusal	Submaxillary gland, sublingual gland
Tangential posteroanterior	Prone or erect; chin and nose in contact with cassette; longitudinal axis of mandibular body perpendicular to film; center angle of mandible to the center of film	Directed perpendicular to midpoint of film	8 × 10 in (20 × 25 cm)	Parotid gland
Tangential anteroposterior	Supine or erect; orbitomeatal line perpendicular to cassette; head rotated slightly toward affected side; center angle of mandible to the film	Directed perpendicular to midpoint of film	8 × 10 in (20 × 25 cm)	Parotid gland
Posteroanterior	Prone or erect; nose and forehead against cassette, centered 2½ in inferior to gonion; head adjusted to true posteroanterior position; orbitomeatal baseline perpendicular to film	Directed perpendicular to midpoint of film	8 × 10 in (20 × 25 cm)	Parotid gland
Anteroposterior	Supine or erect; chin depressed toward chest; orbitomeatal baseline placed perpendicular to film by centering the cassette just below the mouth	Directed perpendicular to midpoint of film	8 × 10 in (20 × 25 cm)	Parotid gland

*MSP: median sagittal plane.

REFERENCES

1. Yune, H. Y., and Klatte, E. C.: Current status of sialography, Am. J. Roentgenol., *115*:420, 1972.
2. Som, P. M., and Khilnani, M. T.: Modification of a butterfly infusion set for sialography, Radiology, *143*:791, 1982.
3. Wackens, G., and De Smedt, E.: Sublingual sialography, Oral Surg., *50*:382, 1980.
4. Rabinov, K. R., and Joffe, N.: A blunt-tip side injecting cannula for sialography, Radiology, *92*:1438, 1969.

SUGGESTED READINGS

Blair, G. S.: Sublingual sialogram, Oral Surg., *42*:540, 1976.
Ellis, H.: Clinical Anatomy, 5th ed., Oxford, Blackwell Scientific Publications, 1973.
Granone, F. G., and Juliani, G.: Submaxillary sialography in combination with pneumoradiography and tomography, Am. J. Roentgenol., *104*:692, 1968.
Gullotta, U., and Schekatz, A.: Digital subtraction sialography, Eur. J. Radiol., *3*:339, 340, 1983.
Kushner, D. C., and Weber, A. L.: Sialography of salivary gland tumors with fluoroscopy and tomography, Am. J. Roentgenol., *130*:941, 1978.
Larsson, S. G., Lufkin, R. B., and Hoover, L. A.: Computed tomography of the submandibular salivary glands, Acta Radiol., *28*:693–696, 1987.
Mancuso, A., Rice, D., and Hanafee, W. N.: Computed tomography of the parotid gland during contrast sialography, Radiology, *132*:211, 1979.
Meine, F. J., and Woloshin, H. J.: Radiologic diagnosis of salivary gland tumors, Radiol. Clin. North Am., *8*:475, 1970.
Som, P. M., and Biller, H. F.: The combined CT-sialogram, Radiology, *135*:387, 1980.
Sterling, S.: Some radiographic considerations in sialography, Radiol. Technol., *42*:57, 1970.
Stone, D. N., et al.: Parotid CT sialography, Radiology, *138*:393, 1981.
Wiesenfeld, D., Ferguson, M. M., and McMillan, N. C.: Simultaneous computed tomography and sialography of the parotid and submandibular glands, Br. J. Oral Surg., *21*:268–276, 1983.
White, I. L.: Sialography: X-ray visualization of major salivary glands, Laryngoscope, *82*:2032, 1972.
Woodburne, R. T.: Essentials of Human Anatomy, 7th ed., New York, Oxford University Press, 1983.

7 Interventional Radiography

twenty-two

Vascular Interventional Procedures

TECHNIQUES USED TO REDUCE BLOOD
  FLOW
Indications and Contraindications
Procedure
    Transcatheter Embolization and
      Balloon Occlusion
    Intravascular Electrocoagulation
    Vasoconstrictor Infusion
Complications
TECHNIQUES USED TO INCREASE BLOOD
  FLOW

Indications and Contraindications
Procedure
    Percutaneous Transluminal
      Angioplasty
    Intravascular Thrombolysis
      (Fibrinolysis)
    Excisional Atherectomy
    Infusion of Vasodilators
Complications
REMOVAL OF INTRAVASCULAR FOREIGN
  BODIES

The term "interventional radiology" was coined by Wallace in 1976 to describe any selective catheter or needle technique used for the diagnosis and treatment of disease.[1] Although the basic techniques had been used for many years, this subspecialty began in 1964 when Dotter and Judkins successfully recanalized arthrosclerotic stenosed femoral arteries.[2] Drawing on their experience as angiographers and using standard equipment, they were able to pass catheters through occluded arterial segments. Their technique used overlapping (coaxial), or telescoping, catheters to compress the plaque. The method improved, and in 1974 Gruntzig developed the double-lumen balloon sheath catheter, which improved the recanalization procedure and reduced trauma to the vascular system at the puncture site.[3] These and other interventional procedures have proven to reduce the cost of treatment without increasing risk to the patient. They have a low mortality rate and, in many cases, are better tolerated by the patient than are more complicated and extensive therapeutic or surgical procedures. In general, interventional radiography encompasses both vascular and nonvascular procedures. The results of an interventional technique can be diagnostic as well as therapeutic. Samples may be taken for diagnosis to provide histological, bacteriological, and biochemical information. Table 22–1 illustrates the present scope of interventional radiography for both vascular and nonvascular procedures.

Vascular interventional radiography procedures use angiography as the primary procedural method. They can be divided into methods that either reduce or increase blood flow. These vascular methods are primarily therapeutic in nature.

Table 22–1. COMPARISON OF INTERVENTIONAL RADIOGRAPHY PROCEDURES

Vascular Studies	Nonvascular Studies
Increase blood flow	Biopsy
Mechanical methods	Thyroid
Dilation of stenotic artery (PTA)	Intracranial tumor
Recanalization of occluded artery	Intraorbital tumor
Removal of embolus	Spinal cord tumor
Intra-arterial method	Pleural
Infusion of vasodilators	Bronchial
	Abdominal mass
Decrease blood flow	Abscess
Mechanical methods	Ureter
Embolization	Renal
Balloon techniques	Retroperitoneal
Intravascular electrocoagulation	Lymph node
Intravascular method	Soft tissue
Infusion of vasoconstrictors (e.g., posterior	Bone
pituitary extract)	
	Drainage of abscesses
Miscellaneous intravascular method	Puncture and drainage of cysts
Infusion of chemotherapeutic agents	
Laser angioplasty	Placement of stents*
Vena cava filtering	
Renin sampling	Removal of calculi
	Renal
	Biliary
	Extracorporeal shock wave lithotripsy
	Endoscopic retrograde
	cholangiopancreatography
	Sinography
	Joint aspiration
	Percutaneous nephrostomy

*A stent is any material used to hold tissue in place while healing is in progress.

TECHNIQUES USED TO REDUCE BLOOD FLOW

Procedures for reducing blood flow include embolization and balloon occlusion, intravascular infusion of vasoconstrictors, and intravascular electrocoagulation. Most of these techniques are performed using percutaneous puncture of the femoral or other superficial arteries. Occasionally, the embolic material is inserted directly into the vessel via an arteriotomy.

Indications and Contraindications

The use of transcatheter embolization is indicated in cases of posttraumatic hemorrhage, for occlusion of the blood supply to highly vascular neoplasms, and for reduction of bleeding during and after surgical procedures. Because transcatheter embolization is presently used in high-risk cases, there are no definitive contraindications to the procedure. Ideally, the embolization method chosen reduces the flow of blood without incurring ischemia of the tissue.

Electrocoagulation can be used to occlude blood vessels in cases of diagnosed tumors, hemangiomas, and arteriovenous fistulas. Definite indications and contraindications have not been determined for this procedure because it is infrequently used and has remained classified as experimental.

Infusions of vasoconstrictors are indicated in cases of suspected upper gastrointestinal bleeding and as an aid to improving the diagnostic capabilities of angiography in certain areas of the body. If vasoconstrictors are administered during hepatic angiography or peripheral angiography, the diagnostic value of the examination is enhanced. In cases of suspected hepatomas and adenomas, the instillation of vasoconstrictors results in an improved visualization of the neoplasms.

Procedure

TRANSCATHETER EMBOLIZATION AND BALLOON OCCLUSION

With this technique, intravascular occlusion is accomplished by placing a foreign substance, tissue, or blood clot into the lumen of a selected vessel. The naturally occurring particulate types of embolic materials have become obsolete with the increased use of percutaneous catheter methods. The following list is a summary of the embolic materials and methods that are used for vascular embolization.

Natural agents (obsolete)
  Autogenous blood clots (regular)
  Autologous blood clots (modified)
  Tissue fragments (muscle, fat, and so on)
Synthetic agents
  Solid (resorbable)
    Gelatin sponge (Gelfoam)
    Oxidized cellulose (Oxycel)
    Occlusion gel (Ethibloc)
    Collagen suspensions
      Microfibrillar bovine collagen (Avitene)
      Equine collagen (Tachotop)
  Solid (permanent)
    Polyvinyl alcohol (Ivalon)
    Silicone beads
    Plastic beads
    Metal beads
    Glass beads
  Solid (mechanical)
    Coils (stainless steel)
      Wool threads
      Silk threads
      Dacron threads
    Springs (stainless steel)
  Solid (balloon systems)
    Nondetachable balloon systems
    Detachable balloon systems
    Controlled-leak balloon catheter systems
  Liquid
    Isobytyl-2-cyanoacrylate (IBCA; Bucrylate)
    Silicone elastomer
    Absolute ethanol
    Barium sulfate
    Hot contrast agents
Chemoembolization
  Micromycin C microcapsules
Electrocoagulation

The search for the "ideal" embolic material has yielded many different products, but none of these exhibits all of the characteristics of an ideal substance. An ideal embolic material is nontoxic, stable, insoluble in the vascular system, radiopaque, and capable of being shaped, sterilized, and introduced via an angiographic catheter.[4] The material used is determined by the pathology, the patient's clotting ability, and the nature of the blood supply. Occasionally, it is necessary to use a combination of more than one type of embolic material to successfully isolate an area.

The substances used to occlude the blood vessels can be categorized by how long they remain in the vessel—they can be temporary or long lasting. Substances such as Gelfoam, autologous blood clots, muscle tissue clots, and balloon catheters are temporary occluders. These substances are either mechanically removable, such as the balloon catheter, or quickly absorbed by the body through intravascular lysis.

Embolic media such as Gianturco coils, detachable balloon catheters, IBCA, and polyvinyl alcohol foam are long-term agents used for permanent occlusion of vessels.

CELLULOSE SPONGE EMBOLIC MEDIA. These include microfibrillar collagen, oxidized cellulose, and Gelfoam, which is the most popular. Gelfoam is manufactured in sheets and in powder (Fig. 22–1). It was first used in 1945 to control hemorrhage during neurosurgery, and it has been successfully used in intravascular occlusion. The powdered form consists of particles ranging from 40 to 60 μm in size. When Gelfoam is used, small fragments (pieces) are cut from the sheet and soaked in normal saline solution, a contrast agent, or both to provide radiopacity. These pieces are then placed into the vessel by injection through an angiographic catheter. The size of the inside lumen of the catheter determines the maximum size of the piece to be used. Gelfoam has the disadvantage of being easily refluxed, causing recanalization of the vessel. This type of embolic medium, when injected into the lumen of a vessel, provides a framework for blood clot formation. Intravascular lysing of this type of material can occur in a relatively short period of time, but it is much more persistent in a vessel than an autologous blood or tissue clot alone.

Gelfoam powder that has been radiopacified by the addition of tantalum powder is used to produce occlusion at the precapillary level. At this level, recanalization by collateral vessel formation is minimized, making Gelfoam powder an excellent choice for tumor treatment.

This type of embolic medium lasts from less than 48 h to 30 days.

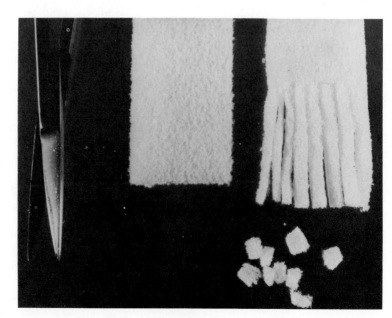

Figure 22–1. Sheet of Gelfoam cut for use. (From Kadir, S., et al.: Selected Techniques in Interventional Radiology, Philadelphia, W. B. Saunders, 1982, p. 31.)

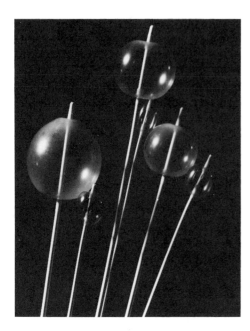

Figure 22–2. Occlusion balloon catheters.

BALLOON CATHETER. Use of the balloon catheter provides a safe temporary method of occluding vessels to control or prevent bleeding, as well as isolating vessels for selective infusion of chemotherapeutic agents or placing other types of embolic media (Fig. 22–2). The advantages of using the balloon catheter are that it is retrievable for removal and the position of the balloon can be changed easily.

Four types of balloon catheters are available. The single-lumen type is used with catheter introduction and exchange sheath sets or coaxial catheters. The double-lumen type is constructed to permit contrast injection and balloon inflation in the same catheter. The double-lumen catheter consists of one catheter within a second, larger catheter. The third type—flow-directed detachable miniature balloon catheters—are used for permanent occlusion of high-flow vascular lesions. The controlled-leak balloon catheter systems are also flow-directed catheters that allow the delivery of a liquid embolic material or contrast agent.

Single- and double-lumen catheters are primarily used as temporary occluders. Detachable balloon catheters are used to provide long-term occlusion, especially in areas in which high blood flow is present. Detachable balloon catheters are equipped with self-sealing valves and are usually filled with contrast medium or another opaque medium when the study is performed. The catheter has a stainless-steel stem that fits into the valve of the balloon. When the balloon is placed in the vessel to be occluded, it can be inflated. The catheter is then withdrawn, disconnecting the stem and leaving the balloon in the vessel. Detachable balloons can also be flow-guided into position. The detachable balloon catheters are used with coaxial catheter systems to facilitate placement of the miniballoon.[5]

A balloon catheter can be used in conjunction with embolic material and in such cases function like a cork to prevent reflux of the particulate material from the target vessel. Once the particulate embolic material has been firmly set in place, the balloon can be removed (Fig. 22–3).

OCCLUDING SPRING EMBOLI AND OTHER MECHANICAL OCCLUDERS. Occluding springs are mechanical devices of stainless-steel coiled wire about 5 cm long and available in 3-, 5-, 8-, 10-, 12-, and 15-mm diameters. Strands of wool, silk, or Dacron are affixed to the wire to provide a framework for clot formation. The wool-tailed coils are primarily used for larger arteries, whereas the silk- or Dacron-tailed coils are used

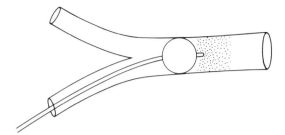

Figure 22–3. Schematic of an occlusion balloon catheter used in conjunction with particulate embolic material.

to occlude smaller arteries. These coils were developed in 1975 by Gianturco, Anderson, and Wallace and are commonly called Gianturco-Anderson-Wallace (GAW) coils (Fig. 22–4).[6]

These devices are supplied uncoiled and braided into an introducer cartridge. To place the coil into the catheter, the introducer cartridge is inserted into the stopcock until it contacts the flared catheter end. The coil is then pushed into the catheter with the stiff end of a guide wire. The distance that the coil should be pushed into the catheter in the loading stage is usually recommended by the manufacturer. In the case of the GAW coil, the manufacturer (Cook, Inc.) recommends leading for a distance of 20 to 30 cm. The guide wire and introducer are removed, and the spring embolus is

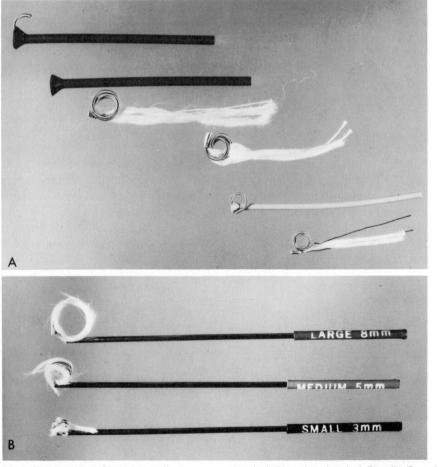

Figure 22–4. Stainless-steel Gianturco coils shown as unloaded *(A)* and preloaded *(B)* units. (From Kadir, S., et al.: Selected Techniques in Interventional Radiology, Philadelphia, W. B. Saunders, 1982, p. 34.)

then pushed through the distal end of the catheter for placement in the vessel. A smaller version of the GAW coil, the minicoil, is also available. This unit is delivered through a 5F catheter.

Occluding spring emboli are considered permanent embolic media because they remain in the vessel for more than 30 days.

The "bristle brush" has also been successfully used to occlude vessels.[7] This device resembles a miniature chimney cleaning brush and has a central core consisting of a stainless-steel coil with nylon pieces threaded through it. These brushes require the use of large-bore catheters for introduction into the target vessel, where they remain to provide a framework for clot formation. They also are considered permanent embolic media.

LIQUID EMBOLIC MEDIA. Substances in this category include tissue adhesives such as IBCA and silicon elastomer. These products are long-term embolic media, lasting more than 30 days. These materials are used primarily in life-threatening cases. They solidify (polymerize) when they come into contact with ionizing solutions. Unlike other embolic materials, these substances do not form the framework on which a blood clot is produced; rather, they form a permanent embolus that seals the vessel almost immediately.

IBCA is used for direct vessel occlusion but has not yet been approved by the Food and Drug Administration for unrestricted use. A permit must be secured for any use of this material in human beings.

The silicon elastomer embolic medium is a low-viscosity substance that exhibits a more controlled polymerization time than IBCA, making it a better choice for occlusion of extensive arteriovenous malformations. Silicon elastomer can be mixed with iron microspheres, which allows an externally applied magnet to control the position of the material until the polymerization process is complete.[8] This procedure was devised to prevent the embolic material from moving to a nontarget vessel.

The technique for placement of these liquid emboli substances requires the use of coaxial catheters. These are specially paired catheters comprising a larger outer catheter and a smaller inner catheter. These sets come with a correctly sized guide wire and are complete for use during intravascular embolization procedures (Fig. 22–5). The large outer catheter is passed through the vessel to the approximate site of occlusion. A small amount of sterile silicon grease can be applied to the tip of the small inner catheter, which is then passed through the outer catheter into the specific vessel to be occluded. The application of the silicon grease helps to prevent adhesion of the catheter tip to the vessel wall after injection of the embolic medium.

The liquid tissue adhesive, mixed with a contrast agent, is then injected into the site. It is important for the inner catheter to be removed as soon as the injection is complete to avoid adhesion of the catheter tip to the vessel wall. Because the substances

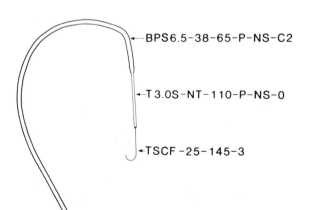

BPS6.5-38-65-P-NS-C2

T3.0S-NT-110-P-NS-0

TSCF-25-145-3

Figure 22–5. Coaxial catheter system. (Available from Cook Incorporated, Bloomington, IN.)

polymerize when in contact with an ionic solution, the catheters cannot be flushed with normal saline solution. The flushing may be accomplished with a 10% solution of dextrose and water.

Embolization by percutaneous catheter delivery of absolute ethanol has proven to be safe and efficient.[9] Its main mode of action is by damaging the endothelium and stimulating the coagulation systems that cause the vascular occlusion. It is generally used with one of the nondetachable balloon systems. The balloon helps to control reflux of the absolute ethanol. This substance has several advantages such as availability, lack of toxicity, low cost, and low complication rate. Ethanol can also be mixed with one of the nonionic contrast agents to monitor and control the embolization procedure.

Routine angiography is usually performed at the beginning of the procedure to localize the site of bleeding and again after injection of the material to confirm occlusion of the vessel. Use of liquid embolic substances can cause a mild histiocytic reaction in the vessel lumen that does not involve the vessel walls or adjoining parenchyma.[10]

INTRAVASCULAR ELECTROCOAGULATION

This technique of vessel occlusion, as the name implies, produces a thrombus in the vessel by an applied electric current. Its use has been limited, however, because of the problems associated with the technique. The procedure itself is rather long and complex, requiring extensive experience for successful occlusion. Thrombus size varies with the voltage, current, and vessel size, and control of the ultimate extent of the thrombus is limited.

The advantages of the procedure are that it can be very precise in localizing and occluding specific vessels, and it does not require the use of foreign substances or materials.

VASOCONSTRICTOR INFUSION

Infusion of certain substances that act as vasoconstrictors is useful in controlling bleeding in some areas of the body. Selective infusion of vasoconstrictors during transcatheter embolization has helped to prevent reflux of the embolic material.

The most popular vasoconstrictor substance is vasopressin, the posterior pituitary extract (Pituitrin and Pitressin). Other substances such as norepinephrine and propranolol have also been tried, but the complication and reaction rates are higher than those with the use of vasopressin.

Vasopressin has been very successful when used to control bleeding in the gastrointestinal tract, primarily because vasopressin can cause bowel constriction as well as artery constriction in this area. Both actions combine to provide a reduction in the flow of blood, allowing clot formation at the site of bleeding. Intra-arterial infusion of vasopressin is usually administered at a rate of 0.2 to 0.4 units/min for 48 to 72 h and is tapered off before termination of the infusion.[4]

Complications

Use of transcatheter vascular embolization produces certain reactions, including localized transient pain accompanied by a mild fever, malaise, increased pulse and respiration rates, restlessness, irritability, loss of appetite, and insomnia for a period of 24 to 48 h after embolization. Other complications may occur, such as embolization of nontarget organs, because of reflux of the embolic medium, ischemia, nerve palsy, infection, and possibly death. It should be remembered that these procedures are performed on patients who present a great surgical risk and on patients who are in life-threatening situations. As in any radiographic procedure, it should be considered that the benefit of performing any interventional procedure outweighs the risks presented by the procedure.

Intravascular electrocoagulation can cause damage to the vessel in which the thrombus is formed. Perforation is another risk associated with this technique.

When a vasoconstrictor such as vasopressin is used to control bleeding, it is important to monitor the patient because vasopressin is a potent diuretic that can cause water retention or have a direct depressive effect on the myocardium.[11]

TECHNIQUES USED TO INCREASE BLOOD FLOW

Interventional procedures can also be applied to increase the flow of blood in a particular vessel. Three types of procedures are used—percutaneous transluminal angioplasty (PTA), intravascular thrombolysis, and intra-arterial infusion of vasodilators. These procedures provide relatively safe methods of increasing blood flow without the necessity of extensive surgery. These studies are usually done using the percutaneous approach. The arterial cutdown approach is occasionally used, and the necessary sterile tray should be available in the radiography suite. Table 22–2 is a summary of some common approaches used for angioplasty.

Indications and Contraindications

Interventional procedures for increasing blood flow are used to either dilate stenotic vessels or recanalize obstructed vessels. PTA encompasses both dilation and recanalization. It is used to treat stenotic arterial disease primarily in medium- to large-sized vessels. Coronary, renal, and peripheral arteries are prime candidates for PTA. The lesions treated are usually localized and contain either fibromuscular or complicated plaque (atheroma). Fibromuscular plaque affects the intima by the production of smooth muscle cells, collagen, elastic fibrils, and some lipids. Complicated plaque is actually a fibromuscular plaque encased in a thin fibrous cap. The lesions should be short (not more than 10 cm) for successful angioplasty. Congenital coarctation, Takayasu's arteritis, and fibromuscular dysplasia can also be treated with PTA.[12]

Intravascular thrombolysis is a technique used to treat arterial thromboemboli. The areas that benefit most from this technique are the coronary, peripheral, visceral, and pulmonary vascular sites.

Infusion of vasodilators is useful in treating cases of vessel spasm or constriction and has been successful in the treatment of arthrosclerosis obliterans, a common cause of vascular occlusion.

There are no defined contraindications to the use of these procedures. In most cases, the patients are usually candidates for surgery, and attempts at treatment with these techniques usually outweigh the risks involved. When percutaneous transluminal coro-

Table 22–2. SUMMARY OF CATHETER APPROACHES FOR ANGIOPLASTY

Approach	Target Vessels
Percutaneous	
Retrograde femoral catheterization	Iliac artery, renal artery
Left axillary catheterization	Visceral vessels, renal artery with acute angle entry
Antegrade femoral catheterization	Superficial femoral artery, popliteal artery
Arterial cutdown	
Retrograde brachial cutdown	Coronary arteries

nary angioplasty is done, a surgical team and an operating room should be available for immediate coronary bypass surgery if complications occur. The only other contraindication is if the anatomy precludes the passage of a dilation catheter.

Procedure

PERCUTANEOUS TRANSLUMINAL ANGIOPLASTY

This procedure was first performed in 1964 by Dotter and Judkins; they used a coaxial catheter system (telescoping catheter) to recanalize a stenosed femoral artery.[2] In 1974, Gruntzig developed the double-lumen balloon catheter, which reduced the complication rate at the puncture site.[3] Currently, there are many different balloon lengths and diameters available for use during PTA (Fig. 22–6).

The objectives of this procedure may be summarized as follows[13]: improvement of blood flow (increase in lumen size), maintenance of long-term vessel patency, creation of a smooth inner surface, production of no distal emboli, and minimal disturbance of the vascular wall structure. Basically, the procedure should permanently improve blood flow in a vessel and result in minimum complications. Obviously, not all of these objectives are achieved in all cases.

Angioplasty has also been used as an adjunct to surgery and can be performed in the operating suite. Intraoperative transluminal angioplasty is useful in reaching lesions that are outside the surgical field.

The technique of catheter introduction during PTA is the same as that used for

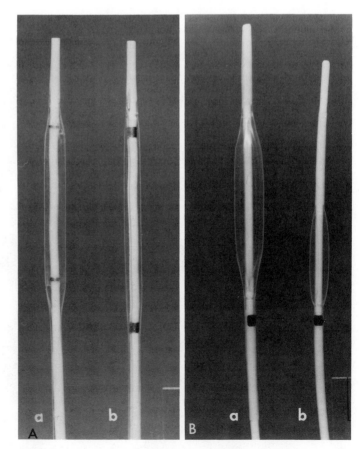

Figure 22–6. Balloon dilation catheters. *(A)* 7F catheter with polyvinyl chloride balloon: *(a)* 3 cm long, 6 mm diameter; *(b)* 4 cm long, 4 mm diameter. *(B)* Polyethylene balloon: *(a)* 8F catheter, 8-mm diameter balloon 2 cm from catheter tip: *(b)* 7F catheter, 2-cm long, 5-mm diameter balloon 3 cm from catheter tip. (From Kadir, S., et al.: Selected Techniques in Interventional Radiology, Philadelphia, W. B. Saunders, 1982, p. 162.)

routine angiography. Usually, a routine angiogram is performed to define the anatomy. Once this has been accomplished, the coaxial or balloon catheters are introduced, at which time the angioplasty guide wire is advanced through the lesion. When the guide wire has successfully traversed the lesion, the appropriate catheter is advanced over it through the lesion. The balloon is then inflated, and dilation of the vessel is accomplished.

The preceding is an oversimplification of the angioplasty procedure. Difficulties may arise in passing the guide wire and catheter through the lesion because of anatomic variations. This is the most critical part of the procedure; most complications occur at this stage. The amount of force required to open the vessel successfully varies with the type of lesion and its flow characteristics. The amount of pressure applied should be sufficient to achieve the objectives of angioplasty, as stated above. The fluoroscopic image of the balloon indicates when a successful dilation has been accomplished—the balloon becomes tube shaped. Pressure gauges are available to monitor the balloon during inflation; these allow the angiographer to stay within the manufacturer's recommended inflation pressure limits (Fig. 22–7).

After dilation, a postprocedural angiogram is usually performed to assess the results. If dilation has been successful, the catheter is then removed.

Antithrombotic medication both before and after the procedure is being used in many institutions. Several medications and methods of administration have been used, as summarized by the following[14]:

1. Aspirin (acetylsalicylic acid) and/or Persantine (dipyridamole) 24 to 48 h before angioplasty
2. Heparin, 5000 units intra-arterially during angioplasty

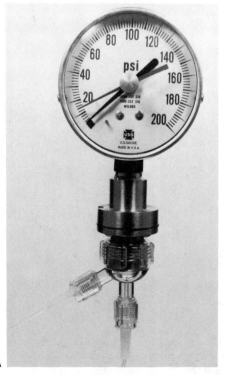 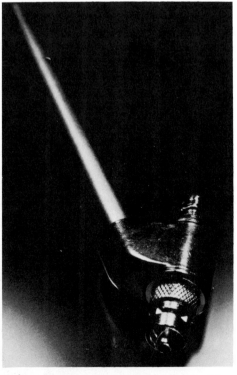

A   B

Figure 22–7. Gauges for monitoring balloon catheter inflation pressure. (*A* from Medi-Tech, Inc. *B* from Cook Incorporated, Bloomington, IN.)

3. Nitroglycerin, 1% lidocaine, or oral calcium antagonists after arterial catheterization
4. Intravenous heparin drip 24 to 48 h after angioplasty
5. Long-term administration (3 to 6 months) of aspirin and/or Persantine
6. Long-term administration (1 to 3 months) of warfarin (Coumadin)

The theory behind the use of these agents is that foreign materials (e.g., catheters, guide wires) introduced into the body are thrombogenic in nature. PTA itself is disturbing to the vascular system, and its flow pattern creates a situation in which complicating thrombosis is a possibility. Preprocedural administration of antithrombotic agents usually reduces the likelihood of thrombus formation. Postprocedural regimens have been recommended for the same reasons as well as to improve long-term patency rates. The physician performing the angioplasty selects the agent or agents to be used.

Balloon PTA has several limitations in permanently treating atherosclerotic disease. Restenosis of the vessel is the major limiting factor to the procedure. The development of adjunct procedures has provided the physician with the means to increase the success rate of this interventional procedure; among these techniques are laser-assisted balloon angioplasty, excisional atherectomy, and percutaneous coronary rotational angioplasty.

PERCUTANEOUS LASER ANGIOPLASTY. Recent innovations in fiberoptical technology have provided the mechanism to link laser systems with angiographic catheter systems. This allows the treatment of vascular lesions that are not amenable to treatment by current technology. Several laser systems are used both clinically and experimentally for this procedure.

The laser system converts light (electromagnetic radiation) into a highly amplified form of radiation that differs from ordinary light in several ways. The laser beam is composed of monochromatic radiation that travels in the same phase. It also possesses a small amount of divergence and therefore tends to travel in a straight line. Laser radiation systems are capable of producing considerable energy. This energy is expressed in watts per square centimeter. Different laser systems vary in wavelength, energy levels, whether they are pulsed or continuous, and the amount of tissue penetration and interaction that they produce. The laser systems currently available can be divided into two categories—thermal and nonthermal.

The thermal laser systems destroy tissues by converting the solid material into a gas. This process is also called thermal vaporization. These systems can cause vascular burn injury and vascular spasm. They are usually equipped with a small orifice, which minimizes the amount of area that can be treated.

The nonthermal laser systems are of the excimer variety and use argon, krypton, or xenon associated with a halogen such as chlorine, bromine, or fluorine. These systems cause vaporization through the ionization of the atoms with subsequent dissociation of the molecules of the tissue. Unlike the thermal systems, they do not cause vascular burn injury or vascular spasms. Table 22–3 is a summary of the laser systems currently in use.

Other components of the system are the optical fibers that transmit the laser beam to its target. The light-transporting portion of the fiberoptical system is usually quartz-enveloped in a refractive coating that reflects light back toward the quartz core. An external sheath of inert material such as Teflon surrounds the fiberoptical system. The fiberoptical component is covered by a heat-generating element at its tip (Fig. 22–8); the tip provides the laser–tissue interaction.

The tip of the optical fiber can be open or capped with metal or a lens; the metal-tipped fiber is used most extensively. For all systems, an external power unit is used to provide energy (Fig. 22–9).

The open-tipped laser system uses tissue absorption of the energy to effect the angioplasty. It has not been as successful as the other systems. The metal-tipped fiber uses the heat produced by the laser energy to interact with the tissue. Temperatures of

Table 22–3. SUMMARY OF LASER SYSTEMS

Neodymium:yttrium aluminum garnet (Nd:YAG) laser system
   Near-infrared spectral emission (1060 nm)
   60 mm depth of tissue penetration
   Much tissue scatter
   High level of thermal vascular trauma
   Continuous wave or pulsed wave application

Argon laser system
   Visible (blue-green) spectral emission (488 to 514 nm)
   1000 mm depth of tissue penetration
   Moderate tissue scatter
   High level of thermal vascular trauma
   Continuous wave or pulsed wave application

CO_2 laser system
   Far-infrared spectral emission (10,600 nm)
   0.03 mm depth of tissue penetration
   Little tissue scatter
   Limited thermal vascular trauma
   Continuous wave or pulsed wave application

Excimer laser system
   Ultraviolet spectral emission (308 nm)
   0.001 mm depth of tissue penetration
   Minimal tissue scatter
   Minimal thermal vascular trauma
   Pulsed wave application

400 to 600° C can be reached in a short period of time. The lens-tipped fiber is able to focus the laser beam for more precise treatment. This type of system is still in the investigative stage.

The procedure can be performed in the angiographic or special procedure suite. It is currently used in conjunction with balloon angioplasty to treat peripheral obstructions that cannot be resolved with conventional PTA.

The percutaneous catheterization procedure is the same as for other interventional procedures. An angiogram is done to localize the site of the obstruction. The laser probe is advanced through the catheter, positioned at the point of occlusion, and confirmed by fluoroscopy. The laser is activated, and the tip is advanced through the occlusion until penetration of the obstruction has been achieved (Fig. 22–10). Angiography confirms the opening of the vessel. Balloon angiography is then performed to further dilate the vessel.

Laser systems have recently been combined with balloon catheter systems to reduce the elastic recoil and cellular proliferation. These factors contribute to the restenosis of the treated vessel that can occur after conventional balloon angioplasty[18] (Fig. 22–11). The complications associated with this procedure are the same as those of conventional angioplasty, and postprocedural treatment of the patient is similar to that of other percutaneous interventional procedures.

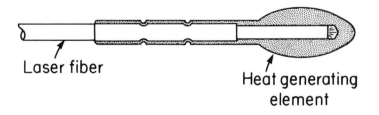

Laser fiber

Heat generating
element

Figure 22–8. The basic laser probe design. (From Topol, E.: Textbook of Interventional Cardiology, Philadelphia, W. B. Saunders, 1990.)

Figure 22–9. Quantronix series 1500 cw Nd:YAG laser system for delivering and coupling 1064-nm radiation to the laser balloon angioplasty catheter. Multiple safety mechanisms, including an automatic thermal shutoff device that terminates laser exposure in the event of fiberoptic fracture, are incorporated into the laser system, the function of which is computer controlled in a "user-friendly" manner. (From Topol, E.: Textbook of Interventional Cardiology, Philadelphia, W. B. Saunders, 1990.)

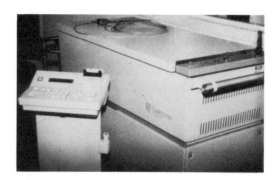

EXCISIONAL ATHERECTOMY

Excisional atherectomy includes directional atherectomy, extraction atherectomy, and percutaneous coronary rotational atherectomy. These procedures have a common objective—to remove the material that obstructs or occludes the vessel. These procedures use the techniques of introducing the catheter system that are used during balloon PTA. The differences lie in the type of removal system.

DIRECTIONAL CORONARY ATHERECTOMY. This type of system has a nonflexible cutting/collecting assembly at the distal portion of the catheter system (Fig. 22–12). The cutting assembly is offset on one side by a balloon. When the balloon is inflated,

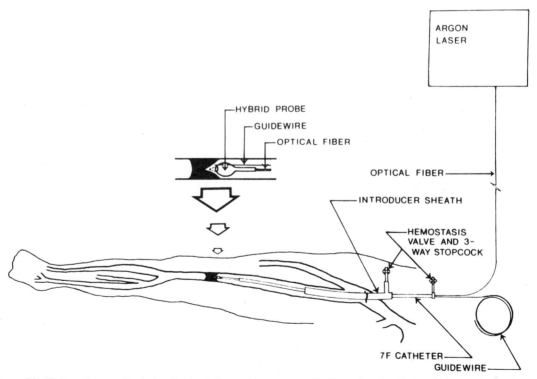

Figure 22–10. The diagram illustrates the technique of laser recanalization using the "hybrid" probe. The probe tip is shown in proximity to a lesion totally occluding the superficial femoral artery. The probe is extended from a 7F catheter that is inserted via a sheath in the common femoral artery. A guide wire is also passed alongside the probe. The 300-μm core optical fiber is connected to the probe from the 7F catheter to the argon laser system. A magnification of the contact site between the probe tip and the arterial occlusion shows the beam vaporizing a channel in the obstruction and widening the vascular lumen. (From Abela G. S., Seeger J. M., Pry R. S., et al.: Percutaneous laser recanalization of totally occluded human peripheral arteries: A technical approach. Dynamic Cardiovasc. Imag. *1*:302–308, 1988.)

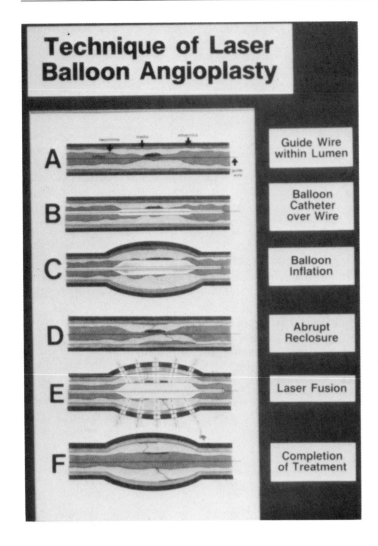

Technique of Laser Balloon Angioplasty

A — Guide Wire within Lumen

B — Balloon Catheter over Wire

C — Balloon Inflation

D — Abrupt Reclosure

E — Laser Fusion

F — Completion of Treatment

Figure 22–11. Schematic drawing of the treatment of acute closure *(D)* after percutaneous transluminal coronary angioplasty *(A to C)* with laser balloon angioplasty *(E)*. Thermal fusion of separated tissue layers, dehydration of thrombus, and reduction of arterial recoil with successful laser balloon angioplasty would result in a relatively wide, smooth, thrombus-free lumen. (From Topol, E.: Textbook of Interventional Cardiology, Philadelphia, W. B. Saunders, 1990.)

the open window of the cutting assembly is forced against the plaque. As this occurs, some of the plaque protrudes into the window of the cutting assembly. The cutter is then advanced by cutting away the material that protrudes into the device (Fig. 22–13). The tip of the assembly, or nose cone, is hollow to collect the material being cut away. The procedure is repeated after rotating the cutting assembly until a sufficient amount of plaque has been removed. Patency of the vessel is confirmed through angiography. Some of the drawbacks of this system are dissection, spasm, and subsequent thrombosis of the vessel resulting from the expansion of the balloon within its lumen.

EXTRACTION ATHERECTOMY. This technique uses a rotational cutting tip at the distal end of the catheter system. The cutting assembly is hollow. Suction is applied to the lumen of the cutter to remove the debris caused by the cutting action of the device (Fig. 22–14). This system is undergoing clinical trials, and its efficacy has not been determined.

PERCUTANEOUS CORONARY ROTATIONAL ANGIOPLASTY. With this procedure, the plaque is mechanically broken up into very small particles by a rotational burr attached to the distal tip of the catheter assembly (Fig. 22–15). The burr assembly is driven by air pressure and rotates at extremely high speeds. It is most effective in the treatment of calcified plaque, which is prone to fragmentation. The particles resulting from the procedure are extremely small and cannot obstruct the capillaries.

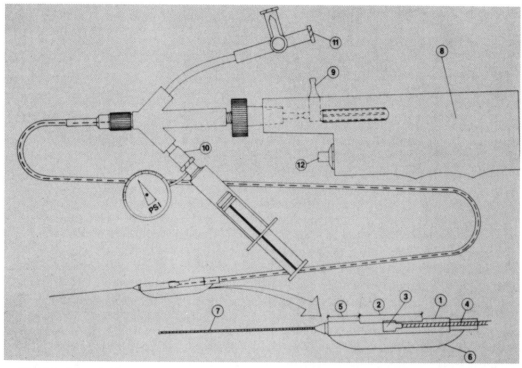

Figure 22–12. Peripheral atherectomy catheter system. The components of the catheter are the (1) cylindric housing, (2) longitudinal opening, (3) cutter, (4) cutter drive cable (to motor), (5) specimen collection area, (6) balloon support mechanism, (7) fixed guide wire, (8) motor, (9) cutter advance lever, (10) balloon inflation port, (11) flush port, and (12) on/off switch for motor. (From Simpson J. B., Selmon M. R., Robertson G. C., et al.: Transluminal atherectomy for peripheral vascular disease. Am. J. Cardiol. *61*:96G–101G, 1988, by permission.)

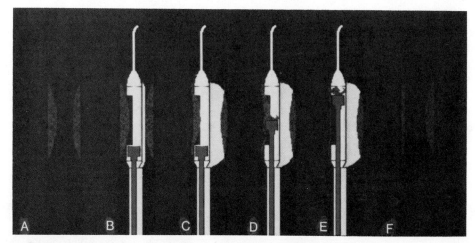

Figure 22–13. Diagram of the atherectomy procedure. *(A)* The lesion before atherectomy; *(B)* atherectomy catheter in position across the lesion; *(C)* the balloon support inflated; *(D)* the cutter advanced; *(E)* the specimen trapped in the housing; *(F)* the balloon deflated, and the catheter removed. (From Topol, E.: Textbook of Interventional Cardiology, Philadelphia, W. B. Saunders, 1990.)

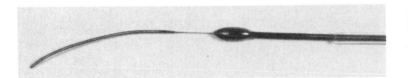

Figure 22–14. Distal part of the Rotablator with the abrasive tip. (From Topol, E.: Textbook of Interventional Cardiology, Philadelphia, W. B. Saunders, 1990.)

INTRAVASCULAR THROMBOLYSIS (FIBRINOLYSIS)

This procedure allows selective infusion of thrombolytic agents to dissolve a vessel obstruction. Use of this procedure was initially limited to the systemic application of thrombolytic agents. It was successful, but the high rate of hemorrhagic complications prevented its widespread use. The technique has recently been modified to provide selective and subselective applications of these substances (local thrombolysis), with a marked decrease in the rate of side effects. It is now primarily used to treat acute myocardial infarction and acute thrombotic occlusion of the peripheral vessels.

The substances available for use in intra-arterial thrombolysis include streptokinase, a nonenzymatic protein derived from β-hemolytic streptococci, and urokinase, which is derived from human kidney tissue cultures. There are differences between the two agents, but these differences do not affect the efficacy of either substance (Table 22–4). Another fibrolytic agent is under investigation—tissue-type plasminogen activator. Its advantage is that it functions only in the presence of fibrin, which limits its action to the area of the thrombus.[16]

The success of treatment is dependent on the age, size, and location of the lesion. Single-vessel clots that are less than 7 days old and located in vessels with a flow pattern that can provide good runoff of the thrombolytic agent are prime targets for this procedure. As the age of the thrombus approaches and exceeds 7 days, it becomes increasingly resistant to treatment by the thrombolytic agent. If the clot is too extensive, complete removal becomes more difficult, and the chance for successful treatment is diminished. In totally occluded vessels that provide no runoff, retrograde clot formation can occur along the path of the catheter.

The procedure involves selective administration of streptokinase at a rate of 5000 to 10,000 units/h for 6 h. At this time, an angiogram is done, and the dosage may be increased. Infusion continues, and the catheter is advanced according to individual requirements. The procedure can be continued for 72 to 96 h or until complete lysis of the clot has been accomplished. If no improvement is seen after 12 h, selective urokinase treatment may be initiated. If no improvement is detected after 24 h, the infusion may be terminated. Bleeding complications may occur that would also result in termination of the procedure.

The patient should be closely monitored for complications and improvement throughout the course of the infusion. Considering the length of the procedure, this is best accomplished in an intensive care unit.[14]

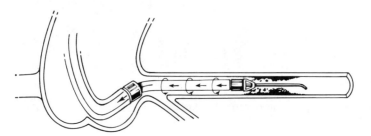

Figure 22–15. Illustration of a coronary artery showing the flexible steerable guide wire through the lesion with simultaneous excision and extraction of the plaque through the center of the TEC torque tube. (From Topol, E.: Textbook of Interventional Cardiology, Philadelphia, W. B. Saunders, 1990.)

Table 22–4. SUMMARY OF DIFFERENCES BETWEEN THROMBOLYTIC AGENTS

Streptokinase	Urokinase
Nonenzymatic	Enzymatic
Derived from β-hemolytic streptococci	Derived from human kidney tissue
Relatively inexpensive	Expensive
Cannot be used in patients with high antistreptococcal antibody titers	No use restriction

INFUSION OF VASODILATORS

Infusion of a vasodilator such as prostacyclin, reserpine, papaverine, prostaglandin E, or sodium nitroprusside is used primarily to treat vascular spasm or nonocclusive acute mesenteric ischemia, although it can be used to dilate stenotic vessels. However, most occlusive vascular problems are managed with one of the techniques previously discussed.

Complications

All of these procedures can have complications. Many reported problems associated with the percutaneous approach are those associated with the catheterization itself, such as flow disturbances, vessel occlusion, localized hemorrhage, and systemic embolization.

PTA presents the risks of vessel dissection or perforation, thrombotic occlusion, distal embolization caused by debris from the lesion, vessel spasm caused by the movements of the catheter, and guide wire and balloon rupture caused by overinflation.

In all of the procedures discussed, the principle of benefit versus risk is applicable. Patient selection is made with the possible hazards in mind, and patients should be closely monitored before, during, and after the study to minimize the risk of complications.

REMOVAL OF INTRAVASCULAR FOREIGN BODIES

In 1964, Thomas described a nonsurgical procedure for the removal of foreign bodies from intravascular locations.[17] Since then, various devices have been developed to remove foreign bodies from these sites. These materials arise from accidental loss or breakage of intravascular equipment such as guide wires or catheters. It is important to remove these from the vascular system before serious complications occur. Before Thomas's use of this technique, they had to be surgically removed.

Several types of devices have been developed, including helical loop basket sets, grasping devices, hook-shaped catheter and guide wire sets, snare loop catheter sets, and balloon-tip retrieval catheters. The helical loop basket catheters, such as the Dotter Intravascular Retriever Set, is used to snare foreign fragments and move them to peripheral vascular locations, where they are easily removed (Fig. 22–16).

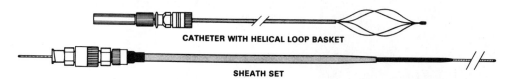

CATHETER WITH HELICAL LOOP BASKET

SHEATH SET

Figure 22–16. The Dotter Intravascular Retriever Set. (Courtesy of Cook Incorporated, Bloomington, IN.)

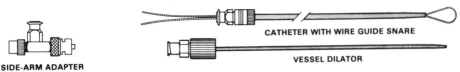

Figure 22–17. The Curry Intravascular Retriever Set. (Courtesy of Cook Incorporated, Bloomington, IN.)

Snare loop catheter sets, such as the Curry Intravascular Retriever Set, are used to retrieve lost catheters (Fig. 22–17). This is accomplished by catching a free end of the lost catheter in the snare loop and maneuvering it to a location from which it can be withdrawn from the vessel. In some cases, both ends of the lost device may be lodged in a vessel, and it is necessary to free one end before using the snare loop catheter. This can be accomplished with a hook-shaped catheter, which pulls one end of the catheter from the vessel.

Balloon-tip retrieval catheters pull fragments from locations when retrieval by one of the other methods is not possible. The balloon tip is passed beyond the fragment, inflated, and then carefully withdrawn under fluoroscopic supervision, moving the fragment along its path. When the foreign body is in a suitable location, one of the other devices is used for complete removal.

Grasping devices are not usually designed for intravascular use and present the risk of vessel trauma, but they can be used, if necessary, to remove fragments through arterial cutdown. These devices are only used when other methods are not successful. Figure 22–18 shows an example of one type of grasping device.

Complications arising from the use of this type of interventional procedure are very rare. The possibility of complications depends on the length of time the foreign body has been in place, the patient's disposition toward mechanical stimulation, and the ultimate location of the foreign body.

SUMMARY

Interventional radiography has proven to be a relatively safe and inexpensive method for treating various vascular problems. In many cases, it has obviated the necessity for complicated surgical procedures.

Vascular interventional radiography can be classified into procedures that either increase or decrease blood flow. Several mechanical devices have been developed that are used in conjunction with basic angiographic techniques to provide the desired therapeutic result.

This field is still in its infancy, and newer techniques and applications are being rapidly developed.

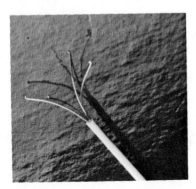

Figure 22–18. MPF 20/55 multipurpose forceps. (From Medi-tech div. of Boston Scientific Corporation.)

REFERENCES

1. Wallace, S.: Interventional radiology, Cancer *37*:517, 1976.
2. Dotter, C. T., and Judkins, M. P.: Transluminal treatment of arteriosclerotic obstruction: Description of a new technique and a preliminary report of its application, Circulation, *30*:654, 1964.
3. Zeitler, E., Gruntzig, A., and Schoop, W.: Percutaneous Vascular Recanalization: Technique, Application, Clinical Results. New York, Springer-Verlag, 1978.
4. Athanasoulis, C. A.: Therapeutic applications of angiography (first of two parts), N. Engl. J. Med., *302*:1117, 1980.
5. Debrun, G., et al.: Detachable balloon and calibrated-leak balloon techniques in the treatment of cerebral vascular lesions, J. Neurosurg., *49*:635, 1978.
6. Gianturco, C., Anderson, J. H., and Wallace, S.: Mechanical devices for arterial occlusion, Am. J. Radium Ther. Nucl. Med., *124*:428, 1975.
7. Gomes, A., et al.: The use of the bristle brush for transcatheter embolization, Radiology, *129*:345, 1978.
8. Mosso, J. A., and Rand, R. W.: Ferromagnetic silicon vascular occlusion: A technique for selective infarction of tumors and organs, Ann. Surg., *178*:663, 1973.
9. Ekelund, L., et al.: Occlusion of renal arterial tumor supply with absolute ethanol: Experience with 20 cases, Acta. Radiol. [Diagn.] (Stockh), *25*:195, 1984.
10. Freeny, P. C., et al.: Long-term radiographic-pathologic follow-up of patients treated with visceral transcatheter occlusion using isobutyl-2-cyanoacrylate (Bucrylate), Radiology, *132*:51, 1979.
11. Fisher, C. H., et al.: Effect of superior mesenteric artery vasopressin infusion on cardiac output and coronary blood flow in dogs, Invest. Radiol., *9*:496, 1974.
12. Fallon, J. T.: Pathology of arterial lesions amenable to percutaneous transluminal angioplasty, Am. J. Radiol., *135*:913, 1980.
13. Abele, J. E.: Balloon catheters and transluminal dilation: Technical considerations, Am. J. Radiol., *135*:901, 1980.
14. Murray, P. D., Garnic, J. D., and Bettmann, M. A.: Pharmacology of angioplasty and intravascular thrombolysis, Am. J. Radiol., *139*:795–803, 1982.
15. Spears, J. R.: Percutaneous transluminal coronary angioplasty restenosis: Potential prevention with laser balloon angioplasty, Am. J. Cardiol., *60*:61B–64B, 1987.
16. Collen, D.: On the regulation and control of fibrinolysis, Hemostasis, *43*:77–89, 1980.
17. Thomas, J., et al.: Nonsurgical retrieval of broken segments of steel spring guide from right atrium to superior vena cava, Circulation, *30*:106, 1964.

SUGGESTED READINGS

INTERVENTIONAL RADIOGRAPHY (GENERAL)

Athanasoulis, C. A.: Therapeutic applications of angiography (first and second parts), N. Engl. J. Med., *302*:1117, 1174, 1980.

VASCULAR OCCLUSION

Anderson, J. H., et al.: Mini-Gianturco stainless steel coils for transcatheter vascular occlusion, Radiology, *132*:301, 1979.
Barth, K. H., et al.: Metrizamide, the ideal radiopaque filling material for detachable silicone balloon embolization, Invest. Radiol., *14*:35, 1979.
Bentson, J., et al.: Unexpected complications following therapeutic embolizations, Neuroradiology, *16*:420, 1978.
Casteneda-Zuniga, W. R., Sanchez, R., and Amplatz, K.: Experimental observations on short- and long-term effects on arterial occlusion with Ivalon, Radiology, *126*:783, 1978.
Doppman, J. L., et al.: Transcatheter embolization with a silicone rubber preparation: Experimental observations, Invest. Radiol., *6*:304, 1971.
Dotter, C. T., et al.: Instant selective arterial occlusion with isobutyl-2-cyanoacrylate [work in progress], Radiology, *114*:227, 1975.

Goldman, M. L., et al.: Transcatheter vascular occlusion therapy with isobutyl-2-cyanoacrylate (Bucrylate) for control of massive upper gastrointestinal bleeding, Radiology, *129*:41, 1978.
Greenfield, A. J., et al.: Transcatheter embolization: Prevention of embolic reflux using balloon catheters, Am. J. Radiol., *131*:651, 1978.
Hilal, S. K., and Michelson, W. J.: Therapeutic percutaneous embolization for extra-axial vascular lesions of the head, neck and spine, J. Neurosurg., *43*:275, 1975.
Kerber, C. W.: Catheter therapy: Fluoroscopic monitoring of deliberate embolic occlusion, Radiology, *125*:538, 1977.
Laitinen, L., and Servo, A.: Embolization of cerebral vessels with inflatable and detachable balloons [technical note], J. Neurosurg., *48*:307, 1978.
Miller, M. D., et al., Clinical use of transcatheter electrocoagulation, Radiology, *129*:211, 1978.
Pevsner, P. H.: Micro-balloon catheter for superselective angiography and therapeutic occlusion, Am. J. Radiol., *128*:225, 1977.
Serbienko, F. A. L.: Balloon catheterization and occlusion of major cerebral vessels, J. Neurosurg., *41*:125, 1974.
White, R. I., et al.: Embolotherapy with detachable silicone balloons: Technique and clinical results, Radiology, *131*:619, 1979.

VASCULAR DILATION

Ahn, S. S., Auth, D. C., Marcus, D. R., and Moore, W. S.: Removal of focal atheromatous lesions by angioscopically guided high speed rotary atherectomy, J. Vasc. Surg., 7:292–299, 1988.

Athanasoulis, C. A.: Percutaneous transluminal angioplasty: General principles, Am. J. Radiol., 135:893, 1980.

Gruntzig, A., et al.: Percutaneous transluminal dilatation of arthrosclerotic renal artery stenosis, Circulation, 58:213, 1978.

Gruntzig, A., and Kumpl, D. A.: Technique of percutaneous transluminal angioplasty with the Gruntzig balloon catheter, Am. J. Radiol, 132:547, 1979.

Katzen, B., et al.: Percutaneous transluminal angioplasty for treatment of renovascular hypertension, Radiology, 131:53, 1979.

Stack, R. S., et al.: Treatment of peripheral vascular disease with the transluminal extraction catheter: Results of a multicenter study, J. Am. Coll. Cardiol., 13:227A, 1989.

Stertzer, S. H.: Brachial approach to transluminal coronary angioplasty, In Angioplasty. New York, McGraw-Hill, 1986, p. 260–294.

Tegtmeyer, C. J., et al.: Percutaneous transluminal dilatation of the renal arteries, Radiology, 135:589, 1980.

Topol, E. J.: Emerging strategies for failed percutaneous transluminal coronary angioplasty, Am. J. Cardiol., 63:249–250, 1989.

Turina, M., et al.: Percutaneous transluminal dilatation of coronary artery stenosis, Thorac. Cardiovasc. Surg., 27:199, 1979.

Wholey, M. H.: Advances in balloon technology and reperfusion devices for peripheral circulation, Am. J. Cardiol, 61:87G–95G, 1988.

Wholey, M. H.: The technology of balloon catheters in interventional angiography, Radiology, 125:671, 1977.

INTRAVASCULAR INFUSION

Athanasoulis, C. A., et al.: Mesenteric arterial infusion of vasopressin for hemorrhage from colonic diverticulosis, Am. J. Surg., 129:212, 1975.

Baum, S.: Angiographic management of postoperative bleeding, Radiology, 113:37, 1974.

Baum, S., and Nusbaum, M.: Control of gastrointestinal hemorrhage by selective mesenteric arterial infusion of vasopressin, Radiology, 98:487, 1971.

Baum, S., et al.: Selective mesenteric arterial infusions in the management of massive diverticular hemorrhage, N. Engl. J. Med., 288:1269, 1973.

Chuang, V. P., et al.: Alterations in gastric physiology caused by selective embolization and vasopressin infusion of the left gastric artery, Radiology, 120:533, 1976.

Conn, H. O., et al.: Selective intra-arterial vasopressin in the treatment of upper gastrointestinal hemorrhage, Gastroenterology, 63:634, 1972.

Davis, G. A., et al.: Advantage of intra-arterial over intravenous vasopressin infusion in gastrointestinal hemorrhage, Am. J. Radiol., 128:733, 1977.

Davis, G. B., et al.: The relative effects of selective intraarterial and intravenous vasopressin infusion, Radiology, 120:537, 1976.

Dorricott, N. J., et al.: Effect of intra-arterial vasopressin on canine gastric mucosal permeability, Gastroenterology, 65:625, 1973.

Johnson, W. C., and Widrich, W. C.: Efficacy of selective splanchnic arteriography and vasopressin perfusion in diagnosis and treatment of gastrointestinal hemorrhage, Am. J. Surg., 131:481, 1976.

Kadir, S., and Athanasoulis, C. A.: Catheter dislodgement: A cause of failure of intra-arterial vasopressin infusions to control gastrointestinal bleeding, Cardiovasc. Radiol., 1:187, 1978.

Rosch, J., et al.: Selective vasoconstrictor infusion in the management of arteriocapillary gastrointestinal hemorrhage, Am. J. Radiol., 116:279, 1972.

Rosch, J., et al.: Selective arterial infusion of vasoconstrictors in acute gastrointestinal bleeding, Radiology, 99:27, 1971.

Sherman, L. M., et al.: Selective intra-arterial vasopressin: Clinical efficacy and complications, Ann. Surg., 189:298, 1979.

Steckel, R. J., et al.: New developments in pharmacoangiography (and arterial pharmacotherapy) of the gastrointestinal tract, Invest. Radiol., 6:199, 1971.

White, R. I., et al.: Pharmacologic control of hemorrhagic gastritis: Clinical and experimental results, Radiology, 111:549, 1974.

twenty-three

Nonvascular Interventional Procedures

NEEDLE BIOPSY
Indications and Contraindications
Guidance Methods
    Ultrasonography
    Computed Tomography
PUNCTURE AND DRAINAGE METHODS
Percutaneous Puncture
    Procedure
    Complications
Percutaneous Drainage
    Procedure for Percutaneous
        Catheter Nephrostomy

Complications of Percutaneous
    Catheter Nephrostomy
PERCUTANEOUS CALCULI REMOVAL
Renal Calculi Removal
Postoperative Biliary Calculi Removal
    Procedure
    Complications
Nonoperative Percutaneous Biliary
    Calculi Removal
    Procedure
    Complications
Extracorporeal Shock Wave Lithotripsy

Nonvascular interventional radiography encompasses a wide range of procedures, and a discussion of all of them is beyond the scope of this text. However, some major areas—notably, percutaneous needle biopsy, puncture and drainage procedures, and percutaneous removal of calculi—require a brief discussion.

NEEDLE BIOPSY

Indications and Contraindications

Needle biopsy is performed for diagnostic purposes in many areas of the body, including the thyroid; intracranial and intraorbital structures; spinal cord; lungs; abdomen; abscessed regions; genitourinary, lymphatic, and biliary systems; soft tissues; and bone. Each technique varies with the anatomy involved and information desired. The specific needles used also vary with the type of anatomic structure being biopsied, as well as with the type of procedure being performed. Two basic methods of biopsy are used—these are classified by the type of needle used to do the biopsy. Specimens are obtained with the large-gauge core-type needle method or the percutaneous fine needle aspiration approach.

With the large-gauge core needle method, a "plug" of tissue is cut for analysis. Its advantage is that it produces a larger specimen for analysis, but use of this method also entails a greater risk of complications than does the use of the fine needle technique. Because of the anatomy, as for bone biopsy, for example, or the type of specimen required, certain procedures or conditions require the use of the cutting or core biopsy method. Histological analysis or study of the tissue structure requires the large-gauge core technique. Specimens for cytologic analysis or the study of tissue cells can be collected with the fine needle aspiration method.

If complications resulting from needle biopsies occur, they are usually nonfatal and cause no permanent damage. Use of computed tomography (CT) or ultrasonic guidance reduces the complication rate if all necessary precautions are taken. Some possible complications are infection, bleeding, formation of fistulas, and tumor seeding. It should be remembered that the percutaneous biopsy procedure replaces surgical biopsy, which has considerably higher complication and mortality rates.

Guidance Methods

To successfully localize the lesion, the procedure must be guided. This guidance is accomplished with ultrasonography, CT, conventional fluoroscopy, and/or magnetic resonance imaging. These modalities are used alone or in combination to provide the maximum diagnostic information about the components of the lesion. Each of the modalities has advantages and disadvantages. The choice of method depends on the physician's preference, equipment availability, and hospital protocol. Table 23–1 is a summary of the types of modalities and some of the anatomic areas where they have been used.

Most needle biopsies require ultrasound or CT to guide the biopsy needles precisely. These techniques pinpoint the lesion's location and allow a high degree of accuracy in sampling. The two guidance methods achieve the same results, but there are some basic differences between them. The use of ultrasound to guide the needle is both more cost-effective and safer for the patient than CT. Ultrasonographic equipment is considerably more economical to purchase and install. This method eliminates the need for exposure

Table 23–1. SUMMARY OF GUIDANCE METHODS USED FOR INTERVENTIONAL RADIOGRAPHIC BIOPSY PROCEDURES

Guidance Method	Anatomic Area
Ultrasonography	Lymph nodes Breast Abdominal viscera Liver Extremities Intrathoracic lesions Vertebral column
Computed tomography	Lymph nodes Brain lesions Abdominal viscera Kidneys Bone lesions Mediastinal masses Breast
Conventional fluoroscopy	Lymph nodes Lung Kidney Mediastinal masses
Magnetic resonance imaging	Brain lesions Bone lesions Breast

to radiation during the localization phase of the procedure. Equipment design also permits faster lesion location and puncture. Specialized puncturing transducers are available that accurately guides the puncture needle. In addition, the use of real-time ultrasonographic equipment permits visual guidance of the needle.

Although the use of ultrasound appears to be the best method of needle guidance, there are situations in which the use of ultrasonography is contraindicated or impossible. Indications for using CT for guided needle biopsy include the following:

1. Extremely obese patients
2. Presence of overlying gas
3. Presence of overlying bone
4. Skin pathology that precludes transducer contact
5. Pathology that contraindicates skin compression
6. Necessity for three-dimensional resolution
7. Unsuccessful ultrasonography guidance

One disadvantage to the use of CT as the guidance method is that the length of the procedure is usually extended. CT requires several manipulations of the needle, especially for small lesions. The specific organ to be biopsied also governs the choice of guidance method.

Magnetic resonance imaging guidance methods have not been widely used clinically and is still undergoing evaluation.[1]

ULTRASONOGRAPHY

Ultrasonic guidance is performed with either the static or the dynamic scanning technique. Static scanning is the older of the two methods. The target lesion is initially located and referenced with two planes perpendicular to each other. The puncture route should always be the shortest distance possible. The scan continues by manipulating the transducer to show on the television monitor the ultrasonic beam running along the chosen puncture path. At this point, the skin surface is marked, the patient is prepped for the puncture procedure, and the physician introduces a local anesthetic. The scan is repeated using a special puncture transducer, which has a central canal that accepts the puncture needle. The central canal allows the needle to follow the direction of the ultrasonic beam. These types of transducers accept several different needle sizes with the use of special adapters. The distance from the skin surface to the lesion is measured from the image on the television monitor. The needle stop is then set for the scan depth plus the length of the transducer. When this is done, the puncture can proceed.[2]

Dynamic scanning has been made possible with the use of real-time ultrasonic scanners. These units show the movement as it is occurring, which increases the accuracy of the puncture considerably because moving target lesions can be continuously monitored during puncture. Small changes in direction or distance can be compensated for with direct visual control of the needle. The basic procedures for lesion location and needle introduction are the same as those for static scanning. Equipment designs for dynamic scanners will have variations, usually in the type of transducer used for the scan.

COMPUTED TOMOGRAPHY

When the use of ultrasonography is contraindicated, CT may be used for localization and needle guidance for lesion puncture. As in ultrasonography, the same basic rule applies to needle puncture with CT assistance, that is, the route chosen should be as short as possible. This pathway is marked on the skin during a preliminary CT scan.

The patient is prepped for the puncture by sterilizing and draping the skin, the local anesthetic is applied, and the needle is inserted along the predetermined pathway to the desired depth. The patient is then rescanned to determine whether the needle has been accurately inserted into the lesion. There are several different methods of needle insertion; the ultimate choice of insertion technique is made by the radiographer performing the procedure.

Once the needle has been successfully placed in the lesion, material may be removed for cytologic analysis. The aspiration technique is the most frequently used biopsy method. This is done by attaching an empty syringe to the needle hub and withdrawing the plunger. A small sample of tissue or fluid is then aspirated into the needle and prepared for cytologic diagnosis.

The same method can be used to facilitate needle placement for cyst and abscess drainage. These studies are usually performed with minor modifications in the equipment and techniques used.

PUNCTURE AND DRAINAGE METHODS

This group of procedures includes the percutaneous needle puncture technique for diagnosis of cystic masses and the percutaneous drainage of fluid accumulations. These have proven to be safe procedures, with relatively low complication rates. The following outline summarizes the types of puncture and drainage procedures currently being performed:

Genitourinary system
  Percutaneous nephrostomy techniques
    Catheter inserted through needles
    Catheter-sheathed needle
    Angiographic system
    Trocar-cannula-catheter system
  Percutaneous catheter drainage of renal and extrarenal fluid collections
  Cyst puncture
  Fluid drainage procedures
Biliary system
  Periductal fluid drainage procedures
    T tube or Penrose drain access
    Percutaneous puncture, dilation, and drainage
  Biliary system drainage
    Percutaneous transhepatic biliary drainage after fine needle transhepatic cholangiography
    Percutaneous choledochoplasty
Abdomen
  Percutaneous abscess drainage techniques
    Angiocatheter system
    Trocar-catheter system
Pelvis
  Percutaneous drainage techniques
    Transvectal approach
    Transperineal approach
    Transsciatic notch approach
Thorax
  Percutaneous fluid drainage techniques
    Trocar method
    Angiocatheter method

Percutaneous Puncture

The percutaneous puncture of identified renal masses is an example of this type of procedure. After the mass has been localized, it must be determined whether it is a cyst or tumor. Several methods of diagnosing the mass are available, including ultrasonography, nephrotomography, arteriography, and needle puncture. Percutaneous needle puncture procedures provide samples of aspirate for cytologic analysis and can help demonstrate the mass radiographically by using a contrast agent. If the mass is shown to be solid when punctured, arteriography is then used to demonstrate it successfully for diagnosis.

PROCEDURE

The percutaneous puncture method is relatively simple and does not require much sophisticated equipment for successful lesion puncture. Ultrasonographic guidance can be used to precisely guide the needle to the mass. The localization requires the use of a special transducer (discussed above). It also necessitates fluoroscopy to demonstrate the mass radiographically.

The setup for a percutaneous puncture examination includes an assortment of syringes, anesthesia and puncture needles, contrast agent, and anesthetic. The actual puncture setup varies slightly with the anatomic area of interest and the puncture method used. A typical equipment grouping for a renal cyst puncture is shown in Figure 23–1. The percutaneous puncture technique is considered a minor operative procedure and should be carried out under aseptic conditions. Preparation of the patient also varies with the location of the lesion.

Renal cyst puncture requires the patient to be in the prone position for preparation and puncture. The lesion is then localized with either fluoroscopy or ultrasonography. If ultrasound is used, the needle follows the path presented by the special puncture transducer. This method shortens the actual procedure time. When fluoroscopy is used, the lesion is first localized and marked, and the needle insertion is then tracked as it is being inserted into the lesion. Once the lesion has been localized by the physician, the puncture needle is inserted through the segment of anesthetized tissue parallel to the path of the x-ray beam. In this method, the needle is advanced slowly with fluoroscopic monitoring of the needle's progress after each advancement. Successful puncture is confirmed by the aspiration of cystic fluid.

Once the cyst has been entered, cytologic analysis of the aspirated fluid and radiographic examination of the interior of the cyst are performed. The contrast agent used for the internal examination of the cyst can be any of the water-soluble preparations. Figure 23–2 shows a cyst after radiographic localization by CT and after the cyst has been punctured and opacified.

Cytologic analysis is essential in the determination of the nature of the cyst. When the diagnostic portion of the examination has been completed, interventional treatment of the cyst can be initiated. In most cases, the cystic fluid is aspirated, and some type of sclerosing agent is then injected. Figure 23–3 shows the cyst pictured in Figure 23–2 after partial evacuation of the cystic fluid.

COMPLICATIONS

Percutaneous puncture procedures do not entail a great risk to the patient. Complications usually occur as a result of the needle insertion procedure—for example, a needle might pass through the wall of the kidney and cause hemorrhaging. Another possible complication is extravasation of the contrast agent when a thin-walled cyst is encountered.

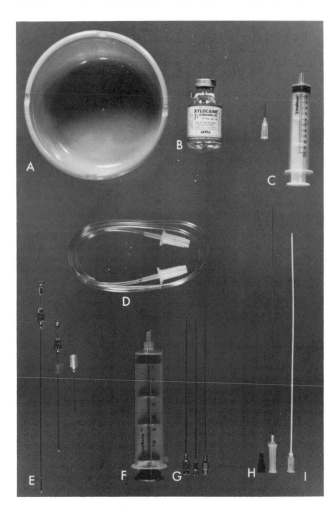

Figure 23–1. Typical grouping of equipment for renal mass puncture. (A) Bowl for contrast material; (B) local anesthetic agent; (C) syringe and 25-gauge needle for skin anesthesia; (D) extension tube; (E) 22-gauge needles for deeper anesthesia and puncture; (F) 35-ml syringe for aspirating and opacifying large cysts; (G) Cuatico needle with side holes; (H) trocar-sleeve assembly; (I) standard 20-gauge and Teflon-sheathed needles. (From Athanasoulis, C. A., et al.: Interventional Radiology, W. B. Saunders, 1982, p. 411.)

Percutaneous Drainage

The drainage of fluid collections—abscesses in the urinary system, biliary system, and abdominal cavity—can be done with the percutaneous catheter drainage method. The use of this technique also enables physicians to dilate stenotic channels, occlude areas of leakage, close off fistulas, infuse substances to dissolve or remove calculi, and perform biopsies. The obvious advantage of this technique is that fewer surgical procedures must be performed to achieve these results. Other benefits to the patient are reduced hospital costs and a reduced complication rate.

A representative method is percutaneous catheter nephrostomy (PCN), which provides for diversion of the renal output. It relies on the placement of a catheter within the kidney by percutaneous insertion. There are four techniques that can be used for the introduction of the catheter; the most popular involves the trocar-cannula unit. This system allows a catheter of relatively large diameter to be passed into the kidney. Once the trocar has been inserted, various procedures can be performed. The following outline is a summary of the applications of PCN[3]:

Drainage
   Generalized obstruction (external drainage)
   Selected obstruction (internal release)
   Leaks and fistulas

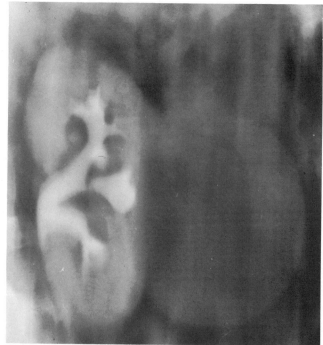

Figure 23–2. *(A)* Cyst localization by CT; *(B)* contrast-filled renal cyst after percutaneous puncture. (From Athanasoulis, C. A., et al.: Interventional Radiology, Philadelphia, W. B. Saunders, 1982, p. 417.)

A

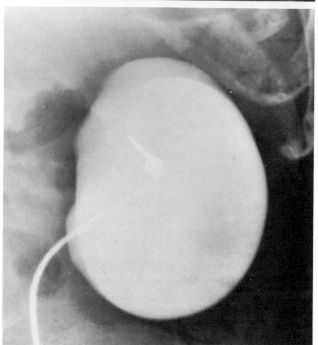

B

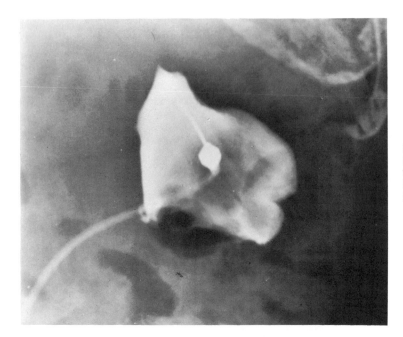

Figure 23–3. Renal cyst partially aspirated, showing collapsed cyst wall. (From Athanasoulis, C. A., et al.: Interventional Radiology, Philadelphia, W. B. Saunders, 1982, p. 417.)

Renal-perirenal fluid collections
   Infected cyst
   Abscess
   Urinoma
   Seroma
   Lymphocele
Drug instillation
   Treatment of bacteria with antibiotics
   Treatment of fungi with antifungal agents
   Chemical dissolution of calculi
   Chemotherapy
Special instrument insertion
   Steerable basket catheters
   Steerable biopsy brushes
   Nephroscope insertion
   Dilating balloon catheters

PROCEDURE FOR PERCUTANEOUS CATHETER NEPHROSTOMY

PCN patients are mildly sedated and well hydrated before beginning the procedure. After the patient is prepared and draped, the kidney is localized by using either intravenously injected contrast agents followed by fluoroscopic localization or ultrasonography or CT. Once the position of the kidney has been determined, a local anesthetic is administered, and the kidney is punctured with a 22-gauge spinal needle (Fig. 23–4). The puncture is done in a manner similar to that used for previously discussed studies—that is, it normally parallels the x-ray beam. When the needle punctures the kidney and enters the collecting system, it can be attached to a flexible connecter tube. Manometric measurements can be made and urine samples taken for analysis.

After these preliminary steps have been completed, an antegrade pyelogram is obtained. This is necessary to determine if a PCN is necessary. It is important to instill an amount of contrast agent equal only to the amount of urine that has been aspirated to avoid the possibility of trauma to the urinary system if an obstruction exists. Radiography during this phase is directed by the radiographer performing the procedure. If the antegrade pyelogram indicates the necessity for PCN, the physician chooses the catheter size as determined from the information obtained with the antegrade pyelogram—usually an 8F or 12F Silastic catheter that is either soft or stiff. The trocar-cannula unit chosen matches the catheter size (Fig. 23–5).

The trocar-cannula unit is inserted somewhat laterally to the previously inserted 22-gauge spinal needle (Fig. 23–6). This is accomplished by making a small nick in the skin (approximately 2 cm deep) with a scalpel. The trocar-cannula unit is then inserted under fluoroscopic monitoring until the kidney is punctured. When the trocar is removed, the appropriate catheter is inserted into the kidney through the cannula (Fig. 23–7). After the catheter position is confirmed, the cannula is removed over the catheter and secured to the skin to prevent accidental removal from the kidney. If other procedures are to be performed, they are done before removal of the cannula. Other therapeutic procedures that can be performed after trocar-cannula puncture of the kidney are shown in Figures 23–8, 23–9, 23–10, and 23–11.

When the catheter has been firmly attached, it is prepared to accept a stopcock assembly and drainage bag. At this time, follow-up radiography can be performed, or decompression treatment can be initiated.

COMPLICATIONS OF PERCUTANEOUS CATHETER NEPHROSTOMY

The complication rate from PCN is relatively low. Possible complications include infections, catheter dislodgement, catheter obstruction, and hemorrhage.

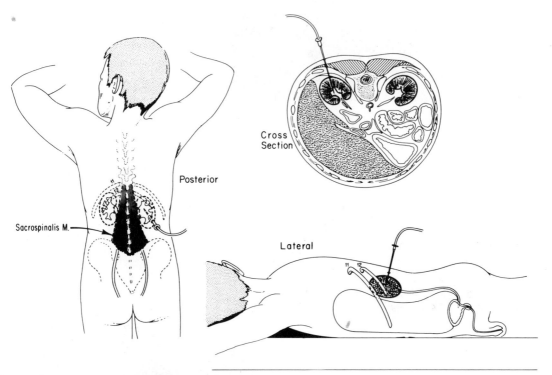

Cross
Section

Posterior

Sacrospinalis M.

Lateral

Figure 23–4. Schematic of anatomy of percutaneous puncture. (From Athanasoulis, C. A., et al.: Interventional Radiology, Philadelphia, W. B. Saunders, 1982, p. 438.)

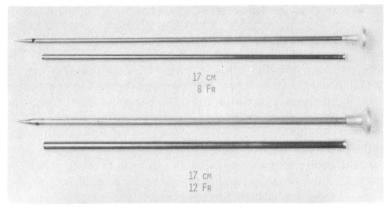

A

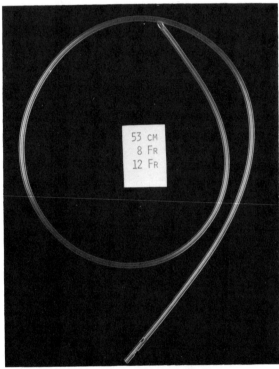

B

Figure 23–5. *(A)* Trocar with cannula units for percutaneous puncture; *(B)* soft flexible silicone catheter used for percutaneous nephrostomy. (From Athanasoulis, C. A., et al.: Interventional Radiology, Philadelphia, W. B. Saunders, 1982, pp. 469, 470.)

Figure 23–6. Schematic of the relation between the fine puncture needle and the trocar-cannula unit. (From Athanasoulis, C. A., et al.: Interventional Radiology, Philadelphia, W. B. Saunders, 1982, p. 476.)

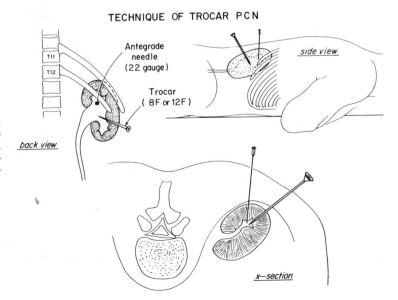

TECHNIQUE OF TROCAR PCN

Antegrade needle (22 gauge)

Trocar (8F or 12F)

side view

back view

x—section

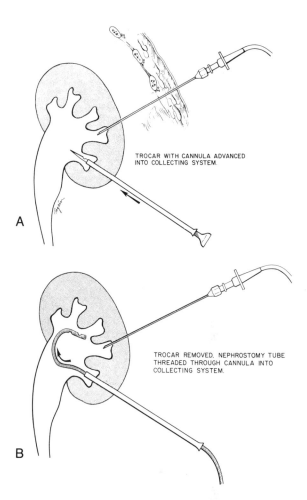

Figure 23–7. Schematic of the kidney, showing trocar-cannula unit placement *(A)* and catheter placement *(B)*. (From Newhouse, J. H., and Pfister, R. C.: Percutaneous catheterization of the kidney and perirenal space. Trocar Technique Urol. Radiol., *2:*157, 1981.)

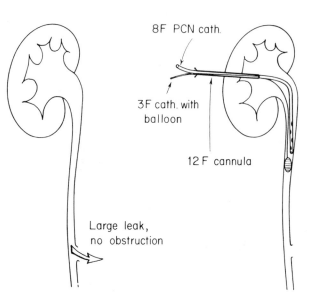

Figure 23–8. Mechanism for diverting the urine in case of a leak in the ureter, using a balloon catheter and an external drainage catheter. (From Athanasoulis, C. A., et al.: Interventional Radiology, Philadelphia, W. B. Saunders, 1982, p. 481.)

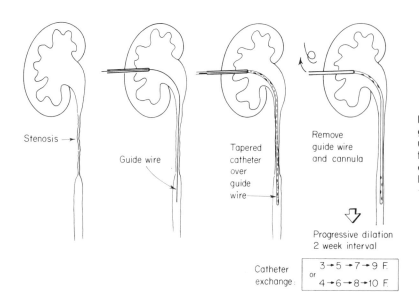

Stenosis →

Guide wire

Tapered catheter over guide wire

Remove guide wire and cannula

Figure 23–9. Mechanism for progressive dilation of a stenosed ureter using graduated catheters. (From Athanasoulis, C. A., et al.: Interventional Radiology, Philadelphia, W. B. Saunders, 1982, p. 483.)

Progressive dilation 2 week interval

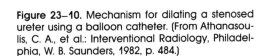

Catheter exchange:

3→5→7→9 F.
or
4→6→8→10 F.

Figure 23–10. Mechanism for dilating a stenosed ureter using a balloon catheter. (From Athanasoulis, C. A., et al.: Interventional Radiology, Philadelphia, W. B. Saunders, 1982, p. 484.)

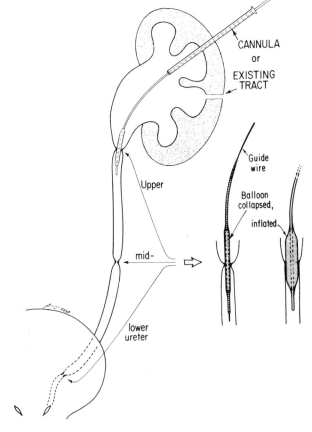

CANNULA
or
EXISTING TRACT

Upper

Guide wire

Balloon collapsed,

inflated

mid-

lower ureter

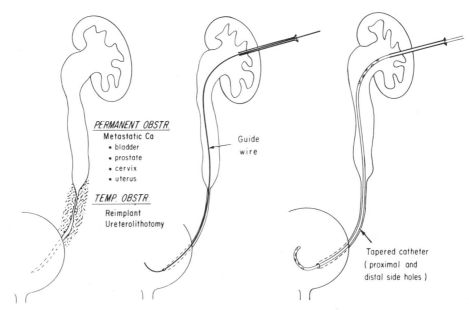

Figure 23–11. Mechanism for stent placement through the trocar-cannula unit in an obstructed or leaky ureter. (From Pfister, R. C., et al.: Percutaneous radiological procedures. Semin. Roentgen., *16*:135, 1981.)

PERCUTANEOUS CALCULI REMOVAL

Residual calculi can be removed percutaneously from either the genitourinary or biliary system, usually after an initial operative procedure. The risks associated with percutaneous calculi removal are minimal compared with those of surgery, and the procedure is usually performed on an outpatient basis.

Renal Calculi Removal

Renal calculi can be removed percutaneously from the renal pelvis, calyx, or ureter with the procedure described above for PCN. Once the percutaneous nephrostomy cannula is positioned, a steerable catheter system with a stone basket can be introduced into the kidney. Many variations of this system are available, and the ultimate choice remains with the radiographer. The catheter with a stone basket is inserted through the cannula and positioned close to the calculus. The stone basket is then advanced in a fully opened position and maneuvered to engage the calculus. The basket is retracted until it contacts the catheter tip, which has the effect of closing the basket over the calculus (Fig. 23–12). Both the catheter and the stone basket are then removed together through the cannula. When all of the calculi are removed, a nephrostomy catheter is placed into the kidney and secured in place. Several days after stone removal, radiographs should be taken, with contrast agent, to determine the patency of the urinary tract and the presence or absence of calculi.

Calculi can be removed from the biliary tree either after surgery through a T-tube or percutaneously after transhepatic biliary drainage. Both methods require the use of a steerable catheter system with a stone basket catheter insert. Percutaneous transhepatic biliary calculi removal is usually performed on patients who are poor candidates for surgery.

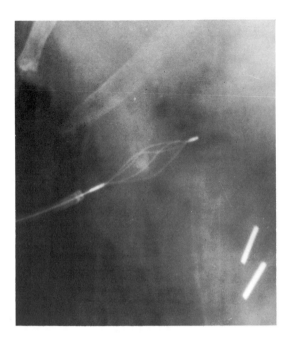

Figure 23–12. Radiograph of a renal calculus caught in a stone basket and ready for removal through the trocar-cannula unit. (From Athanasoulis, C. A., et al.: Interventional Radiology, Philadelphia, W. B. Saunders, 1982, p. 513.)

Postoperative Biliary Calculi Removal

This procedure is performed from 4 to 6 weeks after surgery to allow biliary T-tube tract preparation. Medication is limited to minor doses of drugs to relieve anxiety, such as diazepam, and to an antibiotic regimen to reduce the possibility of infection.

The equipment necessary for this type of study is minimal: a steerable catheter system, stone baskets, syringe, guide wire, and suitable contrast agent. Figure 23–13 shows some basic equipment used during postoperative biliary calculi removal.

PROCEDURE

The procedure begins with a T-tube cholangiogram to determine the location and number of calculi present, as well as to provide the necessary contrast during the procedure (Fig. 23–14A). On completion of the cholangiogram, a guide wire is inserted through the T tube, the T tube is removed, and the guide wire is left in the biliary tract at the lower end of the duct (Fig. 23–14B). The steerable catheter is inserted over the guide wire and positioned close to the calculus to be removed, and the guide wire is removed (Fig. 23–14C). The stone basket is then advanced to the tip of the catheter (Fig. 23–14D). Several positioning methods can be used to ensnare the calculus in the stone basket (Fig. 23–14E and F). The steerable catheter and stone basket are removed, extracting the calculus (Fig. 23–14G).

When multiple calculi are encountered, the steerable catheter must be reinserted and manipulated to remove subsequent stones. In such cases, the radiographer may insert multiple guide wires into the biliary tract through the T tube, which makes reinsertion of the steerable catheter and stone basket easier to accomplish. Occasionally, a small stone in the lower duct can be maneuvered into the duodenum with a Fogarty balloon catheter.

In uncomplicated single calculus removal, the catheter is removed after a repeat cholangiogram. However, in cases of multiple stone removal or if a complication arises, the catheter should be left in the tract to facilitate drainage until a follow-up study is performed.

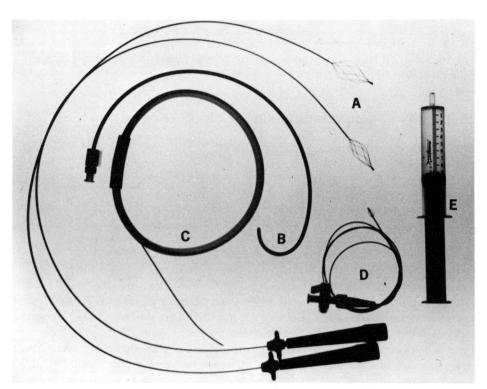

Figure 23–13. Basic equipment for percutaneous biliary calculi removal. (A) 11-mm and 15-mm stone baskets; (B) curved distal tip catheter; (C) guide wire and holder; (D) Fogarty balloon catheter; (E) syringe. (From Athanasoulis, C. A., et al.: Interventional Radiology, Philadelphia, W. B. Saunders, 1982, p. 525.)

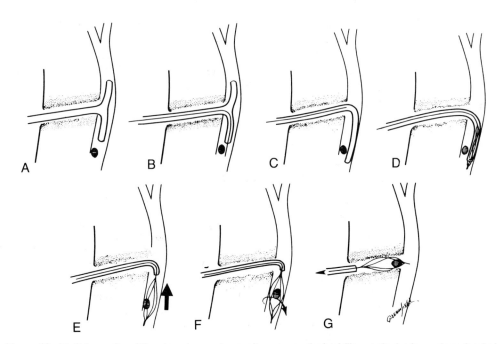

Figure 23–14. Schematic of the stepwise postoperative removal of a biliary calculus by a stone basket. (From Athanasoulis, C. A., et al.: Interventional Radiology, Philadelphia, W. B. Saunders, 1982, p. 526.)

COMPLICATIONS

The risks associated with postoperative biliary calculi removal are minimal. Most problems occur because of improper catheter advancement that results in hemorrhage, periductal leaks, duct perforations, or pancreatitis.

Nonoperative Percutaneous Biliary Calculi Removal

The method of percutaneous biliary calculi removal was developed as a modification of percutaneous transhepatic cholangiography. With angiographic methodology, catheter introduction into the biliary tree became possible. One risk of this procedure is the possibility of peritonitis as a result of the puncture; thus, a prerequisite to its use is antibiotic treatment initiated at least 1 day before the procedure and continued for 2 to 3 days after the puncture. Another means of reducing the incidence of peritonitis is by using a catheter-sheathed needle.

PROCEDURE

When the patient has been prepared, the biliary tract must be opacified by using the fine needle transhepatic cholangiography technique. This procedure involves the percutaneous puncture of the lining with a small-gauge needle. When puncture of the lining has been confirmed, a contrast agent is injected to provide the necessary contrast for visualization of the biliary tree. Percutaneous biliary catheterization can then be done using the opacified biliary tract and fine needle system as reference points. The catheter-sheathed needle is guided by direct radiography or fluoroscopy. When the catheter-needle system has entered the biliary tract, the needle is removed, and a syringe is attached to the catheter sheath. The catheter is manipulated until bile is aspirated, and a small amount of contrast agent is injected to confirm successful intubation. The catheter is then positioned close to the hilum of the lining, and the bile is drained. Figure 23–15 shows the puncture of the lining, followed by guide wire and catheter insertion.

The removal of biliary calculi is usually done several days after the initial intubation to provide adequate drainage for patient stabilization. When this has been determined, the biliary calculi are then removed. The originally placed catheter is exchanged for a nontapered variety, and two guide wires are inserted into the biliary tree. The catheter is removed, and a steerable catheter-stone basket system is introduced over one guide wire. The calculus is removed as described above (see "Postoperative Biliary Calculi

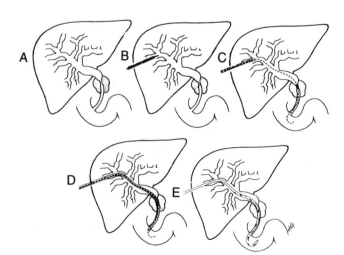

Figure 23–15. Schematic of the percutaneous transhepatic puncture procedure. (a) Obstructed biliary tract; (b) catheter-sheathed needle insertion; (c) needle removed and guide wire inserted through sheath; (d) sheath removed and dilation catheter inserted; (e) dilation catheter replaced by drainage catheter with curved tip. (From Athanasoulis, C. A., et al.: Interventional Radiology, Philadelphia, W. B. Saunders, 1982, p. 536.)

Removal"). Another drainage catheter can then be inserted over the second guide wire, if necessary.

The basic procedure for percutaneous transhepatic biliary drainage allows other interventional procedures to be performed on the biliary tract, including percutaneous transhepatic biliary drainage, fine needle transhepatic cholangiography, percutaneous transhepatic biopsy, percutaneous transhepatic stone extraction, percutaneous transhepatic choledochoplasty, and percutaneous transhepatic stent insertion.

COMPLICATIONS

Percutaneous transhepatic biliary calculi removal, in addition to complications similar to those of postoperative biliary calculi removal (see above), has the added risk of infection caused by the insertion and removal of needles, guide wires, and catheters. Most of these problems can be successfully treated with antibiotic therapy and usually have no long-term effects.

Extracorporeal Shock Wave Lithotripsy

Extracorporeal shock wave lithotripsy is a noninvasive method that is used therapeutically for both urolithiasis and cholelithiasis. Extracorporeal shock wave lithotripsy has been applied to the fragmentation of uroliths since 1980. It has become the method of choice for treatment of most upper tract urinary stones. Recently, the technique has been investigated in the treatment of patients with biliary calculi. It has also been shown to be cytotoxic to certain forms of tumors.[4]

Extracorporeal shock wave lithotripsy is based on the use of high-energy shock waves to fragment the stones without causing significant damage to the normal surrounding structures. The shock waves can be generated by electromagnetic, mechanical, or piezoelectric techniques. The smaller fragments resulting from the procedure can be dissolved by orally administered drugs, can be removed mechanically, or can be passed from the organ physiologically.

Specialized equipment is necessary for performance of the procedure. The equipment is manufactured by several companies, and the designs vary with the method used to produce the shock waves. Depending on the design, the patient is immersed in a water bath (first-generation) or placed in intimate contact with some sort of flexible water-containing device (second-generation), which provides the path for the shock waves to reach the site of pathology. It has evolved into a relatively safe procedure that can be performed on an outpatient basis without the use of anesthesia.

SUMMARY

Nonvascular interventional radiography has advanced to provide a broad spectrum of diagnostic as well as therapeutic procedures. These methods have proven to be more cost-effective than their corresponding surgical interventional procedures, with a considerably lower risk factor.

The use of ultrasonography and CT as guidance systems has allowed more precise percutaneous studies to be done, with lower complication rates. Fluoroscopic guidance is also used to a great extent as a guidance mechanism for cannula insertion.

Percutaneous needle biopsy can be performed in almost all areas of the body and is a safe and efficient means of acquiring samples for pathological study. This is also true for percutaneous puncture and drainage techniques, which have the added benefit of playing both diagnostic and therapeutic roles. The techniques involved in the extraction of calculi have been expanded to include the reestablishment of ductal patency and the placement of endoprosthetic devices, such as stents. Extracorporeal shock wave lithotripsy, the technique of fragmenting kidney stones and gallstones with high-energy shock waves, has gained acceptance as a therapeutic procedure in lieu of surgical intervention.

The contraindications for any of these procedures are minimal. In most cases, percutaneous interventional studies can be carried out on patients who are very poor surgical risks, thus greatly increasing the chance for successful treatment.

REFERENCES

1. Dondelinger, R. F., Rossi, P, Kurdziel, J. C. and Wallace, S. (eds.): Interventional Radiology. New York, Thieme Medical Publishers, Inc., 1990, p. 42.
2. Wilkins, R. A., and Viamonte, H., Jr. (eds.): Interventional Radiology. Boston, Blackwell Scientific Publications, 1982, Chap. 25.
3. Athanasoulis, C. A., et al.: Interventional Radiology. Philadelphia, W. B. Saunders, 1982, p. 470.
4. Kohri, K., Uemura, T., Iguchi, M., and Kurita, T.: Effect of high energy shock waves on tumor cells, Urol. Res., 18:101–105, 1990.

SUGGESTED READINGS

NEEDLE BIOPSY

Brynitz, S., Struve-Christensen, F., Borgeskow, S., and Bertelsen, S.: Transcarinal mediastinal needle biopsy compared with mediastinoscopy, J. Thorac. Cardiovasc. Surg., 90:21, 1985.

Ferrucci, J. T., et al.: Diagnosis of abdominal malignancy by radiologic fine needle aspiration biopsy, Am. J. Radiol., 134:323, 1980.

Gobien, R. P.: Aspiration biopsy of the solitary thyroid module, Radiol. Clin. North Am., 17:543, 1979.

Haaga, J. R., and Alfidi, R. J.: Precise biopsy localization by computed tomography, Radiology, 118:603, 1976.

Lindgren, P. G.: Percutaneous needle biopsy—a new technique, Acta Radiol. [Diagn.] (Stockh.), 23:653, 1982.

Livraghi, T., et al.: Risk in fine needle abdominal biopsy, J. Clin. Ultrasound., 11:77, 1983.

Lufkin, R. B., Peresi, L. M., and Hanafee, W. N.: New needle for MR guided aspiration cytology of the head and neck, Am. J. Roentgenol., 149:380, 1987.

Miller, D. A., et al.: Fine needle aspiration biopsy: The role of immediate cytologic assessment, Am. J. Roentgenol., 147:155, 1986.

Miller, J. M., et al.: Diagnosis of thyroid nodules: Use of fine needle aspiration and needle biopsy, J.A.M.A., 241:481, 1979.

Pagani, J. J.: Biopsy of focal hepatic lesions—comparison of 18 and 22 gauge needles, Radiology, 147:673, 1983.

Weymuller, E. A., Jr., et al.: Aspiration cytology: An efficient and cost effective modality, Laryngoscope, 93:561, 1983.

PUNCTURE AND DRAINAGE PROCEDURES

Deveney, C. W., Lurie, K., and Deveney, K. E.: Improved treatment of intra-abdominal abscess: A result of improved localization, drainage, and patient care, not technique, Arch. Surg., 123:1126, 1988.

Elyaderani, M. K., and Gabriele, O. F.: Brush and forceps biopsy of biliary ducts via percutaneous transhepatic catheterization, Radiology, 135:777, 1980.

Gerzof, S. G., et al.: Percutaneous catheter drainage of abdominal abscesses guided by ultrasound and computed tomography, Am. J. Radiol., 133:1, 1979.

Haaga, J. R., and Weinstein, A. J.: CT guided percutaneous aspiration and drainage of abscesses, Am. J. Radiol., 135:1187, 1980.

Harbin, W. P., and Ferucci, J. T., Jr.: Nonoperative management of malignant biliary obstruction: A radiologic alternative, Am. J. Radiol., 135:103, 1980.

Harrington, D. P.: Teflon sheath placement in the biliary tree using high torque J guide wires, Radiology, 135:248, 1980.

Hellekant, C., Jonsson, K., and Gennell, S.: Percutaneous internal drainage in obstructive jaundice, Am. J. Radiol., 134:661, 1980.

Lurie, K., Plzak, L., and Deveney, C. W.: Intra-abdominal abscess in the 1980s, Surg. Clin. North Am., 67:621, 1987.

MacErlean, D. P., et al.: Radiological management of abdominal abscess, J. R. Soc. Med., 76:256, 1983.

Makuuchi, M., et al.: Ultrasonically guided percutaneous transhepatic bile drainage, Radiology, 136:165, 1980.

Molnar, W., and Stockham, A. E.: Transhepatic dilatation of choledochoenterostomy strictures, Radiology, 129:59, 1978.

Nakayama, T., Ikeda, A., and Okuda, K.: Percutaneous transhepatic drainage of the biliary tract, Gastroenterology, 74:554, 1978.

Ring, E. J., et al.: Therapeutic applications of catheter cholangiography, Radiology, 128:333, 1978.

Rupp, N., et al.: Biliary drainage by Teflon endoprosthesis in obstructive jaundice—experiences in 69 patients treated by PTCD or ERCD, Eur. J. Radiol., 3:42, 1983.

Smith, E. H., and Bartrum, R. J.: Ultrasonically

guided percutaneous aspiration of abscesses, Am. J. Radiol., *122*:308, 1974.

Stephenson, T. F., Guzzetta, L. R., and Tagulinao, O. A.: CT guided Seldinger catheter drainage of a hepatic abscess, Am. J. Radiol., *131*:323, 1978.

Sunshine, J., et al.: Percutaneous abdominal abscess drainage: Portland area experience, Am. J. Surg., *145*:615, 1983.

Van Gansbeke, D., et al.: Percutaneous drainage of subphrenic abscesses, Br. J. Radiol., *62*:127, 1989.

Van Sonnenberg, E., et al.: Periappendiceal abscess: Percutaneous drainage, Radiology, *163*:23–26, 1987.

Van Sonnenberg, E., et al.: Percutaneous drainage of abscesses and fluid collections: Technique, results, and applications, Radiology, *142*:1, 1982.

Wittich, G. R., Karnel, F., Schurawitzki, H, and Jantsch, H.: Percutaneous drainage of mediastinal pseudocysts, Radiology, *167*:51, 1988.

Zuidema, G. D., et al.: Percutaneous transhepatic management of complex biliary problems, Ann. Surg., *197*:584, 1983.

PERCUTANEOUS NEPHROSTOMY

Bigoniari, L. R., et al.: Percutaneous ureteral stent placement for stricture management and internal urinary drainage, Am. J. Radiol., *135*:865, 1979.

Casal, G. L.: Fascial dilator for percutaneous drainage procedures, Radiology, *155*:833, 1985.

Gray, R. R., St. Louis, E. L., and Grosman, H.: Failure in placement of trocar mounted catheters, J. Can. Assoc. Radiol., *37*:102, 1986.

Gunther, R., et al.: Percutaneous nephropyelostomy using a fine needle puncture set, Radiology, *132*:228, 1979.

Gunther, R., et al.: Transrenal ureteral embolization, Radiology, *132*:317, 1979.

Maillet, P. J., et al.: Fistulas of the upper urinary tract: Percutaneous management, J. Urol., *138*:1382–1385, 1987.

Naidich, J. B., Rackson, M. E., Mossey, R. T., and Stein, H. L.: Nondilated obstructive uropathy: Percutaneous nephrostomy performed to reverse renal failure, Radiology, *160*:653, 1986.

Newhouse, J. H., and Pfister, R. C.: Percutaneous catheterization of the kidney and perirenal space: Trocar technique, Urol. Radiol., *2*:157, 1981.

Pfister, R. C., and Newhouse, J. H.: Interventional percutaneous pyeloureteral techniques: II. Percutaneous nephrostomy and other procedures, Radiol. Clin. North Am., *17*:351, 1979.

Sadlowski, R. W., et al.: New technique for percutaneous nephrostomy under ultrasound guidance, J. Urol., *121*:559, 1979.

Smith, A. D., et al.: Percutaneous nephrostomy in the management of ureteral and renal calculi, Radiology, *133*:49, 1979.

Strijk, S. P., et al.: Dissolution of bilateral renal calculi via percutaneous nephrostomy: Report of a case, Acta Radiol. [Diagn.] (Stockh.), *23*:599, 1982.

FOREIGN BODY REMOVAL

Burhenne, H. J.: Percutaneous extraction of retained biliary tract stones: 661 patients, Am. J. Radiol., *134*:889, 1980.

Castaneda-Zuniga, W. R., et al.: Percutaneous removal of kidney stones, Urol. Clin. North Am., *9*:113, 1982.

Cotton, P. B.: ERCP: Progress report, Gut, *18*:316–341, 1977.

Cotton, P. B.: Endoscopic management of bile duct stones (apples and oranges), Gut, *25*:587–597, 1984.

Mason, R.: Percutaneous extraction of retained gallstones via the T-tube tract: British experience of 131 cases, Clin. Radiol., *31*:497, 1980.

Mason, R., et al.: Combined endoscopic and percutaneous trans-cystic approach to a retained common duct stone, Br. J. Radiol., *53*:38, 1980.

Price, H. I., et al.: Ureteral calculus extraction: A nonsurgical percutaneous approach, J. Kansas Med. Soc., *84*:120, 1983.

Smith, P. L.: Percutaneous removal of a biliary stone impacted in a cystic duct, Radiology, *140*:240, 1981.

EXTRACORPOREAL SHOCK WAVE LITHOTRIPSY

Brijendra, R., and Burhenne, H. J.: Extracorporeal shock wave lithotripsy of calcified gallstones (work in progress), Radiology, *175*:667–670, 1990.

Brownlee, N., et al.: Controlled inversion therapy: An adjunct to the elimination of gravity dependent fragments following extracorporeal shock wave lithotripsy, J. Urol., *143*:1096–1098, 1990.

Chaussy, C. H., et al.: First clinical experience with extracorporeal induced destruction of kidney stones by shock waves, J. Urol., *127*:217, 1982.

Ferrucci, J. T.: Biliary lithotripsy: What will the issues be? Am. J. Roentgenol., *149*:227, 1987.

Gravenstein, J. S., and Peter, K.: Extracorporeal Shock Wave Lithotripsy for Renal Stone Disease: Technical and Clinical Aspects. Boston, Butterworths, 1986.

Greiner, L., Munks, C., Heil, W., and Jakobeit, C.: Gallbladder stone fragments in feces after biliary extracorporeal shock wave lithotripsy, Gastroenterology, *98*:1620–1624, 1990.

Keane, F. B. V., and Tanner, W. A.: Extracorporeal lithotripsy for gall stones, Br. J. Surg., *75*:506, 1988.

McGahan, J. P., Gerscovich, E., and Lindfors, K.: Gallbladder disease: Perspectives in diagnosis and treatment, Radiol. Rep., *1*:171–179, 1989.

Rothschild, J. G., Holbrook, R. F., and Reinhold, R. B.: Gallstone lithotripsy vs cholecystectomy: A preliminary cost-benefit analysis, Arch. Surg., *125*:710–714, 1990.

Sackmann, M., et al.: Shock wave lithotripsy of gallbladder stones, N. Engl. J. Med., *318*:393, 1988.

GENERAL

Haaga, J. R., et al.: Interventional CT scanning, Radiol. Clin. North Am., *15*:449, 1977.

Kadir, S., et al.: Selected Techniques in Interventional Radiology. Philadelphia, W. B. Saunders, 1982.

Rosen, R. J.: Interventional biliary radiology, Bull. N. Y. Acad. Med., *58*:795, 1982.

Sagel, S. S.: Special Procedures in Chest Radiology. Philadelphia, W. B. Saunders, 1976.

Yeh, H. C.: Sonography of the adrenal glands: Normal glands and small masses, Am. J. Roentgenol., *135*:1167, 1980.

8   Special Techniques

This segment deals with several specialized techniques used in special procedure radiography—subtraction, serial magnification, and xeroradiography. The basic principles underlying these techniques are discussed, and examples of the specialized equipment are given.

Subtraction is the most widely practiced of these techniques. Both manual and digital methods are used in special procedures, but digital subtraction angiography is equipment dependent and is not available at all institutions.

The use of serial magnification in special procedure radiography is limited to large teaching and research institutions. Its greatest use is during superselective studies to image very small vessels. Specialized equipment, specifically a smaller focal spot x-ray tube, is necessary for the performance of magnification techniques. However, digital subtraction angiography can image smaller vessels because digital manipulation of the data results in enhanced contrast of smaller vessels and is replacing the technique of serial magnification in some areas.

Xeroradiography has been used primarily as a technique for breast examination (mammography). Xerox Corporation has discontinued manufacturing xeroradiographic equipment but supports the existing model 125 and 126 systems still in use. A discussion of the technique for these systems is included in this text to acquaint the student and practicing radiographer with a technique that is still viable in the clinical setting. Xerox has also withdrawn the model 175 system from the market; because this system was not very popular, a discussion on this modality is not included.

twenty-four

Xeroradiography

PLATE CHARGING

X-RAY EXPOSURE OF THE PLATE

DEVELOPMENT OF THE PLATE

IMAGE TRANSFER

IMAGE FIXING

PLATE CLEANING AND CONDITIONING

Xeroradiography is an x-ray imaging system used in certain medical institutions to record some special radiographic procedures. Its most extensive use has been in mammography. However, xeroradiography has also been used in other special procedures, such as arthrography, sialography, and venography. Because this system is a specialized method of image recording that differs from conventional radiography, a discussion of the xeroradiographic process is in order.

The xeroradiographic process involves six steps, which are schematically presented in flow-chart form in Figure 24–1. An electrostatic image is produced by x-rays on an electrically charged plate rather than on silver halide crystals or on intensifying screens, as in conventional radiography. The development process is also considerably different. Conventional radiographic film obviously cannot be used with this system; film is replaced by the xeroradiographic (XR) plate.

The XR plate is the most essential element of the system. It consists of an aluminum sheet with a photoconductive layer of selenium applied to it. The surface of the selenium is coated with a thin layer of plastic to protect it from mechanical damage. The XR plate is reusable after it undergoes cleaning and conditioning. This prepares the plate for subsequent exposure and development.

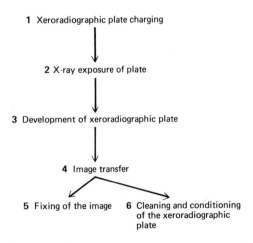

Figure 24–1. Flow chart of the xeroradiographic process.

The system itself consists of an XR plate and cassette, a conditioning unit (Fig. 24–2), and a processing unit (see Fig. 24–2).

All operations, except x-ray exposure of the plate, are performed within the conditioning and processing units. The entire three-stage operation of the system is shown in Figure 24–3. The first stage comprises conditioning, charging, and loading of the plate into a cassette. Then x-ray exposure occurs (image formation stage). Last, the plate is developed, processed, and cleaned, and the image is transferred to paper.

XR plates are prepared for use in the conditioning unit. The plates are loaded into the conditioning unit by a storage-transfer magazine, which is a container that holds a maximum of four plates. The storage-transfer magazine is compatible with both the conditioning and processing units and acts as the receiving and supply magazines for the system. When the storage-transfer magazine is inserted into the conditioning unit, individual XR plates are automatically transported to the relaxation oven. Here, any residual charge left on the plate from a previous exposure is removed. This step is essential because any residual charge retains the image of the previous exposure and can create confusing shadows on subsequent xeroradiographs.

After relaxation, the plates are moved to an internal storage magazine, which can store a maximum of 16 XR plates. Panel lights on the unit indicate the number of plates available for use.

PLATE CHARGING

To initiate the charging process, a cassette must be inserted into the conditioning unit. This energizes the unit, and it automatically transfers an XR plate from the internal storage magazine to the charging station. As the XR plate travels toward the cassette, it passes under an air ion–generating device that deposits a uniform electrostatic charge onto the plate.

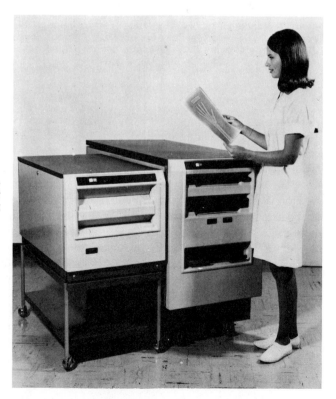

Figure 24–2. The major components of the xeroradiographic system—the conditioning unit *(left)* and the processing unit *(right)*. (From Xerox Corporation.)

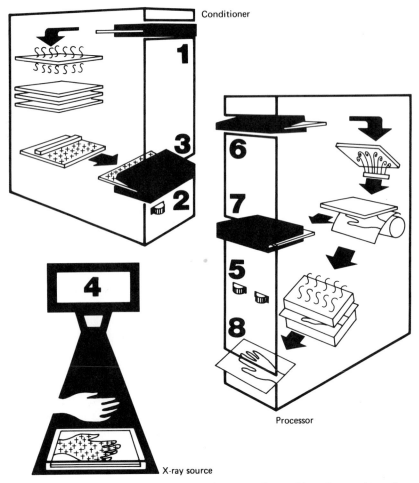

Figure 24–3. Schematic showing the components of the xeroradiographic system and how the operation is carried out. *(1)* Storage and transfer magazine; *(2)* image contrast selector; *(3)* cassette (being loaded); *(4)* x-ray exposure of the plate; *(5)* image density selector; *(6)* cassette (being unloaded in processing unit); *(7)* storage and transfer magazine accepting cleaned plates; *(8)* the finished xeroradiographic print. (From Xerox Corporation.)

The air ion–generating device consists of three wires maintained at a sufficiently high voltage to produce ionization of the immediately surrounding air. These wires are positively biased, which causes the positive air ions to move down toward the selenium layer of the XR plate. This results in a uniform positive charge being deposited onto the plate. As the surface of the selenium layer becomes positively charged, the rigid base on the XR plate supplies an equal number of negative charges to the surface close to the selenium. This operation makes the plate responsive to the effect of x-radiation. While in the charged state, the XR plate is highly sensitive to low-energy radiation. Therefore, the plate should not be exposed to light after the charging process because this will discharge the plate. By adjusting the amount of surface charge applied to the plate, the image contrast can be varied. A higher contrast results if the surface charge is increased.

After passing through the air ion–generating device, the XR plate is moved into the cassette. The cassette is then removed and used like any conventional x-ray cassette.

The cassette is constructed of plastic and measures $15.75 \times 10.25 \times 0.75$ in ($39.38 \times 25.62 \times 1.88$ cm). It is light-tight to prevent accidental discharge of the plate due to exposure to light. It is also compatible with the conditioning and processing units.

X-RAY EXPOSURE OF THE PLATE

Once the plate is charged, it should be used and processed within 30 min to preserve image quality. The charge on the plate begins to dissipate slowly, with a negligible amount being lost within the first 30 min. If the plate is not processed promptly, image quality deteriorates.

The second stage in the xeroradiographic process is x-ray exposure of the prepared plate. The XR plate is used like any conventional cassette containing silver halide x-ray film, but the exposure factors are somewhat different than those for conventional techniques. In general, 120 kV is standard for all body parts. The number of milliampere seconds is variable and can range from 15 mA for a hand to 200 mA for a femur. It is recommended that a grid or Bucky not be used for any of the procedure. Grids are usually unnecessary because the XR plate is not as sensitive to the effects of scattered radiation as conventional film. The use of a grid during, for example, radiography of the hip joint requires 400 mA. This represents a large increase over the conventional method. (See "Appendix," Tables A–2 and A–3, for guides to recommended xeroradiographic technique.)

Xeroradiography is not recommended for all areas of the body. In general, this method is not advised for procedures involving thick body parts such as the trunk or thorax; however, when compared with conventional radiographic methods, there are certain cases in which xeroradiography may be best.

Xeroradiographs exhibit a specific type of image contrast called "edge enhancement." In effect, a sharp demarcation occurs between two broad areas of density. The two broad areas, however, exhibit only slightly different densities. In conventional radiography, the broad areas show a vast difference in density but are not very sharply separated. Edge enhancement makes xeroradiography valuable for demonstrating sharp, abrupt differences in density, whereas conventional radiography is useful for areas with gradually changing differences in density (Fig. 24–4).

The xeroradiograph can be processed in either a positive or a negative image. The negative image exhibits the same density relations as conventional radiographs: Thinner areas appear dark blue (black on conventional x-ray film), and thicker areas appear white (clear on conventional x-ray film). The reverse occurs with the positive image (Fig. 24–5).

When the XR plate is exposed to x-rays, the positively charged plate surface discharges; the more radiation reaching the plate, the greater will be the discharge.

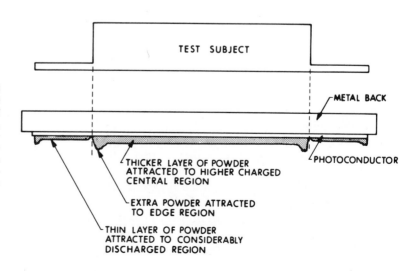

Figure 24–4. Schematic showing how the powder particles are attracted in greater amounts at the edges of areas of density, thus creating the edge enhancement found on xeroradiographs. (From Hayford, R. E.: The Principles of the Xeroradiographic Process, Xerox Corporation, 1971.)

TEST SUBJECT

METAL BACK

PHOTOCONDUCTOR

THICKER LAYER OF POWDER ATTRACTED TO HIGHER CHARGED CENTRAL REGION

EXTRA POWDER ATTRACTED TO EDGE REGION

THIN LAYER OF POWDER ATTRACTED TO CONSIDERABLY DISCHARGED REGION

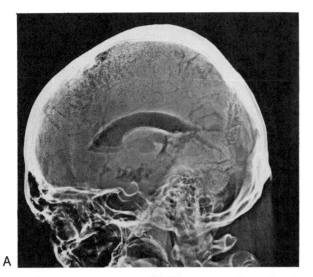

A

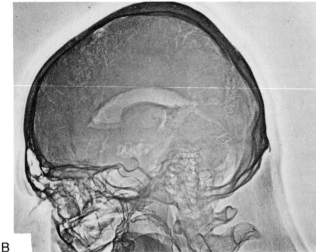

B

Figure 24–5. Normal xeroradiographic pneu-moencephalograms—negative image *(A)* and positive image *(B)*. (From Medical Application Bulletin, Xerox Corporation, 1971.)

Figure 24–6 illustrates the difference in discharge between thick and thin areas. Segments of the XR plate not exposed to x-rays do not lose any surface charge.

DEVELOPMENT OF THE PLATE

After exposure to x-radiation, the plate must be developed to make visible the latent electrostatic image on the plate. This electrostatic image can be equated to the latent image produced on conventional x-ray film.

Development and image transfer are carried out in the processing unit. Development of the XR plate converts the electrostatic image produced by x-ray exposure into a visible image. The visible image is then transferred to a sheet of opaque paper, which can be read and then stored.

The developing process begins when the cassette is inserted into the processing unit. The type of image (positive or negative) is selected before the cassette is inserted. The XR plate is automatically removed from the cassette and transported to the development chamber, where, in the positive mode, it is exposed to a cloud of charged powder particles. The negatively charged powder particles are attracted to the positively charged

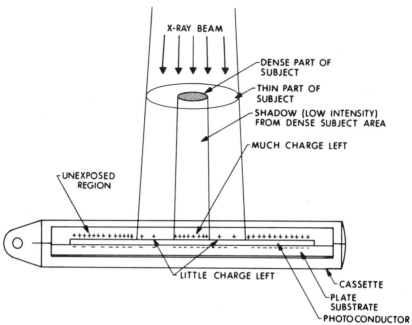

Figure 24–6. Schematic of the exposure of an object using a radiographic plate. This demonstrates the difference in area discharge between a dense section and a thin section of an object. Note that the area outside the collimated beam is not discharged. (From Hayford, R. E.: The Principles of the Xeroradiographic Process, Xerox Corporation, 1971.)

image on the plate in proportion to the amount of charge remaining after the x-ray exposure. In other words, the areas with the most remaining charge attract the most powder, and the areas with less charge attract less powder. The remaining charge on the plate is not sufficient to attract the negatively charged powder cloud (Fig. 24–7).

The development chamber is also equipped with a grid that is positively biased (Fig. 24–8). This tends to uniformly attract the negatively charged particles while repelling the positively charged powder particles. The XR plate backing is also biased positively, which aids in attracting negative particles to the plate surface, where the local charges hold the powder particles to form a visible image. With the grid and plateback positively biased, a positive image is formed on the plate surface.

To produce a negative image, the negative mode is selected. This changes the bias on the grid and plateback. The positively charged powder particles are then attracted

Figure 24–7. The powder deposit that forms the developed image. Highly discharged areas have thinner layers of powder, whereas charged areas have thicker layers. Note how extra powder forms at the edge region. This provides the edge enhancement at the boundaries of large areas of densities. (From Hayford, R. E.: The Principles of the Xeroradiographic Process, Xerox Corporation, 1971.)

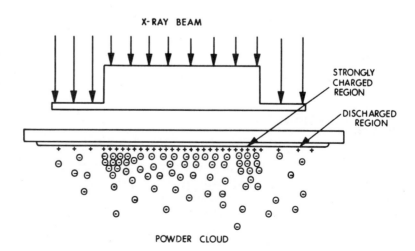

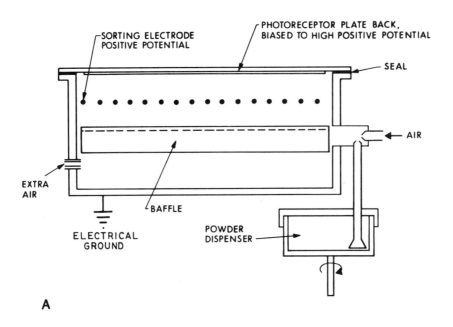

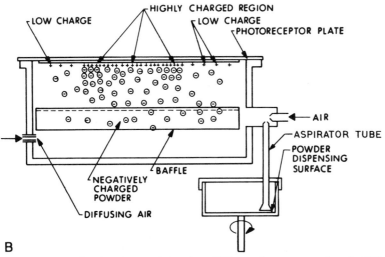

Figure 24–8. Schematics of the development chamber. *(A)* The major component parts; *(B)* the negatively charged powder is attracted toward the highly positively charged plate. (From Hayford, R. E.: The Principles of the Xeroradiographic Process, Xerox Corporation, 1971.)

toward the plate surface, where they are deposited on the most strongly discharged areas.

IMAGE TRANSFER

When development is completed, the plate is transported to the transfer area of the processing unit. Here the visible powder image is transferred to the opaque paper sheet. This is accomplished when the plate and paper come into contact over a transfer-charging device. Most of the powder particles are transferred to the paper and adhere as the plate and paper diverge (Fig. 24–9). The paper containing the powder image is

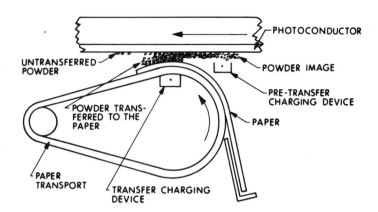

Figure 24-9. Schematic of the image transfer device of the processing unit. Here the image is transferred from the xeroradiographic plate to a sheet of paper. The paper and xeroradiographic plate make contact over the transfer-charging device, and the paper with the image is then separated from the plate and transported to the fixing station. (From Hayford, R. E.: The Principles of the Xeroradiographic Process, Xerox Corporation, 1971.)

moved toward the fixing station while the plate is transported to the cleaning section of the processor.

IMAGE FIXING

The fixing process simply makes the powder image on the paper permanent and resistant to mechanical damage. The special xeroradiography paper that accepts the image is plastic coated. The paper is heated to fix the image; this softens the plastic layer and allows the powder particles to become embedded. As the xeroradiograph is transported toward the output tray, the plastic layer is cooled, which permanently bonds the visible image to the paper. The finished xeroradiograph is then delivered dry within 90 s.

PLATE CLEANING AND CONDITIONING

The XR plate contains some residual powder particles after the transfer process that must be removed mechanically from the surface plate. This is done with a soft mechanical brush that contacts the plate while it is transported to the storage-transfer magazine.

When the storage-transfer magazine is full, it is released from the processing unit, and the plates can again be loaded into the conditioning unit. Here they are heated to restore the conductivity of the plate and remove any traces of the previous image. In this way, the plate is reusable, and the process may be repeated.

SUMMARY

Xeroradiography is a system that has been used in a wide variety of diagnostic procedures, especially mammography. It is a photoelectric rather than a photochemical imaging system. The system uses a photoconductive plate, electrostatic charges, and a specialized developing process to produce either positive or negative images.

The xeroradiographic process consists of three stages—conditioning, exposure, and processing. The first and third stages are carried out in self-contained units using a reusable cassette and opaque paper to record the final image.

The system produces a special type of contrast, edge enhancement, which tends to demonstrate sharp density differences such as fractures, microcalcifications, soft tissue detail, and foreign bodies.

Xeroradiographic exposure technique differs from conventional x-ray film technique in that a relatively high kVp is used. The overall exposure for most studies is usually greater than that of conventional radiographic diagnostic methods.

SUGGESTED READINGS

Bedrossian, C. W., and Martin, J. E.: Xeroradiography of the lung. Radiology, *107*:217, 1973.

Dessaur, J. H., and Clark, H. E.: Xerography and Related Processes. New York, Focal Press, 1965.

Feig, S. A., and McLelland, R.: Breast Carcinoma: Current Diagnosis and Treatment. New York, Masson, 1983.

Henny, G. C.: Effect of roentgen ray quality on response in xeroradiography, Am J. Roentgenol., *79*:158, 1958.

Nagami, H.: Discussion of the x-ray characteristics of xeroradiographic plates, Electrophotography, *4*:3, 1962.

Pagani, J. J., et al.: Efficacy of combined film-screen/xeromammography: Preliminary report, Am. J. Roentgenol., *135*:141, 1980.

Phillips, C. W., Lutterbeck, E. F., and Wilkholm, L.: Xeroradiography of the breast, Int. Surg., *58*:607, 1973.

Sickles, E. A.: Mammographic detectability of breast microcalcifications, Am. J. Roentgenol., *139*:913, 1982.

Speiser, R. C., and Carlson, R. A.: Dose comparisons for mammographic systems, Med. Phys., *13*:667, 1986.

Woesner, M. E., and Sanders, I.: Xeroradiography, a significant modality in the detection of non-metallic foreign bodies in soft tissues, Am. J. Roentgenol., *115*:636, 1972.

Wolfe, J. N.: Xeroradiography: Image content and comparison with film roentgenograms, Am. J. Roentgenol., *117*:690, 1973.

Wolfe, J. N.: Xeroradiography of bones, joints and soft tissues, Radiology, *93*:583, 1969.

Wolfe, J. N.: Xeroradiography of the Breast, 2nd ed. Springfield, IL, Charles C Thomas, 1983.

Wolfe, J. N., et al.: Atlas of Xeroradiographic Anatomy of Normal Skeletal Systems. Springfield, IL, Charles C Thomas, 1978.

twenty-five

Serial Magnification in Special Procedures

PRINCIPLES OF MAGNIFICATION   EQUIPMENT

Magnification in radiography is a normal occurrence. In every radiograph, there are various degrees of inherent magnification because structures within the body are located at different levels. Therefore, in any radiographic projection, different structures are at different distances from the film, which creates a number of magnifications on a single radiograph. This can be detrimental when it is necessary to visualize structures at their normal sizes, or without the effect of magnification. Therefore, in most cases of routine radiography, magnification is avoided and considered a distortion of the recorded image if present to any great degree.

If the principles underlying magnification are understood, it can be a valuable tool in producing radiographs that can be used to make more accurate diagnoses of pathology. The field of special radiographic procedures is currently using this technique during various angiographic procedures, resulting in an improvement in image resolution. The use of magnification during angiography is not an innovation, but with advances in x-ray tube and equipment design, this technique has only recently been fully exploited. Before a discussion of serial magnification radiography can be undertaken, a review of the basic principles and prerequisites for proper magnification technique is necessary.

PRINCIPLES OF MAGNIFICATION

There are two basic types of magnification—geometric and photographic. The latter is the magnification of images from an existing radiograph. Photographic magnification, however, does not offer an improvement in the amount of resolution obtained. In this method, there is also enlargement of the grain of the original radiograph and of the grain of the intensifying screen used, which tends to offset any possibility of improved resolution of the image. On the other hand, when geometric or direct x-ray magnification is performed, the structure itself is enlarged and recorded directly on film. This results in a significant improvement in not only the resolution but also the overall radiographic contrast. Geometric magnification, therefore, is the technique of choice when an increase in resolution is desired during specific procedures.

Geometric magnification is controlled by the source-image distance (SID) and the object-image distance (OID). If the OID is small, the per cent enlargement is also

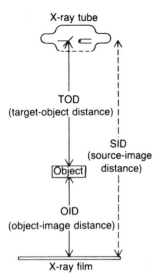

Figure 25–1. Schematic of an object placed a distance from the film and the tube. This also demonstrates the division of the SID into a TOD and an OID.

small. As the OID increases, the per cent enlargement also increases. The SID is inversely related to magnification; as the SID decreases, the magnification increases. Changes in the SID do not influence magnification as much as do changes in the OID. Radiographs taken at longer SIDs are produced by the parallel rays of the primary beam. At shorter distances, the divergent rays, which are the weaker rays, are used to produce a portion of the image. Many of these divergent rays, being weaker, are absorbed by the patient. It is an accepted practice in radiography departments to use 40 in (100 cm) as the standard SID for tube-over-table radiography. At this distance, the radiographs are produced by the more energetic parallel rays. Therefore, the factor that is usually manipulated to produce functional geometric magnification is the OID. It is necessary to understand the effects of manipulating this factor to produce consistent results when using the magnification technique.

If the object to be radiographed is moved away from the film, the total SID can be divided into two separate measurements—the target-object distance (TOD) and the OID (Fig. 25–1). When the OID equals the TOD, there is a 1:1 ratio. This produces a resultant linear magnification of two times the original size (2 ×). For example, if the object were a 1- × 1-in square (2.5 × 2.5 cm), its linear dimensions after a 2 × direct x-ray enlargement would be 2 × 2 in (5 × 5 cm). Comparing the area enlargement in this particular case (Table 25–1), it can be seen that there is an area enlargement of 4 ×. The area enlargement should be kept in mind when performing direct enlargement because enlargements of even relatively small segments result in greatly increased projected radiographic areas. This illustrates the fact that it would be impractical to

Table 25–1. LINEAR AND AREA COMPARISON OF AN OBJECT 1 × 1 IN (2.5 × 2.5 CM) AT VARIOUS ENLARGEMENT RATIOS

SID:TOD	Magnification	Object Linear Measurement (l × w)		Relative Linear Enlargement	Object Area Measurement		Relative Area Enlargement
		in	*cm*		*in²*	*cm²*	
40:40	0	1 × 1	2.5 × 2.5	1	1	6.25	1
40:20	2×	2 × 2	5 × 5	2×	4	25	4×
40:13	3×	3 × 3	7.5 × 7.5	3×	9	56.25	9×
40:10	4×	4 × 4	10 × 10	4×	16	100	16×
40:8	5×	5 × 5	12.5 × 12.5	5×	25	156.25	25×
40:6.66	6×	6 × 6	15 × 15	6×	36	225	36×

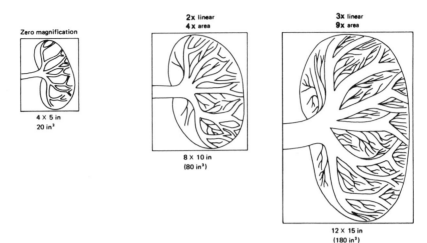

Figure 25–2. Schematic showing the area increase produced by magnification techniques over conventional methods.

attempt enlargement radiography on large areas of the body because of the great amount of area enlargement. Another important consideration regarding area enlargement is that the magnified image may be too large for specific recording systems (Fig. 25–2).

The degree of magnification can be calculated from the ratio of the SID to the TOD:

$$\text{Magnification} = \frac{\text{SID}}{\text{TOD}}$$

If a 40-in SID were being used and the degree of magnification desired was $3\times$, the TOD could be easily calculated from the formula above as follows:

$$\text{Magnification} = \frac{\text{SID}}{\text{TOD}}$$

$$3 = \frac{40}{\text{TOD}}$$

$$\text{TOD} = \frac{40}{3} = 13.3, \text{ or } 13 \text{ in}$$

If the OID is required, it is necessary to subtract the TOD from the SID.

$$\text{OID} = \text{SID} - \text{TOD}$$

In the example above, the OID would be:

$$\text{OID} = \text{SID} - \text{TOD}$$
$$= 40 - 13 = 27 \text{ in}$$

Most direct serial radiographic enlargement is performed with a degree of magnification of from $2\times$ to $3\times$. In selected cases, greater degrees of magnification may be desired; however, unless the proper equipment and techniques are used, it is impractical and could result in an error in diagnosis.[1]

EQUIPMENT

Specific equipment requirements necessary to properly use the magnification technique include the x-ray tube, intensifying screens, radiographic tables, and rapid sequence changers.

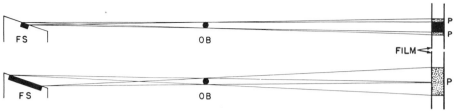

Figure 25–3. Schematic of the blurring that occurs when the focal spot is larger than the object size during a magnification procedure. (From Fuchs, A. W.: Principles of Radiographic Exposure and Processing. Springfield, IL, Charles C Thomas, 1969.)

The proper radiographic tube is the most important prerequisite for direct magnification radiography. Specifically, the focal spot size is the critical factor. It is essential that the x-ray tube have a focal spot of no more than 0.3 mm. The primary reason for the use of a fractional focal spot of this order is the increase in geometric sharpness; another term for this is "penumbra." The penumbra appears as a blurred or fuzzy region that surrounds the image. The greater the penumbra, the greater will be the lack of clarity of the image. This fact becomes critical during magnification radiography because objects that are smaller than the size of the focal spot are obliterated by the penumbra and disappear on the radiograph (Fig. 25–3). Because the purpose of the magnification technique is to improve the resolution of fine details, extremely small focal spots are essential.

A great amount of heat is produced when an electron stream is converted to x-rays. This heat must be distributed over the focal spot area and dispersed, or damage to the target occurs. It follows that larger focal spots have larger heat accumulation capacities before this damage occurs. Fractional focal spot tubes make efficient use of the line focus principle to allow for greater heat loading yet provide extremely small focal spots.

The actual focal spot size is determined by the size and shape of the filament. The anode face is angled so that the x-ray beam is projected at 90° to the long axis of the tube. This incline produces a smaller effective focal spot. By varying this angle over a certain range, it is possible to produce various focal spot sizes. The smaller the anode angle, the smaller will be the effective focal spot size. This is true to a point dictated by the heel effect, the cutoff point. The anode angle may vary from 7° to a maximum of 20°. The anode angles commonly found in high-resolution fractional focus tubes are 7° and 10°. The heel effect is critical when these tubes are used. For example, the Varian A272 high-resolution 0.3-mm fractional focus tube, with a 7° target angle, will cover a 9.8- × 9.8-in (24.5- × 24.5-cm) maximum field size at an SID of 40 in (see Fig. 1–7). Accurate positioning becomes necessary to avoid loss of the image because of the heel effect.

Because the focal spot is such a critical factor in image resolution, especially during the magnification technique, it is important to accurately determine its effective size. This is especially essential when the magnification technique is performed routinely.

Methods of determining the focal spot size include measurement with a pinhole camera, measurement with a Buckbee-Meers resolution plate, and the Francke star method.[2, 3]

The pinhole method does not allow for an accurate demonstration of the distribution of the radiation. Differences can occur in the distribution of the x-rays emitted (one may be emitted from the center and another from the periphery), even though external dimensions are the same. This can cause a discrepancy in the image resolution of the tubes.[2]

A more accurate method is the use of the Buckbee-Meers resolution plate. This method measures the effective size of the focal spot while considering the distribution of the emitted radiation. With this method, lines and spaces wider than half of the focal spot size are defined on a radiographic image of the plate. If the lines and spaces are smaller, they overlap and cannot be well defined. The point at which the lines are no longer defined can be located on the radiograph of the Buckbee-Meers resolution plate. This is the point at which the interval between lines and spaces approximates half of the focal spot size. To determine the effective focal spot size, this interval is multiplied by 2.

The star method uses a phantom that contains converging lead lines. By radiographing the phantom, a resolution pattern of the focal spot can be obtained.

Magnifications on the order of $3\times$ and $4\times$ can be attained with x-ray tubes equipped with electrostatic biasing. These tubes provide a negative voltage to the cathode, which results in increased resolution. Nonbiased conventional x-ray tubes demonstrate a double-peaked intensity distribution that acts as two separate sources of radiation. This arrangement tends to produce pseudoresolution, or double-image formation (Fig. 25–4A). With biasing, the intensity distribution becomes more homogeneous and circular, providing for reductions in the effective focal spot size and improved resolution capabilities (Fig. 25–4B).

The use of fractional focus tubes demands a strict adherence to tube rating and cooling charts. If not calculated, the total heat units generated during a serial magnification procedure may be excessive and subsequently damage the tube. An important procedural step in any angiographic examination should be determination of the heat-loading capacity of the x-ray tube. Although heavy-duty special procedure tubes are equipped with rhenium-tungsten-faced molybdenum anodes that possess increased heat-loading capacities, it is still necessary to calculate the maximum number of heat units that can be applied during the procedure.

The stepwise procedure used to determine the maximum angiographic exposure sequence may be summarized as follows:[4]

1. Determine if the desired individual exposure factors are within the ratings permitted for the tube type and focal spot used.
2. Determine the total time of each filming sequence ("on" time plus "off" time).

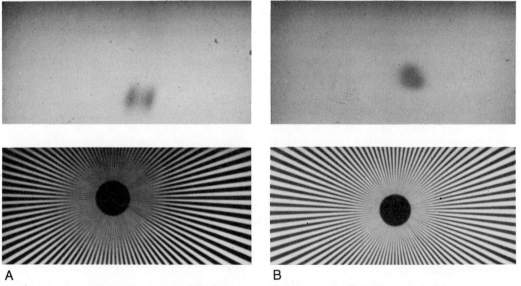

A   B

Figure 25–4. Pinhole images and star resolution test patterns showing double-peak intensity distribution resulting from unbiased tubes *(A)* and the same focal spot after a 75-V bias was applied *(B)*. This demonstrates the resolution enhancement of biased x-ray tubes. (Machlett Laboratories.)

3. Determine the maximum number of heat units that can be applied to the tube for the total time determined above.
4. Compare this maximum heat input with the heat input from the desired technique.

Manufacturers of x-ray tubes supply various angiographic rating charts and tables. Figure 25–5 illustrates the angiographic rating chart for the Varian A282 0.3-mm focal spot x-ray tube. By using the chart, the radiographer can determine the maximum number of kilowatts allowed for each exposure. This is translated into any combination of milliamperes multiplied by kVp, yielding that number of kilowatts. It should be remembered that the combination of factors must fall within the parameters allowed by the radiographic and filament emission charts that accompany the tube.

It is important when using these charts to accurately estimate the number of exposures in the series. The number of exposures per series should be those exposures that are made in succession during one injection of contrast medium. When determining exposure rate, it should be assumed that all of the exposures will be made using the maximum number of films per second in that series. It is advisable, however, to use the lowest possible combination of parameters that produces the desired result to ensure a long tube life.

The screen-film combination is not as critical when the magnification technique is used. During conventional radiography, it is necessary to use either nonscreen radiographic film or detail screens with a small focal spot to overcome the various inherent magnifications described earlier. By the use of the magnification technique, the resolution demanded by the intensifying screen diminishes as the level of magnification increases. In other words, as the object increases in size, it is possible to use a faster screen with larger crystals without a corresponding loss of detail. Magnification produces a reduction in the frequency of information presented to the screen (Fig. 25–6). In general, with the limitations imposed by the x-ray tube, a combination of a high-speed screen and fast film is used during magnification angiography, although any screen-film combination may be used that produces the best possible contrast with the least possible exposure to the patient. It is imperative that good screen-film contact be maintained, because any loss of detail is damaging to the magnified image.

Grids are not essential to magnification radiography. It is essential, however, that scatter radiation be eliminated to preserve the radiographic contrast necessary to demonstrate small objects. Because the object is placed at some distance from the film, an air gap is created. This air gap can be used effectively to clear up the scatter radiation produced by the object. Although some scatter is absorbed by the air, most of this radiation is dispersed and completely misses the film. A 2× magnification technique with a 40-in SID and a 20-in OID would prevent as much radiation from reaching the film as a 15:1 ratio grid.[5] Because most rapid serial changers contain stationary grids, it is necessary to remove them during magnification radiography so that their presence does not detract from any improvement in resolution.

The recording system used for serial magnification angiography must be some type of rapid sequence changer (see Chapter 2). If the purchase of a special angiographic table for magnification radiography is contemplated, one should be chosen that is equipped with an elevating top. Any of the available changers can be adapted for magnification with this type of table.

Existing installations can be used with the Puck film changer. This changer has a small vertical height, and the necessary OIDs can be achieved with a standard angiographic table. Regardless of the type or brand of rapid sequence changer used, the motion of film transport in the changer must be eliminated to avoid any possibility of motion distortion.

It is also important to attempt to eliminate any cause of motion blurriness. Very short exposure times must be used to minimize motion. Some exposure times have

ANGIOGRAPHIC RATINGS

A282   0.3 mm   **10 Degrees   3 PHASE   150/180 HZ**

EXPOSURE RATE PER SECOND	TUBE LOAD (KW) AS A FUNCTION OF THE EXPOSURE TIME (SEC.) OF THE INDIVIDUAL RADIOGRAPHS OF THE SERIES															NUMBER OF EXPOSURES IN SERIES
	.010	.020	.030	.040	.050	.060	.080	.100	.120	.140	.160	.180	.200	.225	.250	
1	11.8	11.6	11.4	11.2	11.1	11.0	10.8	10.6	10.5	10.3	10.2	10.0	9.9	9.8	9.6	
2	11.8	11.5	11.3	11.2	11.0	10.9	10.7	10.5	10.4	10.2	10.0	9.9	9.8	9.6	9.5	
3	11.8	11.5 .	11.3	11.1	11.0	10.9	10.6	10.4	10.3	10.1	9.9	9.8	0.0	0.0	0.0	
4	11.8	11.5	11.3	11.1	10.9	10.8	10.6	10.3	10.2	10.0	0.0	0.0	0.0	0.0	0.0	20
8	11.8	11.4	11.2	10.9	10.8	10.6	0.0	0.0	0.0	0.0	0.0	0.0	0.0	0.0	0.0	
15	11.7	11.3	11.0	10.7	0.0	0.0	0.0	0.0	0.0	0.0	0.0	0.0	0.0	0.0	0.0	
30	11.5	11.0	0.0	0.0	0.0	0.0	0.0	0.0	0.0	0.0	0.0	0.0	0.0	0.0	0.0	
1	11.8	11.4	11.2	11.0	10.8	10.7	10.4	10.1	9.9	9.7	9.5	9.3	9.1	8.9	8.7	
2	11.8	11.4	11.2	11.0	10.8	10.6	10.3	10.0	9.8	9.6	9.4	9.2	9.0	8.8	8.6	
3	11.8	11.4	11.1	10.9	10.7	10.5	10.2	10.0	9.7	9.5	9.2	9.0	0.0	0.0	0.0	
4	11.7	11.4	11.1	10.9	10.7	10.5	10.2	9.9	9.6	9.3	0.0	0.0	0.0	0.0	0.0	40
8	11.7	11.3	11.0	10.7	10.5	10.2	0.0	0.0	0.0	0.0	0.0	0.0	0.0	0.0	0.0	
15	11.6	11.1	10.7	10.4	0.0	0.0	0.0	0.0	0.0	0.0	0.0	0.0	0.0	0.0	0.0	
30	11.4	10.8	0.0	0.0	0.0	0.0	0.0	0.0	0.0	0.0	0.0	0.0	0.0	0.0	0.0	
1	11.7	11.3	11.0	10.8	10.6	10.4	10.0	9.7	9.4	9.2	8.9	8.7	8.5	8.2	8.0	
2	11.7	11.3	11.0	10.7	10.5	10.3	10.0	9.6	9.3	9.1	8.8	8.6	8.3	8.1	7.8	
3	11.7	11.3	11.0	10.7	10.5	10.3	9.9	9.5	9.2	8.9	8.7	8.4	0.0	0.0	0.0	
4	11.7	11.3	10.9	10.7	10.4	10.2	9.8	9.4	9.1	8.8	0.0	0.0	0.0	0.0	0.0	60
8	11.6	11.2	10.8	10.5	10.2	9.9	0.0	0.0	0.0	0.0	0.0	0.0	0.0	0.0	0.0	
15	11.5	11.0	10.5	10.2	0.0	0.0	0.0	0.0	0.0	0.0	0.0	0.0	0.0	0.0	0.0	
30	11.3	10.6	0.0	0.0	0.0	0.0	0.0	0.0	0.0	0.0	0.0	0.0	0.0	0.0	0.0	
1	11.7	11.2	10.9	10.6	10.4	10.1	9.7	9.3	9.0	8.7	8.4	8.2	7.9	7.6	7.4	
2	11.6	11.2	10.8	10.6	10.3	10.1	9.6	9.2	8.9	8.6	8.3	8.0	7.8	7.5	7.2	
3	11.6	11.2	10.8	10.5	10.2	10.0	9.5	9.2	8.8	8.5	8.2	7.9	0.0	0.0	0.0	
4	11.6	11.1	10.8	10.5	10.2	9.9	9.5	9.1	8.7	8.4	0.0	0.0	0.0	0.0	0.0	80
8	11.6	11.0	10.6	10.3	10.0	9.7	0.0	0.0	0.0	0.0	0.0	0.0	0.0	0.0	0.0	
15	11.5	10.9	10.4	10.0	0.0	0.0	0.0	0.0	0.0	0.0	0.0	0.0	0.0	0.0	0.0	
30	11.2	10.5	0.0	0.0	0.0	0.0	0.0	0.0	0.0	0.0	0.0	0.0	0.0	0.0	0.0	
1	11.6	11.1	10.7	10.4	10.1	9.9	9.4	9.0	8.6	8.3	8.0	7.7	7.4	6.7	6.0	
2	11.6	11.1	10.7	10.4	10.1	9.8	9.3	8.9	8.5	8.2	7.9	7.6	7.3	6.7	6.0	
3	11.6	11.1	10.7	10.3	10.0	9.7	9.2	8.8	8.4	8.1	7.7	7.4	0.0	0.0	0.0	
4	11.6	11.0	10.6	10.3	10.0	9.7	9.2	8.7	8.3	8.0	0.0	0.0	0.0	0.0	0.0	100
8	11.5	10.9	10.5	10.1	9.7	9.4	0.0	0.0	0.0	0.0	0.0	0.0	0.0	0.0	0.0	
15	11.4	10.7	10.2	9.8	0.0	0.0	0.0	0.0	0.0	0.0	0.0	0.0	0.0	0.0	0.0	
30	11.2	10.4	0.0	0.0	0.0	0.0	0.0	0.0	0.0	0.0	0.0	0.0	0.0	0.0	0.0	
1	11.5	10.9	10.4	10.0	9.6	9.3	8.7	8.2	7.8	7.1	6.3	5.6	5.0	4.4	4.0	
2	11.4	10.8	10.3	9.9	9.6	9.2	8.6	8.1	7.7	7.1	6.3	5.6	5.0	4.4	4.0	
3	11.4	10.8	10.3	9.9	9.5	9.2	8.6	8.0	7.6	7.1	6.3	5.6	0.0	0.0	0.0	
4	11.4	10.8	10.3	9.8	9.5	9.1	8.5	8.0	7.5	7.1	0.0	0.0	0.0	0.0	0.0	150
8	11.4	10.7	10.1	9.6	9.2	8.9	0.0	0.0	0.0	0.0	0.0	0.0	0.0	0.0	0.0	
15	11.2	10.5	9.9	9.3	0.0	0.0	0.0	0.0	0.0	0.0	0.0	0.0	0.0	0.0	0.0	
30	11.0	10.1	0.0	0.0	0.0	0.0	0.0	0.0	0.0	0.0	0.0	0.0	0.0	0.0	0.0	
1	11.1	10.2	9.5	8.9	8.4	7.9	6.3	5.0	4.2	3.6	3.1	2.8	2.5	2.2	2.0	
2	11.1	10.1	9.4	8.8	8.3	7.9	6.3	5.0	4.2	3.6	3.1	2.8	2.5	2.2	2.0	
3	11.0	10.1	9.4	8.8	8.3	7.8	6.3	5.0	4.2	3.6	3.1	2.8	0.0	0.0	0.0	
4	11.0	10.1	9.4	8.7	8.2	7.8	6.3	5.0	4.2	3.6	0.0	0.0	0.0	0.0	0.0	300
8	11.0	10.0	9.2	8.6	8.0	7.6	0.0	0.0	0.0	0.0	0.0	0.0	0.0	0.0	0.0	
15	10.8	9.8	9.0	8.3	0.0	0.0	0.0	0.0	0.0	0.0	0.0	0.0	0.0	0.0	0.0	
30	10.6	9.4	0.0	0.0	0.0	0.0	0.0	0.0	0.0	0.0	0.0	0.0	0.0	0.0	0.0	

NOTES

1. (kW) of Exposure Equals mA x kV
   For example - 70 kV x 300 mA = 21 kW
2. Exposures less than .010 seconds will have a kW Rating same as 0.10 seconds.

Figure 25–5. The angiographic rating chart for the Varian A282 0.3-mm focal spot x-ray tube. To use the chart, *(1)* determine the number of exposures in the series. *(2)* Select the maximum rate per second to be used for the series. *(3)* Select the desired time in seconds for each exposure. *(4)* The maximum number of kilowatts allowed for each exposure is found at the intersection of the exposure rate and the exposure time that were chosen. (From Varian.)

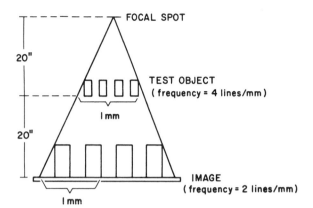

Figure 25–6. Schematic showing that in magnification studies the amount of resolution demanded of the intensifying screen decreases as the magnification increases. Higher speed screens can therefore be used without the accompanying loss of detail. (From Christensen, E. E., Curry, T. S., and Nunally, J.: An Introduction to the Physics of Diagnostic Radiology. Philadelphia, Lea & Febiger, 1972. Reproduced with permission.)

been suggested by Eisenberg and Holland for selected areas of investigation;[6] these are 100 to 200 ms for cerebral vasculature, 50 to 80 ms for abdominal viscera, 20 ms for pulmonary angiography, and 3 to 7 ms for coronary angiography. In any case, the exposure time should never exceed 1/10 s. A high kilovoltage ranging from 83 to 110 kV can be used, if necessary, because of the effective scatter cleanup of the air gap technique. The use of high kilovoltage technique has the added advantage of reducing the radiation dosage to the patient. Milliamperage of 100 mA and higher should be used. The factors used should be within the x-ray tube rating. Another factor that assists in maintaining the high level of contrast necessary for magnification is proper collimation of the x-ray beam.

SUMMARY

Magnification radiography is an important diagnostic tool for visualization of very small anatomic structures, especially during serial angiography. With the principles of geometric magnification and the proper equipment, it is possible to achieve resolution of very small structures on 3× and 4× enlargements.

The important criteria for successful magnification angiography include use of a fractional focus tube with a focal spot no greater than 0.3 mm (preferably equipped with a bias unit), a rapid sequence changer and table combination capable of achieving the necessary object-film distances required, and fast film and high-speed screens in combination with the air gap principle to provide the necessary scatter cleanup.

Exposure factors should be chosen to eliminate motion blurriness. They must fall within the maximum parameters for the specific x-ray tube used. Preferably, a high-kilovoltage technique should be used to decrease radiation dosage to the patient.

REFERENCES

1. Cullinan, J. E.: Illustrated Guide to X-Ray Technics. Philadelphia, J. B. Lippincott, 1980.
2. Bookstein, J. J., and Steck, W.: Effective focal spot size, Radiology, *98*:31, 1971.
3. Spiegler, P., and Breckinridge, W. C.: Imaging of focal spots by means of the star test pattern, Radiology, *102*:679, 1972.
4. Calculation of cinefluorographic and angio-graphic exposure duration from a full-wave rating chart, Cathode Press, 1962.
5. Hale, J., and Mishkin, M. M.: Serial direct magnification cerebral angiography, Am. J. Roentgenol., *107*:616, 1969.
6. Eisenberg, H., and Holland, W. P.: Magnification arteriography with grid biased focal spot x-ray tubes, Cathode Press, (Suppl.), 1973.

SUGGESTED READINGS

Bloom, W. L., et al.: Medical Radiographic Technic, 3rd ed., Springfield, IL, Charles C Thomas, 1979.

Castro, V. G., and Kopenhaver, J. F.: Simple rigid system for accurate measurement of the dimensions of focal spots of x-ray tubes, Am. J. Roentgenol., *13*:376, 1971.

Cope, C.: In vivo magnification angiography, C. R. C. Crit. Rev. Radiol. Sci., *2*:253, 1971.

Curry, T. S., et al.: Christensen's Introduction to the Physics of Diagnostic Radiology, 3rd ed., Philadelphia, Lea & Febiger, 1984.

Friedman, P. J., and Greenspan, R. H.: Observations on magnification radiography, Radiology, *92*:549, 1969.

Greenspan, R. H., and Simon, A.: Magnification coronary arteriography, J. Norm. Clin. Radiol., *16*:414, 1965.

Greenspan, R. H., et al.: In vivo magnification angiography, Invest. Radiol., *2*:419, 1967.

Hallock, A. C.: Machlett Laboratories: A review of methods used to calculate heat loading of x-ray tubes, Cathode Press, *15*:1958.

Hayt, D. B., et al.: Direct serial magnification radiography using a film changer of standard height and a tilting radiographic table, Radiology, *108*:209, 1973.

Heinz, E. R., Fenn, J. O., and Chandler, N.: Resolution of small vessels in angiography, Acta Radiol., *9*:58, 1964.

Hilal, S. (ed.): Small Vessel Angiography, St. Louis, C. V. Mosby, 1972.

Isard, H. J., and Cullinan, J. E.: Roentgenographic enlargement techniques, J.A.E.M.C., *15*:201, 1967.

Jacobi, C. A., and Paris, D. Q.: Textbook of Radiologic Technology, 6th ed., St. Louis, C. V. Mosby, 1977.

Leeds, N. E., et al.: Serial magnification cerebral angiography, Radiology, *90*:117, 1968.

Mahn, G. C.: Machlett Laboratories: Enlargement radiography: A bibliography, Cathode Press, *24*:1967.

Moseley, R. D., and Rust, J. H. (eds.): Diagnostic Radiologic Instrumentation: Modulation Transfer Function, Springfield, IL, Charles C Thomas, 1965.

O'Hara, A. E.: Macroradiography in the pediatric patient, C.R.C. Crit. Rev. Radiol. Sci., *3*:11, 1972.

Rao, G. U. V., and Clark, R. L.: Radiographic magnification vs. optical magnification, Radiology, *94*:196, 1970.

Sakuma, S., et al.: Determination of focal-spot characteristics of microfocus x-ray tubes, Invest. Radiol., *4*:335, 1969.

Seeman, H. E.: Physical and Photographic Principles of Medical Radiography, New York, John Wiley & Sons, 1968.

Spitzer, R. M., Olsson, H. E., and Gibson, B. J.: Modification of a serial film changer for frontal magnification angiography, Radiology, *117*:481, 1975.

Stein, H. L.: Direct serial magnification renal arteriography: A clinical study, J. Urol., *109*:967, 1973.

Takahasi, S., et al.: Angiography at fourfold magnification with special reference to the examination of tumors, Acta Radiol., *4*:206, 1966.

Takaro, T., and Scott, S. M.: Angiography using direct roentgenographic magnification in man, Am. J. Roentgenol., *91*:448, 1964.

Wende, S., and Schindler, K.: Technique and use of x-ray magnification in cerebral arteriography, Neuroradiology, *1*:117, 1970.

Wosolowski, W. E.: The basic concepts of serial direct roentgen enlargement, Radiol. Technol., *45*:237, 1974.

twenty-six

Subtraction

DIRECT X-RAY METHOD
PHOTOGRAPHIC METHOD

ELECTRONIC SUBTRACTION
SUBTRACTION BY COLOR ADDITION

Subtraction is a specialized technique that allows clear visualization of certain information on a radiograph through removal of nonessential images. The procedure does not add new information to a radiograph but renders the diagnostically important images more visible. A subtraction film is actually an image of the differences between two similar films.

In institutions equipped for digital subtraction angiography, the other subtraction techniques have become obsolete. However, these techniques and principles are still viable in clinical settings that lack the necessary hardware for computer-assisted (digital) radiography. The basic principles presented form the basis for all types of subtraction performed today.

Subtraction is used primarily during angiographic procedures. The completed images usually show confusing bone shadows superimposed over contrast-filled vessels. This renders small opacified vessels virtually invisible and makes diagnosis difficult. Subtraction, whether radiographic, photographic, electronic, or digital, eliminates nonessential bone shadows and allows small vessels to stand out against a relatively homogeneous background.

In this chapter, the basic principles of subtraction using radiographic, photographic, and electronic methods are discussed to provide both historical and technical familiarity with these procedures. This discussion should also serve to reinforce the basis for digital subtraction angiography presented in Chapter 6.

To perform subtraction, at least two separate radiographs of the same anatomic region are required. One, the scout film, contains all of the information normally available radiographically concerning that specific region. The second film, the angiogram film, contains all of the information found in the scout film plus that found in the contrast-filled vessels. One other specific criterion is necessary to perform a "perfect" subtraction: There must be no change of position (or motion) by the patient between exposures of the scout and angiogram films. Unfortunately, as the contrast medium is injected, the patient invariably exhibits a slight involuntary reflex motion that precludes the attainment of "perfect" subtraction films. However, this slight motion does not produce objectionable subtraction results, and unless the reflex movement is severe, it can be ignored.

The subtraction procedure is relatively simple and may be accomplished in the following five steps (Fig. 26–1):

1. Expose the scout film.

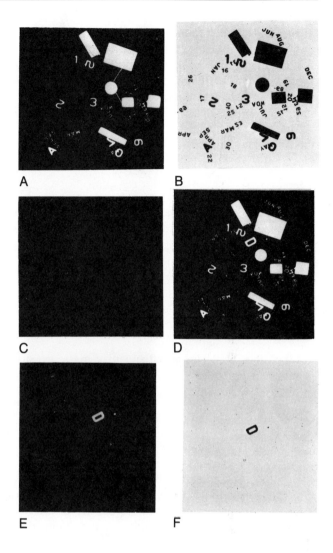

Figure 26–1. Flow representation of the subtraction technique. *(A)* The base, or scout, film. This is usually the initial film of a series. *(B)* The mask. This is produced by making a reversed image of the density differences found on the scout film. *(C)* The mask superimposed over the scout film. When this is done, there should be no resultant density differences seen, and a black image of a single density should then be produced. *(D)* The angiogram film containing the same information present on the scout film plus some added information. *(E)* The mask and the angiogram films superimposed. All information on the angiogram that is the same as that found on the scout film will be obliterated (the same effect produced in *c)* while the added information becomes enhanced. *(F)* The final permanent print of the image produced by the superimposition of the mask and the angiogram film. (From Principles of Subtraction in Radiology, Wilmington, DE, E. I. du Pont de Nemours & Company, Inc., 1971.)

2. Prepare the diapositive mask.
3. Expose the angiogram films.
4. Superimpose the mask and angiogram films.
5. Make the final subtraction print.

Steps 1 and 3 are routinely done during any angiographic procedure and require no further comment. Remember that to produce adequate subtraction prints, there must be no discrepancy in position between the scout film and the angiogram film.

Preparation of the diapositive mask is the most critical step of the subtraction procedure. If the mask is not properly prepared, the final subtraction prints will be of poor quality. During discussion of this step, we review the theory behind the subtraction method.

A diapositive mask is an exact copy of the scout film, with the densities exactly reversed. This is the basis for the theory behind the subtraction methods. It is well known that details are visible on a radiograph because of contrast, with contrast defined as the difference of blackness between adjacent areas. In other words, details are visible because there are density differences on a radiograph. A film that possesses only one density does not show an image. The diapositive mask, which is a reversed image of the scout film, produces a radiograph of a single density when superimposed over the scout film. Because there is no contrast, there is no image.

If the diapositive mask is superimposed over an angiogram film, any information that was the same as that recorded on the scout film should be obliterated. Only the structures filled with contrast media should exhibit contrast. These structures should stand out and be clearly seen without confusing shadows.

This principle is illustrated as follows. Assume that a particular scout film possesses the following densities:

	Area A	Area B	Area C
Scout film	0.6	1.2	2.0

To produce a positive diapositive mask, it is important to produce reversed density differences that correspond exactly to the density differences on the scout film. In other words:

	Area A	Area B	Area C	
Scout film	0.6	1.2	2.0	
Diapositive mask	1.9	1.3	0.5	
Density difference be-tween areas			0.6	
			0.8	

When the scout film and diapositive mask are superimposed, the resultant densities should be equal:

	Area A	Area B	Area C
Scout film	0.6	1.2	2.0
Diapositive mask	1.9	1.3	0.5
Scout film plus diapo-sitive mask	2.5	2.5	2.5

Because the angiogram film is made using the same exposure factors as the scout film, the density differences of areas A, B, and C should equal those on the scout film. Also on the angiogram film is the density of area D, the contrast-filled vessels. If the angiogram film is superimposed over the diapositive mask, it can be readily seen that the only contrast that exists is between the contrast-filled vessels (area D) and the densities from areas A, B, and C. The contrast-filled vessels stand out clearly against the homogeneous background.

	Area A	Area B	Area C	Area D
Diapositive mask	1.9	1.3	0.5	0.0
Angiogram film	0.6	1.2	2.0	0.3
Diapositive mask plus angiogram film	2.5	2.5	2.5	0.3

It is important that the film used to prepare the diapositive mask produce a negative complementary to that of the scout film. In other words, it must neither exaggerate nor lessen the density differences. This property is a function of the film gamma ($\tilde{G}$), a sensitometric measurement that corresponds to the maximum slope, or gradient, of the characteristic curve of the film. This gamma is calculated by the use of a characteristic curve and by the following formula:

$$\text{Gamma} = \frac{D_2 - D_1}{\log E_2 - \log E_1}$$

where log E is the logarithmic value of the relative exposure and D is density.

Film used for subtraction must have a gamma of 1 (Fig. 26–2). The subtraction films

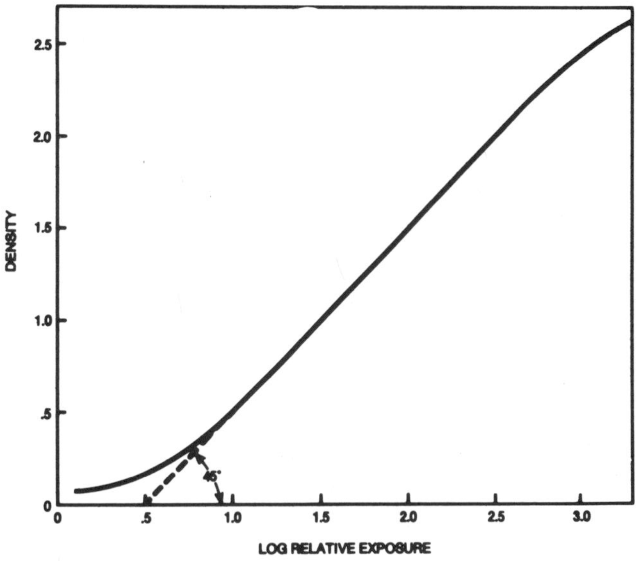

Figure 26–2. A sensitometric curve of du Pont Cronex subtraction film, showing that the curve forms a 45° angle with the base line. This produces a gamma of 1, a property necessary for all film used to make subtraction prints. (From Principles of Subtraction in Radiology, Wilmington, DE, E. I. du Pont de Nemours & Company, Inc., 1971.)

available are designed to yield a gamma of 1 when processed automatically. In general, subtraction films possess only one emulsion side, which should be remembered when preparing the diapositive mask.

If a permanent record of the superimposed diapositive mask and angiogram film is required, a copy of the superimposed films can easily be made.

Now that the theory of subtraction has been discussed and we are familiar with the general procedure, a presentation of the various techniques is in order. Subtraction can be performed by the direct x-ray, photographic, electronic, computer-assisted (digital) (see Chapter 6), and color addition methods.

DIRECT X-RAY METHOD

This is by far the simplest technique involving equipment normally found in any radiology department. An ordinary cassette is used to prepare the diapositive mask, eliminating the necessity for any commercial printing device. The mask is prepared by placing the following items into the cassette in sequential order from the front screen to the rear screen: scout film, unexposed subtraction film (emulsion side up), and opaque (black) paper.

The cassette is closed and receives x-ray exposure to produce the mask film, which is then processed. The mask is superimposed over the angiogram film and placed into the cassette replacing the scout film (front to rear—mask, angiogram film, and subtraction film), and the procedure is repeated to produce the final subtraction print. Although simple, this method has an important disadvantage: It does not produce quality subtraction prints because of radiation fog.

PHOTOGRAPHIC METHOD

The photographic method of subtraction is the method of choice for producing accurate diagnostic subtraction prints. It can be done using a homemade printing frame, a commercial photographic printing frame, or one of the mechanical printers available for duplication and subtraction (Fig. 26–3).

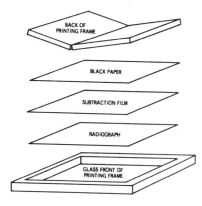

Figure 26–3. Schematic of a photographic printing frame that can be used for subtraction. (From Eastman Kodak Company.)

If a commercial printing frame is used, the procedure is essentially the same as that previously described for the direct x-ray method (Fig. 26–4). The major difference is that with the photographic method, the mask is produced by exposing the sandwich to an external light source. The light source for a homemade device or printing frame is usually a 25-W bulb at a distance of 6 ft from the printing frame. The usual exposure is approximately 3 s, depending on the density of the original film. The main advantage of this method is that the loss of detail resulting from radiation fog is eliminated. Other problems can be encountered, however, such as poor film contact and variability of the light exposure. These problems are usually overcome when a mechanical duplicator/subtraction device is used.

Occasionally, the original mask does not completely subtract all of the scout film images. When this occurs, it is possible to perform a second-order subtraction (composite-mask subtraction) to improve the quality of the final subtraction print. Second-order subtraction simply involves the preparation of a second mask from the combination of the scout film plus the original mask. This has the effect of destroying the density differences not subtracted by the first mask. The final subtraction print is made by superimposing the angiogram film and both masks and by substituting these for the scout film in the original subtraction sandwich (neutral density absorber, scout film

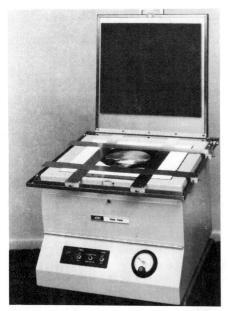

Figure 26–4. Du Pont Cronex duplicator subtractor. (From E. I. du Pont de Nemours & Company, Inc.)

taped to subtraction film, unexposed subtraction film emulsion side up, and opaque paper). Second-order subtraction is not achieved without some difficulty because perfect superimposition of three films is rather difficult and the combined density of the three films is high, which requires greater exposure or a brighter light source. The results of a second-order subtraction, however, are well worth the additional time involved in its preparation.

The duplicator/subtractor printers are equipped with three separate light sources—one for duplicating radiographs, one for subtraction, and a third for viewing the superimposed mask-angiogram combinations before a final print is prepared. The combination printers have greater capabilities for the subtraction process, and second-order subtractions are rarely, if ever, necessary. The actual subtraction can be performed much more quickly than by any of the methods previously discussed.

The diapositive mask is prepared by placing the scout film on the glass plate of the printer. The unexposed subtraction film is then placed over the scout film. The cover is closed, the subtraction mode is selected, the desired exposure time is set (recommended setting is approximately 1 s), and the unit is energized.[3] After the diapositive mask is developed, a final subtraction print is prepared. To do this, the mask is placed against the glass plate of the printer with the emulsion side up. The angiogram is placed over the mark, and by using the viewing light, accurate superimposition can be achieved. The viewing light is then turned off, and a sheet of unexposed subtraction film is placed with the emulsion side down over the superimposed films. The cover is closed, and the appropriate exposure setting is chosen (approximately twice that required to prepare the mask). The unit is then energized, and the print is exposed.

ELECTRONIC SUBTRACTION

Electronic subtraction is the most efficient of the methods discussed so far. It uses two vidicon cameras to record images of the scout film and of the angiogram phase. One radiograph is transmitted as a positive image, and the other is transmitted as a negative image. The signals are mixed and then transmitted to a television monitor, in which the similarities are subtracted out and the differences are accentuated. The image contrast can be adjusted to provide the viewer with the best possible subtraction image. If a permanent record of the electronic subtraction is desired, a cine or 35-mm camera may be attached to the unit to record the image. This type of system is useful when a great number of subtractions are routinely done. It can also accomplish subtraction more accurately and quickly than the direct x-ray and photographic methods. Compared with the other manual systems, electronic subtraction is much more costly. However, the advantage of this system is that it produces more highly detailed subtractions than the manual methods without the cost and installation required for digital subtraction systems. Figure 26–5 illustrates the equipment used for electronic subtraction.

SUBTRACTION BY COLOR ADDITION

Another method of subtraction that has been used in the past is subtraction by addition. This system depends on the addition of primary colors to increase the contrast of differences between two radiographs. This method was developed in 1965 by Wise and Ganson and requires that a simple viewer be constructed (Fig. 26–6).[2] The viewer consists of two light sources—one incandescent and one fluorescent—at right angles to each other and separated by a beam-splitting mirror. A red filter is placed in front of the incandescent source, and a blue filter is placed in front of the fluorescent source.

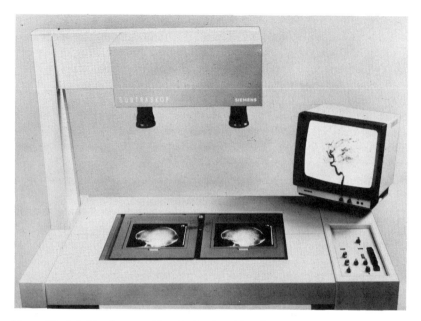

Figure 26–5. Subtraskop used for electronic subtraction. (From Siemens-Elema AB.)

The theory of subtraction by color addition is simple. The primary colors blue and red combine to produce a near-white light when transmitted in equal amounts from areas of similarity on the two radiographs. The images that are similar on the scout and the angiogram films transmit equal amounts of blue or red light. These produce a near-white light that shows up these portions in their normal black, gray, and white tones. The portions of the angiogram film that are different from the scout film transmit a higher percentage of red light. The result appears as an image in which the similarities

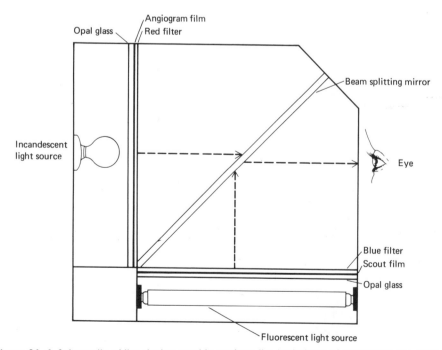

Figure 26–6. Schematic of the device used to perform the technique of subtraction by color addition.

are presented in normal tones, whereas the contrast-filled vessels stand out in red. To show the vessels contrasted in blue, the angiogram film must be placed behind the blue filter.

Combinations of other primary color filters may be used in this device to produce contrast in other colors. For example, yellow and green filters may be used during subtraction of the urinary or biliary systems. If the venous phase of an angiogram is placed under a blue filter and the arterial phase is placed under a red filter, the resultant subtracted image shows the arteries in red and the veins in blue.

Permanent records of color subtraction are made by photographing the resulting image with suitable color film; this can be accomplished with a 35-mm camera and Kodachrome II (daylight) or comparable film.

The advantages to color subtraction by addition are that it can be done quickly and accurately, with minimal expense.

SUMMARY

Enhancement of images of contrast-filled structures on a radiograph is possible with subtraction. The technique is useful during any contrast study but especially during angiography.

Successful subtraction depends on the preparation of a correctly exposed diapositive mask from the scout film, accurate superimposition of the mask and the angiogram, and no movement or position change between the exposure of the scout film and the angiogram.

There are five methods by which subtraction can be performed—direct x-ray, photographic, electronic, digital, and subtraction by addition. In the manual methods, such as the direct x-ray and photographic methods, first-order subtraction is usually sufficient; however, second-order subtraction may be occasionally required to further enhance detail. Subtraction by the addition of color is a simple and efficient method of enhancing detail during contrast radiography; a specialized viewing device is necessary for the proper performance of this technique.

REFERENCES

1. Principles of Subtraction in Radiology. Wilmington, DE, E. I. du Pont de Nemours & Company, 1971.
2. Wise, R. E., and Ganson, J.: Subtraction of radiographic images by color addition, an inexpensive improved method, Lahey Clin. Found. Bull., *14*:131, 1965.

SUGGESTED READINGS

Curry, T. S., Dowdey, J. E., and Murry, R. C.: Christensen's Introduction to the Physics of Diagnostic Radiology, 4th ed. Philadelphia, Lea & Febiger, 1990.
Frey, H. S., and Norman, A.: Radiographic subtraction by color addition, Radiology, *84*:123, 1965.
Joyce, J. W., et al.: Improved contrast in subtraction technique, Radiology, *94*:157, 1970.
Olendorf, W. H.: A modified subtraction technique for extreme enhancement of angiographic detail, Neurology, *15*:336, 1965.

Seeman, H. E.: Physical and Photographic Principles of Medical Radiography. New York, John Wiley & Sons, 1968.
Sweeny, R. J.: Subtraction technique in retrospect and an innovative device for making subtraction, duplication and slide copies of medical radiography, Radiol. Technol., *45*:249, 1973.
Wise, R. E., and Ganson, J.: Subtraction technique: Video and color methods, Radiology, *86*:814, 1966.

Appendix

Table A–1. MANUFACTURERS OF SPECIAL PROCEDURES EQUIPMENT

Company and Address	Product Type*
Ackrad Laboratories 70 Jackson Drive P. O. Box 1085 Cranford, NJ 07016	J (hysterosalpingography catheter)
A. D. A. C. 255 San Geronimo Way Sunnyvale, CA 94086	M
American Edwards Laboratories P. O. Box 11150 Santa Ana, CA 92711	I
Becton Dickinson and Company Becton Dickinson Division Rutherford, NJ 07070-1598	I
Berlex Imaging 300 Fairfield Road Wayne, NJ 07470	K
Blu-Ray, Inc. P. O. Box 337 Essex, CT 06426	H
Cook, Inc. P. O. Box 489 Bloomington, IN 47402	I
Cordis Corporation P. O. Box 525700 Miami, FL 33152	E, I
Eastman Kodak Company Rochester, NY 14650	G
E. I. Du Pont De Nemours & Company, Inc. Wilmington, DE 19898	G, H
Electro-Catheter Corporation 2100 Felver Court Rahway, NJ 07065	I
E. R. Squibb & Sons, Inc. P. O. Box 4000 Princeton, NJ 08540	F
Firma AB Kifa Solna, Sweden	I
Fonar Corporation 110 Marcus Drive Mellville, NY 11747-4292	K

Table continued on following page

Table A–1. MANUFACTURERS OF SPECIAL PROCEDURES EQUIPMENT *Continued*

Company and Address	Product Type*
General Electric Medical Systems 780 N. Fifth Avenue King of Prussia, PA 19406	K
Hitachi 1993 Case Parkway Twinsberg, OH 44087	K
Ilford, Inc. West 70 Century Road Paramus, NJ 07652	G
Imatron, Inc. 389 Oyster Point Boulevard South San Francisco, CA 94080	L
International Imaging Electronics, Inc. 901 S. Kay Addison, IL 60101	J (multiformat imaging devices)
Liebel-Flarsheim Company 2111 East Galbraith Road Cincinnati, OH 45215	C
Mallinckrodt Chemical Works 675 Brown Road Hazelwood, MO 63042	F, J (contrast agent warmer)
MCB Reagents E M Science 480 Democrat Road Gibbstown, NJ 08027	J (vital dyes)
Medi-Tech, Inc. 480 Pleasant Street P. O. Box 7407 Watertown, MA 02172	I, J (Van Sonnenberg sump)
Medrad, Inc. 566 Alpha Drive Pittsburgh, PA 15238	E, I
NAMIC Hospital Supply Division Pruyns Island Glens Falls, NY 12801	J (lymph duct cannulator)

Table **A–1**. MANUFACTURERS OF SPECIAL PROCEDURES EQUIPMENT *Continued*

Company and Address	Product Type*
Olympic Medical Corporation 4400 7th Avenue South Seattle, WA 98101	J (cassette holder and head immobilizer)
Phillips Medical Systems 5170 Campus Drive Plymouth Meeting, PA 19462	K
Picker International 595 Miner Road Cleveland, OH 44143	A, B, K, L, M
Resonex 81 Fayette Avenue Staten Island, NY 10350	K
Siemens Corporation 186 Wood Avenue South Iselin, NJ 08830	A, B, C, I, K, M
Unipoint Industries 1701 Prospect Street High Point, NC 27263-8580	J (polyvinyl alcohol sponge)
United States Catheter and Instrument Corporation P. O. Box 566 Billerica, MA 01821	I
Varian 1698 South Pioneer Road Salt Lake City, UT 84104	D
Winthrop Laboratories 90 Park Avenue New York, NY 10016	F
Xerox Medical Systems 125 N. Vinedo Avenue P. O. Box 5786 Pasadena, CA 91107	J (xeroradiography equipment)

*A: x-ray generating apparatus; B: x-ray tables; C: rapid sequence changers; D: x-ray tubes; E: automatic injection systems; F: contrast media; G: x-ray films; H: duplicators and subtractors; I: catheters, guide wires, needles, and accessories; J: specialty items (in parentheses); K: MRI equipment; L: CT equipment; M: digital radiography equipment.

Table A–2. XERORADIOGRAPHY TECHNIQUE GUIDE (NEGATIVE MODE)

THE FOLLOWING GUIDE IS FOR SINGLE-PHASE, FULL-WAVE RECTIFIED X-RAY EQUIPMENT USING A TUNGSTEN TARGET AND 2-MM ALUMINUM FILTRATION

Part	View	kVp	mA* Small	mA* Medium	mA* Large	Distance (in)	Bucky Grid 8:1	Tunnel	Contrast†	Density†
Hand	PA	120	15	20	25	36	No	No	B	C
	Oblique	120	15	20	25	36	No	No	B	C
	Lateral	120	20	25	25	36	No	No	B	C
Wrist	PA	120	20	25	30	36	No	No	B	C
	Lateral	120	20	25	30	36	No	No	B	C
Forearm	AP	120	20	25	30	36	No	No	C (B)	C
	Lateral	120	20	25	25	36	No	No	B	C
Elbow	AP	120	20	25	30	36	No	No	C	C
	Lateral	120	20	25	30	36	No	No	C	C
	Oblique	120	20	25	30	36	No	Yes	C	C
Humerus	AP	120	30	35	40	36	No	No	C	C
	Lateral	120	30	35	40	36	No	No	C	C
Shoulder	AP	120	60	75	90	36	No	Yes	C	C
Clavicle	Tangential	120	60	70	75	36	No	Yes	B	C
Cervical spine	AP	120	70	80	90	36	No	Yes	C	C
	Lateral	120	70	80	90	36	No	Yes	B	C
	Odontoid	120	70	80	90	36	No	Yes	B	C
Skull	All AP-PA	120	110	120	130	36	No	Yes	D	C
	All lateral	120	90	100	110	36	No	Yes	D	C
Ribs	AP	120	60	75	90	36	No	Yes	C	C
	Oblique	120	60	75	90	36	No	Yes	C	C
Hip	AP	120	400	500	600	40	Yes	Yes	D	D
	Lateral	120	400	500	600	40	Yes	Yes	D	D
Femur	AP	120	200	300	400	40	Yes	Yes	D	D
	Lateral	120	150	200	250	40	Yes	Yes	D	D
Knee	AP	120	35	40	45	36	No	Yes	C	C
	Lateral	120	40	45	50	36	No	Yes	C	C
Patella	Axial	120	30	35	40	36	No	Yes (optional)	B	C
Leg	AP	120	20	25	30	36	No	Yes	C	C
	Lateral	120	20	25	30	36	No	Yes	C	C
Ankle	AP	120	20	25	30	36	No	Yes	C	C
	Lateral	120	20	25	30	36	No	Yes	C	C
Foot	AP	120	20	25	30	36	No	Yes	B	C
	Oblique	120	20	25	30	36	No	Yes	B	C
	Lateral	120	20	25	30	36	No	Yes	B	C
Toes	AP	120	12	15	18	36	No	Yes	B	C
	Oblique	120	12	15	18	36	No	Yes	B	C

*For dry cast, increase mA 20 to 25%; for wet cast, increase mA 40 to 50%; with three-phase generation, reduce mA 30 to 40%.
†Last two columns show machine settings.
PA: posteroanterior; AP: anteroposterior.

Table A–3. XERORADIOGRAPHY TECHNIQUE GUIDE (NEGATIVE MODE)
FOR THE XR-100 XERORADIOGRAPHY CASSETTE
THE FOLLOWING GUIDE IS FOR SINGLE-PHASE, FULL-WAVE RECTIFIED X-RAY EQUIPMENT (XR-100 XERORADIOGRAPHY CASSETTE) USING TUNGSTEN TARGET AND 2-MM ALUMINUM FILTRATION

Part	View	kVp	mA* Small	Medium	Large	Distance (in)	Bucky Grid 8:1	Contrast†	Density†
Hand	PA	120	15	20	25	36	No	B	C
	Oblique	120	15	20	25	36	No	B	C
	Lateral	120	20	25	25	36	No	B	C
Wrist	PA	120	20	25	30	36	No	B	C
	Lateral	120	20	25	30	36	No	B	C
Forearm	AP	120	20	25	30	36	No	C (B)	C
	Lateral	120	20	25	25	36	No	B	C
Elbow	AP	120	20	25	30	36	No	C	C
	Lateral	120	20	25	30	36	No	C	C
	Oblique	120	20	25	30	36	No	C	C
Humerus	AP	120	30	35	40	36	No	C	C
	Lateral	120	30	35	40	36	No	C	C
Shoulder	AP	120	60	75	90	36	No	C	C
Clavicle	Tangential	120	60	70	75	36	No	B	C
Cervical spine	AP	120	70	80	90	36	No	C	C
	Lateral	120	70	80	90	36	No	B	C
	Odontoid	120	70	80	90	36	No	B	C
Skull	All AP-PA	120	110	120	130	36	No	D	C
	All lateral	120	90	100	110	36	No	D	C
Ribs	AP	120	60	75	90	36	No	C	C
	Oblique	120	60	75	90	36	No	C	C
Hip	AP	120	400	500	600	40	Yes	D	D
	Lateral	120	400	500	600	40	Yes	D	D
Femur	AP	120	200	300	400	40	Yes	D	D
	Lateral	120	150	200	250	40	Yes	D	D
Knee	AP	120	35	40	45	36	No	C	C
	Lateral	120	40	45	50	36	No	C	C
Patella	Axial	120	30	35	40	36	No	B	C
Leg	AP	120	20	25	30	36	No	C	C
	Lateral	120	20	25	30	36	No	C	C
Ankle	AP	120	20	25	30	36	No	C	C
	Lateral	120	20	25	30	36	No	C	C
Foot	AP	120	20	25	30	36	No	B	C
	Oblique	120	20	25	30	36	No	B	C
	Lateral	120	20	25	30	36	No	B	C
Toes	AP	120	12	15	18	36	No	B	C
	Oblique	120	12	15	18	36	No	B	C

*For dry cast, increase mA 20 to 25%; for wet cast, increase mA 40 to 50%; with three-phase generation, reduce mA 30 to 40%.
†Last two columns show machine settings.
PA: posteroanterior; AP: anteroposterior.

Index

Note: Page numbers in *italics* refer to illustrations; page numbers followed by *t* refer to tables.

A

Activation system–triggering reactions, to contrast agents, 69
Additive iterative reconstruction of image, in CT, 113
Analgesics, preangiographic, 160
Analog data, definition of, 96
Analog-to-digital (A/D) conversion, in digital subtraction angiography, 101
Analytic reconstruction of image, in CT, 113
Anaphylactic reactions, to contrast agents, 69
Angiocardiography, 214–228
  anatomic considerations on, 214, *215*, 216, *216–218*, 218–222
  contraindications to, 222
  contrast media for, 222–223
  equipment for, 225, 227
  indications for, 222
  parameters for, with automatic injectors, 57*t*
  patient positioning for, 228
  procedure for, 223–224
  selective, 223, 224
Angiogram film, in subtraction, 390, 392
Angiographic tube rating charts, 7–8, *9–10*
  for magnification techniques, 386, *387*
Angiography, 155–212
  care before, 161–162
  cerebral, 232–249. See also *Cerebral angiography.*
  consultation on, 158
  contrast injection and filming in, 166
  definition of, 156
  digital subtraction, 96–108. See also *Digital subtraction angiography (DSA).*
  equipment preparation for, 161
  historical perspective on, 157–158
  informed consent for, 158
  magnetic resonance, 147, *153*
  patient discharge following, 167
  patient instruction for, 161–162
  postprocedural care and instructions in, 166–167
  preangiographic pharmacological agents for, 159–161
  preexamination history for, 158
  principles of, 156–167
    general, 158
  procedures for, parameters for, 56*t*–58*t*
  renal, 202–212. See also *Renal angiography.*
  venous, 179–192. See also *Venous angiography.*
  vessel access establishment in, 162–166
Angioplasty, percutaneous, coronary rotational, 344, *346*

Angioplasty *(Continued)*
  transluminal, 339–342
Aorta, abdominal, 171, *173*
  ascending, 169, *170*
  descending, 171, *172*, *173*
Aortic arch, 169, *170*
  branches of, 232–233
Aortic flush method, of arteriography, 224
Aortic sinuses, 218
Aortography, 169–178
  anatomic considerations for, 169, *170*, 171, *172*, *173*
  contraindications to, 173
  contrast media for, 174
  definition of, 169
  equipment for, 176
  indications for, 171–173
  parameters for, with automatic injectors, 56*t*, 58*t*
  patient positioning for, 176, *177*, 178
  percutaneous catheter, 175
  procedure for, 174–175
  translumbar, 174–175
Aqueduct of Sylvius, 253
Arcuate veins, 205
Arrhythmias, ECG evaluation of, automatic injector in, 44–47
  major, characteristics of, 445*t*
Arterial puncture techniques, for angiography, 163–165
Arteriography, coronary, 223–224
  femoral, 193–200. See also *Femoral arteriography.*
  parameters for, with automatic injectors, 56*t*, 57*t*
Artery(ies), anterior interventricular branch, 218–219
  atrioventricular node, 221
  axillary, puncture of, for angiography, 163–164
  basilar, 235, *237*
  brachial, puncture of, for angiography, 163, 164
  carotid, internal, 233–234
  cerebellar, 235
  cerebral, 232–233
    anterior, 233–234
    middle, 233, 234
  conus, 220
  coronary, 218, *219*
    left circumflex, 219
    left main, 218–220
    right main, 220–221
  direct exposure of, for angiography, 166
  femoral, 193
    puncture of, for angiography, 163

Artery(ies) *(Continued)*
  iliac, 193
  in femoral arteriography, 193, *194*, 194*t*, 195
  inferior suprarenal, 203
  interlobular, 205–206
  left circumflex branch, 218
  marginal, left, 219–220
    right, 220
  paramedian, 235
  popliteal, 193
  posterior descending, 220
  posterior interventricular branch, 220
  renal, 203, 205–206
  right main, 220–221
  tibial, 195
  translumbar puncture of, for angiography, 164, *165*
  vertebral, 234–235
Arthrography, 309–317
  anatomic considerations on, 309–310, 312
  contraindications to, 313
  contrast media for, 313
  double-contrast, 314
  equipment for, 314–315
  fluoroscopic method of, 314
  indications for, 312–313
  patient positioning for, 315, *316*, 317, 318*t*
  procedure for, 313–314
Aspiration bronchography, 305–306
Atherectomy, directional coronary, 343–344, *345*
  excisional, 343–344
  extraction, 344, *346*
Atrioventricular node artery, 221
Atrium, 214, 216, *216–217*
Atropine, preangiographic, 161
Automatic injection devices, 38–65
  automatic injectors as, 39–54. See also *Automatic injectors.*
  CT injectors as. See *CT injectors.*
  lymphangiographic injectors as, 63–65
Automatic injectors, 39–54
  basic components of, 39, *40*, 41, *42*
  control panel of, 39, *40*
  detachable injector head of, 48–49
  double-syringe assembly of, 49
  electrocardiogram triggering device in, 41, 43, 44*t*
  heating device of, 41
  high-pressure mechanism in, 41, *42*
  in arrhythmia evaluation, 44–47
  injection pressure of, 34
  operation of, 49, 51–54
    constant flow rate in, 51–52
    constant pressure in, 53–54
  optional components of, 41, *42*, 43–49
  safety devices of, 49, *50–51*
  strip chart recorders and/or oscilloscope monitors of, 48
  syringe for, 39, 41, *42*
Axillary artery puncture, for angiography, 163–164
Azygos system, venous angiography for, 186

B

Back projection image reconstruction, in CT, 113
Ball-and-socket joint, 310
Balloon occlusion, to reduce blood flow, 334, *335*
Basilar artery, 235, *237*
Benadryl, preangiographic, 159–160

Biliary calculus removal, nonoperative
  percutaneous, 366–367
  postoperative, 364, *365*, 366
Binary and decimal systems, relationship between, 101*t*
Binary digit, 100
Biopsy, needle, 351–354
Biplane operation, of rapid sequence changers, 25, *26*
Bit, 101
Blood flow, techniques to increase, 338–348
  contraindications to, 338–339
  indications for, 338
  procedures for, 339–347
    excisional atherectomy as, 343–344
    infusion of vasodilators as, 347
    intravascular thrombolysis as, 346
    percutaneous transluminal angioplasty as, 339–342
  techniques to reduce, 331–338
    complications of, 337–338
    contraindications to, 331–332
    indications for, 331–332
    procedure for, 332–337
      intravascular electrocoagulation as, 337
      transcatheter embolization and balloon occlusion as, 332–337
      vasoconstrictor infusion as, 337
Blood vessels, establishing access to, for angiography, 162–166
Brachial artery puncture, for angiography, 163, 164
Brachiocephalic vein, 239
Brain, anatomy of, 252–254
  magnetic resonance imaging of, 269, *272*
Brainstem, 252
Bristle brush, to occlude blood vessels, 336
Bronchi, 299–300
  lobar, 301–302
  segmental, 301–303
Bronchography, 299–308
  anatomic considerations on, 299–303
  aspiration, 305
  catheter insertion method of, 305
  contraindications to, 303
  contrast media for, 304
  equipment for, 306
  indications for, 303
  patient positioning for, *307*, 307*t*, 308
  patient preparation for, 304
  percutaneous transtracheal puncture of intercricothyroid membrane for, 305
  procedure for, 304–306
Bronchopulmonary segments, 302–303
Buckbee-Meers resolution plate, in focal spot size determination, 384–385
Byte, 101

C

Calculi, biliary, nonoperative percutaneous removal of, 366–367
  postoperative, 364, *365*, 366
  renal, removal of, 363, *364*
Camera(s), serial spot film, 30–31
  television, for digital subtraction angiography, 105
Cardiac cycle, 218
  coronary arteriography and, 223–224
Cardiovascular reactions, to contrast agents, 69

Carotid artery, internal, 233–234
Cartilage, hyaline articular, 310
Cassette, receiving, of cut film changers, 21
Cassette changers, rapid sequence, 24
Catheter(s), 77–93
    accessories for, 87–88, 89*t*, *89–90*
    balloon, to occlude blood vessels, 334, *335*
    custom-shaping of, 79–82
    diameter of, effect of, on constant pressure injectors, 53
    distal end of, custom-shaping of, *80*, 81
    guide wires for, 84, 87
    length of, effect of, on constant pressure injectors, 53
    needles for, 87–88
    procedure trays and sets for, 88, 91–93
    proximal end of, forming of, *81*, 82
    shape of, 83–84, *85–86*
    side holes in, effect of, on constant pressure injectors, 53–54
        placement of, *81*, 82
    size of, 82–83
    tip of, cutting of, *80*, 91
        preparation of, 79–81
    utility of, 83–84, *86–87*
Catheter insertion method, of bronchography, 305
Catheterization, angiographic, 162–163
    risks of, 167
    cardiac, 213–228. See also *Angiocardiography*.
    percutaneous, for renal angiography, 208–209
Cellulose sponge embolic media, to occlude blood vessels, 333
Central nervous system radiography, 251–269
    anatomic considerations on, 252–256
        in brain, 252–254
        in spinal cord, 254–256
    magnetic resonance imaging of brain in, 269, *272*
    myelography in, 256–267. See also *Myelography*.
    pneumoencephalography as, 267–269
    ventriculography as, 267–269
Cerebellar arteries, 235
Cerebellum, 252
Cerebral angiography, 232–249
    anatomic considerations on, 232–239
        arterial supply in, 232–238
        circle of Willis in, 236, *237*, 238
        internal carotid artery in, 233–234
        venous drainage in, 238–239
        vertebrobasilar system in, 234–235
    contraindications to, 240
    contrast media for, 241
    equipment for, 242–244
    indications for, 240
    patient positioning for, 244, *245–248*, 248–249, 249*t*
    procedure of, 241–242
Cerebral artery, anterior, 233–234
    middle, 233, 234
Cerebrum, 252
Cervical myelography, opaque, patient positioning for, 266–267
Cineangiographic tube rating charts, 8, 11–12
Cinefluorographic systems, 31, *34–35*, 35, *36*
Circle of Willis, 236, *237*, 238
Circulus arteriosus, 236, *237*, 238
Circumflex branch, left, 218
Cisternae, subarachnoid, 253–254
Cisternal pneumoencephalography, 268
Cisternal puncture method, of myelography, 259, *260*

Cleaning, of room, room design considerations for, 6
Coils, occluding, for blood flow reduction, 334–336
Color addition, subtraction by, 395–397
Compression table, of cut film changers, 21
Computed tomography (CT), 110–131
    for needle biopsy guidance, 353–354
    of spine, 259, *261*
    standard, 110–124
        attenuation values in, 113, *114*
        equipment for, 117, *118–120*, 120–121, *122*, 123
        historical perspective on, 110
        image reconstruction methods in, 113
        patient preparation for, 124
        physical principles of, 112–113
        room design for, 113, 117
        technical considerations for, 123
        windowing in, 113, *115–116*
    ultrafast, 124–131
        equipment for, 129
        physical principles of, 124–125, 127
        room design for, 127, *128*
        technical considerations on, 129–131
Computer group, of CT systems, 117, 121
Computer units, in MRI, 145
Condylar joint, 310
Consent, informed, for angiography, 158
Constant flow rate injectors, 51–52
Constant pressure injectors, 53–54
Consultation, on angiography, 158
Continuous digital fluorography, for digital subtraction angiography, 105, 107
Contrast agents, 66–75. See also *Contrast media*.
Contrast media, 66–75
    characteristics of, 68*t*, 71–75
    for aortography, 174
    for arthrography, 313
    for bronchography, 304
    for cerebral angiography, 241
    for femoral arteriography, 197
    for hysterosalpingography, 279–280
    for lymphangiography, 289–290
    for myelography, 257–258
    for pneumoencephalography, 268
    for renal angiography, 207–208
    for ventriculography, 268
    injection of, for angiography, 166
    iodine concentration of, 73–74
    ionic organic iodine compounds as, 72
    low osmolality, 73
    miscibility of, 74
    negative, 66–67
    nonionic, 71, 72–73
    overdose of, 67, 69
    persistence of, 74
    positive, 67
    precautions to take before and after administration of, 70–71
    reactions to, 67, 69–71
    specialty, 74–75
    types of, 66–67
    viscosity of, 73
Control-display system, in MRI, 145
Control group, of CT systems, 117, 121, *122*, 123
Control panel, of automatic injectors, 39, *40*
Conus arteriosus, 216
Conus artery, 220
Coronary arteriography, 223–224

Coronary artery, 218, *219*
  left circumflex, 219
  left main, 218–220
  right main, 220–221
Coronary sinus, 221
Cortex, renal, 202
CT injectors, 54, 58, *59*, 60t–63t
Cubital vein puncture, for angiography, 165
Cut film changers, 19, *20*, 21, *22–23*, 24

D

Data, analog, 96
  digital, 96
Decimal and binary systems, relationship between,
  101t
Demerol, preangiographic, 160
Descending artery, posterior, 220
Detachable injector head, of automatic injectors,
  48–49
Detector system, 117
Diapositive mask, in subtraction, 391–393
Diazepam, preangiographic, 161
Diencephalon, 252
Digital data, definition of, 96
Digital subtraction angiography (DSA), 96–108
  advantages of, 198
  basic principles of, 98–102
  contrast media for, 197
  disadvantages of, 198
  energy, 107
  equipment for, 102–105
  hybrid, 107
  image in, processing of, 100–102
    storage of, 102
  imaging capabilities of, 105, *106*, 107–108
  intra-arterial, 97–98
  intravenous, 97
  medical aspects of, 97–98
  projections for, 200
  temporal, 107
Digital-to-analog (D/A) conversion, in digital
  subtraction angiography, 101–102
Diphenhydramine, preangiographic, 159–160
Direct puncture technique, for cerebral
  angiography, 241–242
Direct x-ray method, of subtraction, 393
Directional coronary atherectomy, 343–344, *345*
Discharge, postangiographic, 167
Double-syringe assembly, of automatic injectors, 49
Drainage, percutaneous, 356, 358–359, *359–363*
Drainage methods, for needle biopsy, 354–359,
  359–363
Dura mater, spinal, 255
Dural sinuses, 238–239

E

Edge enhancement, in digital subtraction
  angiography, 108
Elastomer, silicon, to occlude blood vessels, 336
Electrocardiogram (ECG), normal, 44t
Electrocardiogram triggering device, of automatic
  injectors, 41, 43, 44t
Electrocoagulation, intravascular, to occlude blood
  vessels, 337
Electronic subtraction, 395, *396*
Ellipsoidal joint, 310

Embolic media, cellulose sponge, to occlude blood
  vessels, 333
  liquid, 336–337
Embolization, transcatheter, to reduce blood flow,
  332–337
Energy subtraction, in digital radiography, 107
Equipment, for angiocardiography, 225, 227
  for angiography, preparation of, 161
  for aortography, 176
  for arthrography, 314–315
  for bronchography, 306
  for cerebral angiography, 242–244
  for computed tomography, 117, *118–120*, 120–
    121, *122*, 123
  for digital subtraction angiography, 102, *103–104*,
    105
  for femoral arteriography, 197–199
  for hysterosalpingography, 281–282
  for lymphangiography, 292, *293–294*
  for magnetic resonance imaging, 143, *144–145*,
    145, *146*
  for magnification, 383–386, *387–388*, 388
  for myelography, 260, 263, 263t
  for renal angiography, 210–211
  for sialography, 323
  for ultrafast computed tomography, 129
  for venous angiography, 189, 192
  manufacturers of, 399t–401t
  room design considerations for, 6–7
Excisional atherectomy, 343–344
Exposure field, of cut film changers, 21
External iliac artery, 193
Extracorporeal shock wave lithotripsy, 367
Extraction atherectomy, 344, *346*
Extremity, lower, venous angiography for, 187, 189
  upper, venous angiography for, 185, *188*

F

Fallopian tubes, 276
Femoral arteriography, 193–200
  anatomic considerations on, 193, *194*, 194t, 195–
    196
  contraindications to, 197
  contrast media for, 197
  equipment for, 197–199
  indications for, 196–197
  patient positioning for, 199–200
  procedure for, 197
  serial filming method of, 198
  single-film technique of, 198
Femoral artery, 193
  puncture of, for angiography, 163
Femoral vein puncture, for angiography, 165
Fentanyl, preangiographic, 160
Fibrinolysis, 346
Film changers, cut, 19, *20*, 21, *22–23*, 24
  for magnification techniques, 386
  mounting stand assembly and, 16–17, 19, *20*, 21
  rapid serial, 15–24
  roll, 16–17, *18*, 19
Film coverage, calculation of, 12, *13*
Film processing, room design considerations for, 6
Filming, for angiography, 166
Fluorography, continuous digital, for digital
  subtraction angiography, 105, 107
  pulsed digital, for digital subtraction angiography,
    105
Fluoroscopic method of arthrography, 314

Focal spot size determination, for magnification
    techniques, 384–385
Focal spot tubes, fractional, for magnification
    techniques, 384
Foramen, of Luschka, 253
    of Magendie, 253
    of Monro, 253
Foreign bodies, intravascular, removal of, 347–348
Fractional focal spot tubes, for magnification
    techniques, 384
French gauge scale, for catheter sizes, 82–83
Frequency encoding, in MRI, 140

G

Gadolinium diethylenetriaminepenta-acetic acid
    (Gd-DTPA), as contrast agent in MRI, 74–75
Gas ionization detector, for CT system, 117, 120–
    121
Gelfoam, to occlude blood vessels, 333
Geometric magnification, 381–383
Glands, parotid, 320–321
    sublingual, 321
    submandibular, 321
Gliding joint, 309
Glomerulus, 202, 205
Gradient coil system, in MRI, 145
Gradient-echo sequence, in MRI, 139
Great cardiac vein, 221
Grid, and screens, intensifying, in roll film
    changers, 17
Guide wires, for catheters, 84, 87

H

Heart, 214, 215, 216–217
    rhythm of, ECG evaluation of, 45
Heat units, room design considerations for, 7
Heating device, of automatic injectors, 41
    of lymphangiographic injectors, 63, 65
Hemiazygos system, venous angiography for, 186
Henle's loop, 203, 205
High-pressure mechanism, of automatic injectors,
    42
Hindbrain, 252
Hinge joint, 309
Hyaline articular cartilage, 310
Hybrid subtraction, in digital radiography, 107
Hydroxyzine hydrochloride, preangiographic, 159
Hysterosalpingography, 276–284
    anatomic considerations on, 276–277
    contraindications to, 279
    contrast media for, 279–280
    equipment for, 281–282
    indications for, 277–279
    patient positioning for, 282, 283, 283t, 284
    patient preparation for, 280
    procedure for, 280–281

I

Image, in CT, reconstruction methods for, 113
    in digital subtraction angiography, magnification
        of, 108
        processing of, 100–102
        storage of, 102
Image fixing, in xeroradiography, 379

Image intensification, in indirect imaging systems,
    27–28
Image intensifier, for digital subtraction
    angiography, 105
Image recording systems, 15–37
    basic operational considerations for, 24–25
    biplane operation of, 25, 26
    cut, 19, 20, 21, 22–23, 24
    indirect, 27–31, 32–35, 35, 36. See also Indirect
        imaging systems.
    rapid sequence cassette changers as, 24
    rapid serial film changers as, 15–24
Image reproduction devices, in CT, 123
Image zoom, in digital subtraction angiography, 108
Imaging capabilities, of digital subtraction
    angiography, 105, 106, 107–108
Imaging group, of CT systems, 117, 118–120, 120–
    121
Indirect imaging systems, 27–35
    image intensification in, 27–28
    laser, 2
    photofluorographic systems of, 30–35. See also
        Photofluorographic systems.
    videodisc system in, 28–29
    videotape system in, 28
Inferior suprarenal artery, 203
Inferior vena cava, 182, 206–207
    venous angiography for, 186, 190
Informed consent, for angiography, 158
Infusion, of vasoconstrictors, to occlude blood
    vessels, 337
    of vasodilators, to increase blood flow, 347
Injection devices, automatic, 38–65. See also
    Automatic injection devices.
Injection pressure, in automatic injectors, 54, 55
Injectors, automatic, 39–54. See also Automatic
    injectors.
    CT, 54, 58, 59, 60t–63t
    lymphangiographic, 63, 64, 65
Innominate vein, 239
Instructions, patient, postangiographic, 166–167
    preangiographic, 161–162
Intercricothyroid membrane, percutaneous
    transtracheal puncture of, for bronchography,
    305
Interlobar veins, 205
Interlobular artery, 205–206
Internal carotid artery, 233–234
Internal iliac artery, 193
Internal jugular vein puncture, for angiography, 166
Interventional radiography, 329–369
    nonvascular, 351–368. See also Nonvascular inter-
        ventional procedures.
    room and suite design for, 5–6
    vascular, 330–348. See also Vascular interven-
        tional procedures.
Interventional radiology, definition of, 330
Interventricular branch, anterior, 218–219
    posterior, 220
Interventricular veins, 221
Intravascular electrocoagulation, to occlude blood
    vessels, 337
Intravascular foreign bodies, removal of, 347–348
Intravascular thrombolysis, 346
Inversion-recovery sequence, in MRI, 138
Iodine compounds, ionic organic, as contrast
    agents, 72
Iodine concentration, of contrast agents, 73–74
Ionic organic iodine compounds, as contrast agents,
    72

Island of Reil, 234
Isobutyl-2-cyanoacrylate (IBCA), to occlude blood vessels, 336
Iterative reconstruction, of image in CT, 113

J

Joint(s), cartilaginous, 309
    fibrous, 309
    synovial, 309–310
Joint capsule, 310
Jugular vein, internal, 239
    puncture of, for angiography, 166

K

Kidneys, 202
Knife, film cutoff, manual, 16

L

Landmarking, surgical, in digital subtraction angiography, 108
Large-format camera, 30–31
Laser angioplasty, percutaneous, 341–342
Laser imaging systems, 29
Leptomeninges, 253
    spinal, 256
Liquid embolic media, to occlude blood vessels, 336–337
Lithotripsy, extracorporeal shock wave, 367
Low osmolality contrast agents, 73
Lumbar myelography, opaque, patient positioning for, 263–264, *265*, 266
Lumbar pneumoencephalography, 268
Lumbar puncture method, of myelography, 258–259
Lung(s), 300–303
    left, 301–303
    right, 300–301
Lymph nodes, 287, *288*
Lymph vessels, 286–287
Lymphangiographic injectors, 63, *64*, 65
Lymphangiography, 285–297
    anatomic considerations on, 286–287
    contraindications to, 289
    contrast media for, 289–290
    equipment for, 292, *293–294*
    indications for, 289
    patient positioning for, 292, *295–296*, 297, 297*t*
    patient preparation for, 290
    procedure for, 290–291

M

Magazine, receiving, in roll film changers, 17
    supply, in cut film changers, 21
    in roll film changers, 17
Magnet system, in MRI, 143
Magnetic resonance angiography (MRA), 147, *153*
Magnetic resonance imaging (MRI), 133–147
    equipment for, 143, *144–145*, *146*
    Gd-DTPA in, 74–75
    gradient system of, 139–140
    of brain, 269, *272*
    of spine, 260, *262*
    physical principles of, 133–139
    room design for, 140–141, *142*, 143

Magnetic resonance imaging (MRI) *(Continued)*
    technical considerations on, 145, 147, *148–152*
Magnification, equipment for, 383–386, *387–388*, 388
    geometric, 381–383
    photographic, 381
    principles of, 381–388
    serial, 381–388
    types of, 381–382
Manual film cutoff knife, 16
Manufacturers, of special procedures equipment, 399*t*, 401*t*
Marginal artery, 219–220
Marginal veins, 221
Medulla, 252
    renal, 203
Medullary vein, 205
Meglumine salts, as contrast agents, 72
Membrane, intercricothyroid, percutaneous transtracheal puncture of, for bronchography, 305
    synovial, 310
Meninges, cerebral, 253–254
    spinal cord, 254–256
Meperidine, preangiographic, 160
Mesencephalon, 252
Miscibility, of contrast agents, 74
Monitor, for digital subtraction angiography, 105
Morphine sulfate, preangiographic, 160
Mounting stand, of cut film changers, 21
Myelography, 251, 256–267
    contraindications to, 256
    contrast media for, 257–258
    equipment for, 260,`263
    indications for, 256
    opaque, cervical, patient positioning for, 266–267
        lumbar, patient positioning for, 263–264, *265*, 266
        thoracic, patient positioning for, 266
    patient positioning for, 263–264, 266–267
    patient preparation for, 256–257
    procedure of, 258–260

N

Naloxone, preangiographic, 161
Narcan, preangiographic, 161
Needle biopsy, 351–354
    contraindications to, 352
    guidance methods for, 352–354
    indications for, 351–352
Needles, for catheters, 87–88
Nembutal, preangiographic, 159
Nephrons, 202, 203, *205*
Nephrostomy, percutaneous catheter, 356, 358–359, *359–363*. See also *Percutaneous catheter nephrostomy (PCN)*.
Neuroradiography, 231–273
    central nervous system radiography in, 251–272. See also *Central nervous system radiography*.
    cerebral angiography in, 232–249. See also *Cerebral angiography*.
Nonionic contrast agents, 71, 72–73
Nonoperative percutaneous biliary calculi removal, 366–367
Nonvascular interventional procedures, 351–368
    needle biopsy as, 351–354. See also *Needle biopsy*.

Nonvascular interventional procedures *(Continued)*
  percutaneous calculi removal as, 363–667. See
    also *Percutaneous calculi removal.*
  puncture and drainage methods as, 354–359, *359–
    363*

O

Object-image distance (OID), in geometric
    magnification, 381–383
Occipital sinuses, 239
Occluding spring emboli, to occlude blood vessels,
    334–336
Occlusion, balloon, to reduce blood flow, 334, *335*
Opaque myelography, cervical, patient positioning
    for, 266–267
  lumbar, patient positioning for, 263–264, *265*, 266
  thoracic, patient positioning for, 266
Oscilloscope monitors, of automatic injectors, 48
Ovaries, 276
Overdose, of contrast agents, 67, 69
Oviduct, 276
Oxygen, centralized supply of, room design
    considerations for, 6

P

Paramedian arteries, 235
Parotid glands, 320–321
Pelvis, venous angiography for, 186
Penumbra, in magnification techniques, 383
Percutaneous biliary calculus removal,
    nonoperative, 366–367
Percutaneous calculus removal, 363–367
  complications of, 366
  for postoperative biliary calculi, 364, *365*, 366
  for renal calculi, 363, *364*, *365*
Percutaneous catheter aortography, 175
Percutaneous catheter nephrostomy (PCN), 356,
    358–359, *359–363*
  applications of, 356, 358
  complications of, 359
  procedure for, 358–359, *359–363*
Percutaneous catheterization, for renal
    angiography, 208–209
Percutaneous coronary rotational angioplasty, 344,
    346
Percutaneous drainage, 356, 358–359, *359–363*
Percutaneous puncture, for needle biopsy, 356,
    357–358
Percutaneous transluminal angioplasty (PTA), 339–
    342
Percutaneous transtracheal puncture, of
    intercricothyroid membrane, for
    bronchography, 305
Persistence, of contrast agents, 74
Phase encoding, in MRI, 140
Phase-in time, in rapid sequence changers, 24–25
Phenergan, preangiographic, 159
Phenobarbital, preangiographic, 159
Photofluorographic systems, 30–31, *32–34*, 35, *36*
  cinefluorographic, 31, *34–35*, 35, *36*
  serial spot film cameras in, 30–31, *32–33*
Photographic magnification, 381
Photographic method, of subtraction, 393–395
Pia mater, spinal, 256
Pinhole method, of focal spot size determination,
    384, *385*

Pivot joint, 309
Plane joint, 309
Plate, in xeroradiography, charging of, 373–374
  cleaning and conditioning of, 379
  development of, 376–378
  x-ray exposure of, 375
Pneumoencephalography, 251, 267–269
  cisternal, 268
  contrast media for, 268
  lumbar, 268
  patient positioning for, 269, *269*, *270*, 271t
  procedure for, 268
Pneumomyelogram, 257
Pons, 252
Popliteal artery, 193
Positioning of patient, for angiocardiography, 228
  for aortography, 176, *177*, 178
  for arthrography, 315, *316*, 317, 318t
  for bronchography, 305, *307*, 307t
  for cerebral angiography, 244, *245–248*, 248–249,
    249t
    for anteroposterior view, 244, *245–246*, 249t
    for lateral view, 244, *247*, 249t
    for supine oblique view, 244, 248, *248*, 249t
    for tangential projection, 248–249, *249*, 249t
    for transorbital projection, 248, *248*, 249t
  for femoral arteriography, 199–200
  for hysterosalpingography, 282, *283*, 283t, 284
  for lymphangiography, 292, *295–296*, 297, 297t
  for myelography, 263–264, *265*, 266–267
  for pneumoencephalography, 269, *269*, *270*, 271t
  for renal angiography, 211
  for sialography, 324–326, 327t
  for venous angiography, 192
  for ventriculography, 269
PR intervals, ECG in evaluation of, 45
PR ratio, ECG in evaluation of, 45
Preangiographic pharmacological agents, 159–161
Precession, in MRI, 136–137
  steady-state free, 139
Preexamination history, for angiography, 158
Pressure mechanism, of lymphangiographic
    injectors, 65
Pressure plate, in roll film changers, 17
Procedure trays, of sets, 88, 91–93
Procedures, special, 2–14. See also *Special
    procedure(s).*
Program selector, in roll film changers, 17, 19
  of cut film changers, 21, *23*, 24
Progressive scan, for digital subtraction
    angiography, 105
Promethazine hydrochloride, preangiographic, 159
Psychogenic reactions, to contrast agents, 69
Pulsed digital fluorography, for digital subtraction
    angiography, 105
Puncture, axillary artery, 163–164
  brachial artery, 163, 164
  cubital vein, 165
  femoral artery, 163
  femoral vein, 165
  internal jugular vein, 165
  methods of, for needle biopsy, 354–359, *359–363*
  percutaneous, for needle biopsy, 356, *357–358*
  percutaneous transtracheal, of intercricothyroid
    membrane for bronchography, 305
  translumbar, 164, *165*

Q

QRS complex interval, ECG in evaluation of, 45

R

Radiographic tube, for magnification techniques, 384
Radiography, central nervous system, 251–269. See also *Central nervous system radiography.*
Rapid sequence camera, 30–31
Rapid sequence cassette changers, 24
  for magnification techniques, 386
Rapid serial film changers, 15–24
  roll, 16–17, *18*, 19
Receiving cassette, in cut film changers, 21
Receiving magazine, in roll film changers, 17
Reil, island of, 234
Relaxation, in MRI, 136
Renal angiography, 202–212
  anatomic considerations on, 202–207
  contraindications to, 207
  contrast media for, 207–208
  equipment for, 210–211
  indications for, 207
  patient positioning for, 211–212
  procedure for, 208–210
Renal artery, 203
Renal calculi removal, 363, *364*
Renal sinus, 205
Renal vein, 205
Renal venography, 210
Resonance, definition of, 135
RF synthesizer, in MRI, 143
Roll film changers, 16–17, *18*, 19
Room, computed tomography, design of, 113, 117
  magnetic resonance imaging, design of, 140–141, *142*, 143
  special procedure, design of, 3, *4*, 614
  ultrafast computed tomography, design of, 127, *128*

S

Sacral hiatus puncture method, of myelography, 259, *261*
Saddle joint, 310
Saddle type coil, in MRI, 143
Safety devices, of automatic injectors, 49, *50–51*
Sagittal sinuses, 238
Salivary glands and ducts, radiographic visualization of, 320–326
Saturation-recovery sequence, in MRI, 138
Scintillation detector, for CT system, 117, 120–121
Scout film, in subtraction, 390, 392
Screens, and grids, intensifying, in roll film changers, 17
Sedatives, preangiographic, 159–160
Seldinger approach, to percutaneous arterial puncture, 175
Selective angiocardiography, 223, 224
Serial spot film cameras, 30–31
Sets, procedure, 88, 91–93
Shadowing, 101
Shimming coil system, in MRI, 145
Sialography, 320–326
  anatomic considerations on, 320–321
  contraindications to, 322
  contrast media for, 322
  equipment for, 323–324
  indications for, 321–322
  patient positioning for, 324, 326
    in anteroposterior projection, 324, *325*

Sialography *(Continued)*
    in inferosuperior projection, 326
    in lateral oblique projection, 326
    in lateral projection, *325*, 326
    in modified lateral projection, 326
    in posteroanterior projection, 324
    in standard anteroposterior projection, 324
    in standard posteroanterior projection, 324
    in tangential anteroposterior projection, 324
    in tangential posteroanterior projection, 324
    in true lateral projection, 326
  patient preparation for, 322
  procedure for, 322–323
Sigmoid sinuses, 239
Silicon elastomer, to occlude blood vessels, 336
Sinus(es), coronary, 221
  dural, 238–239
  occipital, 239
  renal, 205
  sagittal, 238
  sigmoid, 239
  transverse, 239
Sodium salts, as contrast agents, 72
Solenoidal coil, in MRI, 143
Source-image distance (SID), in geometric magnification, 381–383
Spatial encoding, in MRI, 139–140
Special procedure(s), definition of, 2
  room for, design of, 3, *4*, 6–14
    equipment in, 6–7
    for film processing, 6
    for ultimate operation, 6
    heat units in, 7
    oxygen supply in, 6
    x-ray generator in, 7
    x-ray tube in, 7–14
  suite design for, 3, *4*
Spinal cord anatomy, 254–256
Spine, computed tomography of, 259, *261*
  magnetic resonance imaging of, 260, *262*
Spin-echo sequence, in MRI, 138–139
Spin-lattice relaxation process (T_2), in MRI, 138
Spin-spin relaxation process (T_2), in MRI, 138
Spot film camera, 30–31
Spring, occluding, to reduce blood flow, 334–336
Star method, of focal spot size determination, 385
Steady-state free precession, in MRI, 139
Strip chart recorders, of automatic injectors, 48
Subarachnoid cisternae, 253–254
Subarachnoid space, 253, 255–256
Subclavian vein, 239
Sublimaze, preangiographic, 160
Sublingual glands, 321
Submandibular glands, 321
Submaxillary glands, 321
Subtraction, 390–397
  by color addition, 395–397
  definition of, 390
  direct x-ray method of, 393
  electronic, 395, *396*
  photographic method of, 393–395
  procedure for, 390–393
Superior vena cava, 180, 239
  venous angiography for, 185
Supply magazine, in cut film changers, 21
  in roll film changers, 17
Suprarenal artery, inferior, 203
Surface coils, in MRI, 143, 145
Surgical landmarking, in digital subtraction angiography, 108

Synovial fluid, 310
Synovial joints, 309–310
Synovial membrane, 310
Syringe, of automatic injectors, 3, 41, *42*
    of lymphangiographic injectors, 63

T

Table, compression, of cut film changers, 21
Target-object distance (TOD), in geometric
    magnification, 382–383
Television camera, for digital subtraction
    angiography, 105
Temporal subtraction, in digital radiography, 107
Thebesian veins, 222
Thoracic myelography, opaque, patient positioning
    for, 266
Three-dimensional encoding, in MRI, 140
Thrombolysis, intravascular, 346
Tibial artery, 195
Tomography, computed, 110–131. See also
    Computed tomography (CT).
    definition of, 112
Trachea, 299
Transcatheter embolization, to reduce blood flow,
    332–337
Translumbar aortography, 174–175
Translumbar puncture, for angiography, 164, *165*
Transverse sinuses, 239
Trays, procedure, 88, 91–93
Trigone, 253

U

Ultrasonography, for needle biopsy guidance, 353
Uterine tubes, 276
Uterus, 277, *279*

V

Valium, preangiographic, 161
Valsalva's sinuses, 218
Vascular interventional procedures, 330–348
    for removal of intravascular foreign bodies, 347–
        348
    to increase blood flow, 338–347. See also *Blood
        flow, techniques to increase*.
    to reduce blood flow, 331–338. See also *Blood
        flow, techniques to reduce*.
Vasoconstrictor infusion, to occlude blood vessels,
    337
Vasodilator infusion, to increase blood flow, 347
Vasopressin infusion, to occlude blood vessels, 337
Vein(s), antebrachial, median, 179
    arcuate, 205
    axillary, 180
    azygos, 180
        venous angiography for, 186
    basilic, 179, 180
    brachiocephalic, 180, 239
    cephalic vein, 179
    cerebral, 238–239
    cubital, median, 179–180
        puncture of, for angiography, 165
    direct exposure of, for angiography, 166
    femoral, 182, 195
        puncture of, for angiography, 165
    great cardiac, 221

Vein(s) *(Continued)*
    hemiazygos, 180–181
        venous angiography for, 186
    iliac, 182, 196
    in femoral arteriography, 195–196
    innominate, 239
    interlobar, 205
    internal jugular, 239
        puncture of, for angiography, 166
    interventricular, 221
    marginal, 221
    median, 180
    medullary, 205
    popliteal, 182, 195
    renal, 205, 206–207
    saphenous, 181–182, 195
    subclavian, 180, 239
    thebesian, 222
Vena cava, inferior, 182, 196, 206–207
        venous angiography for, 186, *190*
    superior, 180, 239
        venous angiography for, 188
Venae cordis minimae, 222
Venography, 179–192. See also *Venous
    angiography*.
    parameters for, with automatic injectors, 56*t*, 58*t*
    renal, 210
Venous angiography, 179–192
    anatomic considerations for, 179–182
    contraindications to, 185
    contrast media for, 115
    equipment for, 189, 192
    indications for, 185
    procedure for, 185–189
Venous puncture techniques, for angiography, 165–
    166
Ventricles, cardiac, 214
    cerebral, 252–253
Ventricular system of brain, 252–253
Ventriculography, 251, 267–269
    contrast media for, 268
    patient positioning for, 269
    procedure for, 268–269
Vertebral arteries, 234–235
Vertebrobasilar system, 234–235
Videodisc, imaging systems, 28–29
Videotape, imaging systems, 28
Vieussen's ring, 21
Viscosity, effect of, on constant pressure injectors,
    53
Vistaril, preangiographic, 159

W

Willis, circle of, 236, *237*, 238
Windowing, in CT, 113, *115–116*
Wires, guide, for catheters, 84, 87

X

Xeroradiography, 372–379
    development of plate in, 376–378
    image fixing in, 379
    image transfer in, 378–379
    plate charging in, 373–374
    plate cleaning and conditioning in, 379
    technique guide for, 402*t*–403*t*
    x-ray exposure of plate in, 375

X-ray exposure of plate, in xeroradiography, 375
X-ray generation, room design considerations for,
    7
X-ray generator, for CT system, 117
    for digital subtraction angiography, 102, 105
X-ray tube(s), for CT system, 117
    for digital subtraction angiography, 102, *104*

X-ray tube(s) *(Continued)*
    room design considerations for, 7

Z

Zero time, in rapid sequence changers, 24